Control of
Communicable
Diseases
in Man

Control of Communicable Diseases in Man

Eleventh Edition
1970

An Official Report of the
American Public Health Association
Prepared under the Auspices of the
Program Area Committee on
Communicable Diseases

Abram S. Benenson, M.D.
EDITOR

Published by
The American Public Health Association
1740 Broadway, New York, N.Y. 10019

This report has been approved in principle by the United States Public Health Service and the Surgeons General of The United States Army, Navy, and Air Force, and has been endorsed by the Association of State and Territorial Health Officers.

The substance of this report has been accepted by the Department of Health and Social Security, England; the Scottish Home and Health Department; and the Department of National Health and Welfare, Canada; Commonwealth Department of Health, Australia; with certain reservations to meet international commitments and agreements and differences in legislative and administrative practice.

EDITORIAL BOARD

ALEXANDER D. LANGMUIR, M.D.
  Director, Epidemiology Program
  National Communicable Disease Center, USPHS
PHILIP E. SARTWELL, M.D., M.P.H.
  Chairman and Professor of Epidemiology
  School of Hygiene and Public Health
  Johns Hopkins University
BRIG. GEN. WILLIAM D. TIGERTT, MCUSA Ret.
  Professor of Experimental Medicine
  University of Maryland School of Medicine
FRANKLIN H. TOP, SR., M.D.
  Professor and Head
  Department of Preventive Medicine and Environmental Health
  University of Iowa College of Medicine
ROBERT J. WILSON, M.D., Dr.P.H.
  Assistant Director
  Connaught Medical Research Laboratories
  Willowdale, Ontario, Canada
THEODORE E. WOODWARD, M.D.
  Professor and Head
  Department of Medicine
  University of Maryland School of Medicine

LIAISON REPRESENTATIVES

ALFREDO NORBERTO BICA, M.D.   Pan American Health Organization
W. CHARLES COCKBURN, M.D., D.P.H.   World Health Organization
H. BRUCE DULL, M.D.   U. S. Public Health Service
K. W. EDMONDSON, M.D.   Department of Health
                                          Canberra, Australia
HERSCHEL E. GRIFFIN, M.D., M.P.H.   U. S. Department of Defense
PROFESSOR NORMAN R. GRIST
                        Scottish Home and Health Department
                                          Edinburgh, Scotland
JACOB KOOMEN, JR., M.D., M.P.H.
            Association of State and Territorial Health Officers
BASIL D. B. LAYTON, M.D., M.P.H.
                Department of National Health and Welfare
                                                    Canada
ANTHONY T. RODEN, M.D.
                Department of Health and Social Security
                                          London, England
JAMES H. STEELE, D.V.M., M.P.H.
                Conference of Public Health Veterinarians

FRANKLIN H. TOP, SR., M.D.
                        American Academy of Pediatrics

vi

PREFACE TO THE ELEVENTH EDITION

The first edition of *Control of Communicable Diseases in Man* was published by the American Public Health Association in 1917; it contained 30 pages and covered 38 diseases. The Eleventh Edition covers 117 diseases in 296 pages, maintaining the tradition established over its first fifty years of providing guidance to health officers and others who are concerned with actual problems in disease control. It presents succinct information on the clinical and laboratory features which help in the recognition of specific communicable diseases, as well as salient features for their control. It is intended to supplement, but not replace, standard textbooks, but because the textbook might not always be at hand, sufficient information is given to guide intelligent action in treatment, especially of those diseases for which any delay in instituting proper therapy may be hazardous to the patient.

Improvements in living conditions, in immunization practices, and in the treatment of communicable diseases have happily led to a low incidence over most of the globe of most of the epidemic diseases of the past, but these do still persist in underdeveloped areas where appropriate insanitary conditions or specific vectors and reservoirs permit infection to occur. The physician educated in the western world today often has had no personal contact with most of the infectious diseases. Modern jet travel, eliminating geographic barriers, has produced the paradoxical situation where any disease may be seen anywhere on the globe, and the patient probably will visit a physician who has never before seen this disease. This pocket manual presents communicable diseases globally in order to help this physician and the health authorities supporting him.

Since the drugs needed for the treatment of exotic diseases, especially for the management of the parasitic diseases, are not generally available, positive action is necessary to assure their availability. Within the United States, this situation has been met by establishment of the Parasitic Disease Drug Service by the Director of the National Communicable Disease Center (NCDC), which makes available to the practicing physician the necessary but usually unavailable drugs. Physicians may telephone Atlanta, Ga., 404-633-3311, extension 3676; the drugs provided by this service are indicated in the section on specific treatment (Paragraph 9B7) of the diseases for which their use is indicated. The NCDC also furnishes special immunoprophylactic or immunotherapeutic materials; these also are mentioned in discussion of the diseases for which their use is appropriate. For management of the complications of smallpox vaccination, vaccinia immune globulin (VIG) has been stockpiled in several American Red Cross blood centers (see Smallpox 9A4, p. 226).

Any attack on communicable diseases must be global; indeed, the time has come when global projects directed toward the eradication of specific diseases (malaria and smallpox) can be mounted. Such efforts have been coordinated by the World Health Organization; in addition, WHO has established a group of international reference centers which form an important worldwide network of institutions able to provide for their national counterparts some or all of the following services: consultations; collection and analysis of information; assistance in the establishment of standards; production and distribution of standard or reference materials; exchange of information; training; and organization of collaborative research. Centers are maintained on enteric, gonococcal, meningococcal, staphylococcal and streptococcal infections; leprosy; plague; treponematosis; tuberculosis; filariasis; leishmaniasis; malaria; schistosomiasis; trypanosomiasis; arboviruses; enteroviruses; influenza; mycoplasma; respiratory virus diseases other than influenza; human rickettsioses; smallpox; trachoma; brucellosis; leptospirosis; rabies; cell cultures; and vector biology and control. WHO should be approached for further details of the services available.

This, the Eleventh Edition, has benefited by representation from the Commonwealth of Australia, so that the consultant group now provides representation from the major English-speaking countries, from WHO and the Pan American Health Organization, as well as from the official and unofficial agencies in the United States concerned with the control of communicable diseases. The editorial group has collaborated to bring this edition abreast of current scientific information, so that the control measures recommended are rational, generally applicable, and effective.

The present edition reflects the strong men who served as its editors in the past. Haven Emerson, its editor for the first seven editions, and John E. Gordon for the next three, developed this publication into a document that has been compared to the dictionary as not necessarily interesting reading, but providing the answer to many questions. Over a time span of more than half a century, it has evolved from a manual concerned with the control measures to be taken in the face of epidemics to one concerned with preventing the development of an epidemic, that is, recognizing the individual case and preventing any spread.

This edition represents no radical revision; it perpetuates the format, and often even the words originally written under the aegis of Dr. Emerson and Dr. Gordon remain. The text has been updated to the present state of knowledge so that recommended practices conform with current information. New chapters have been added on angiostrongyliasis, balantidiasis, intestinal capillariasis, giardiasis, pneumocystis pneumonia, mucormycosis, cytomegalic disease, herpes simplex, viral carditis, and Wolhynian fever (trench fever); melioidosis has been added and glanders has been downgraded to a subsection. Nomenclature has followed that of the 8th Revision of the International Classification of Diseases unless these were too inconsistent with prevailing American usage (e.g., cryptococcosis is used instead of European blastomycosis).

Purposes of the manual—The aim is to provide an informative text for public health workers of official and voluntary health agencies, to include physicians, dentists, veterinarians, sanitary engineers, public health nurses, social workers, health educators and sanitarians; and for physicians, dentists and veterinarians in private practice who have a concern with the control of communicable diseases. The book is also designed for military physicians and others serving with the armed forces at home and abroad, and for health workers stationed in foreign countries. It enters into plans for anticipating the health risks attendant on natural and man-made disasters, and serves as a guide to control of the disease situations such emergencies create. School administrators and students of medicine and public health also find use for the material. The need for a handy reference determines the format of the manual and its pocket size.

A second general purpose is to serve public health administrators as a guide and as a source of materials in preparing regulations and legal requirements for the control of the communicable diseases, in developing programs for health education of the public, and in the administrative acts of official health agencies toward management of communicable disease. The needs of field workers have been given special attention.

The intent is to present factual knowledge in brief fashion and to advance opinion consistent with those facts as a basis for intelligent management of communicable disease, unhampered by local custom and not restricted to prevailing practices. Recommendations for standard administrative or technical procedures are avoided. The emphasis is on principle, because local conditions and interrelated problems commonly require variation in practices from state to state within the United States, and between countries. Because differences in procedure are often due to incomplete knowledge of recent advances and of practices proved successful under other and similar conditions, the attempt has been made to keep facts and opinions reasonably current by revising the manual every five years.

Scope and Content—The presentation is standardized. Each disease is briefly identified with regard to clinical nature, laboratory diagnosis, and differentiation from allied or related conditions. Occurrence, infectious agent, reservoir, mode of transmission, incubation period, period of communicability, and susceptibility and resistance are next presented. Methods of control are described under the following four headings:

A. **Preventive measures:** Applicable generally to individuals and groups when and where the particular disease may occur in sporadic, endemic or epidemic form, and whether or not the disease is an active threat at the moment, e.g., vaccination against smallpox, chlorination of water supplies, pasteurization of milk, control of rodents and arthropods, animal control, immunization, and health education of the public.

B. **Control of patient, contacts, and the immediate environment:** Those measures designed to prevent infectious matter present in the person and the environment of the infected individual from being conveyed in a way to spread the disease to other persons, arthropods or animals; and also the means to keep contacts under surveillance during the assumed period of incubation of the disease, and carriers under control until they are found to be free of the infectious agent. Specific treatment is outlined to limit the period of communicability and to minimize morbidity and mortality.

C. Epidemic measures: Those procedures of emergency character designed to limit the spread of a communicable disease which has developed widely in a group or community or within an area, state or nation, such measures being unnecessary or not justified when the disease occurs sporadically among widely separated individuals or separated by considerable intervals.

D. International measures: Such controls of international travelers, immigrants, goods, animals, and animal products, and their means of transport, as may arise from provisions of international health regulations, conventions, intergovernmental agreements or national laws; also, any controls that may protect populations of one country against the known risk of infection from another country where a disease may be present in endemic or epidemic form.

Reporting of Communicable Diseases—The first step in the control of communicable disease is its rapid identification, followed by notification to the local health authority that a case of communicable disease exists within the particular jurisdiction. Administrative practice as to what diseases are to be reported and how they should be reported varies greatly from one region to another because of different conditions and different frequencies of disease. This manual presents a basic scheme of reporting directed toward practical working procedure rather than ideal practice. The purpose is encouragement of uniformity in morbidity reporting, to permit comparison of data within a country and between nations.

A system of reporting functions at four stages. The first is collection of the basic data in the local community where disease occurs. The data are next assembled at district, state or provincial level. The third stage is the collection of total information under national auspices. Finally, for certain prescribed diseases, report is made by the national health authority to the World Health Organization.

Consideration is here limited to the first stage of a reporting system—the collection of the basic data at the local level; first, because that is the fundamental part of any scheme, and second because this manual is primarily for local health workers. The basic data sought at local level are of two kinds (Definition 36, Report of a disease, p. 293).

1. REPORT OF CASES: Each local health authority, in conformity with regulations of higher authority, will determine what diseases are to be reported as a routine and regular procedure, who is responsible for reporting, the nature of the report required, and the manner in which reports are forwarded to the next superior jurisdiction.

Physicians are required to report all notifiable illnesses which come to their attention; in addition, the statutes or regulations of many localities require reporting by hospital, householder, or other person having knowledge of a case of a reportable disease.

Case Report of a communicable disease provides minimal identifying data of name, address, diagnosis, age, sex, and date of report for each patient and in some instances, suspects; dates of onset and of diagnosis are useful.

Collective Report is the assembled number of cases, by diagnosis, occurring within a prescribed time and without individual identifying data—e.g., 20 cases of malaria, week ending October 6.

2. REPORT OF EPIDEMICS: In addition to requirement of individual case report, any unusual or group expression of illness which may be of public concern (Definition 11, Epidemic) should be reported to the local health authority by the most expeditious means, whether subject to routine report or not specified in the list of diseases officially reportable in the particular locality; and whether a well-known or an indefinite or unknown clinical entity (see Class 4 below).

The communicable diseases listed in this manual are distributed among the following 5 classes, according to practical benefit presumably to be derived from reporting. These classes are referred to by number throughout the text, under Section 9B1 of each disease. The purpose is to provide a scheme on the basis of which each health jurisdiction may determine its list of regularly reportable diseases.

Class I: Case Report Universally Required by International Health Regulations

This class is limited to the internationally quarantinable diseases and to the *Diseases under Surveillance by WHO*. After January 1, 1971, the former will include cholera, plague, smallpox, and yellow fever. After this date, louse-borne relapsing fever and typhus fever, presently quarantinable diseases, will become *Diseases under Surveillance by WHO*, together with poliomyelitis, malaria and influenza.

Obligatory case report to local health authority by telephone, telegraph, or other rapid means; in an epidemic situation, collective reports of subsequent cases in a local area on a daily or weekly basis may be requested by the next superior jurisdiction—as for example, in an influenza epidemic. The local health authority forwards the initial report to next superior jurisdiction by expeditious means if it is the first recognized case in the local area or is the first case outside the limits of a local area already reported; otherwise, weekly by mail or telegraphically in unusual situations.

Class 2: Case Report Regularly Required Wherever the Disease Occurs

Two subclasses are recognized, based on the relative urgency for investigation of contacts and source of infection, or for starting control measures.

A. Case report to local health authority by telephone, telegraph, or other rapid means. These are forwarded to next superior jurisdiction weekly by mail, except that the first recognized case in an area or the first case outside the limits of a known affected local area is reported by telegraph; examples—typhoid fever, diphtheria.
B. Case report by most practicable means; forwarded to next superior jurisdiction as a collective report, weekly by mail; examples, brucellosis, leprosy.

Class 3: Selectively Reportable in Recognized Endemic Areas

In many states and countries, diseases of this class are not reportable. Reporting may be prescribed in particular regions, states or countries by reason of undue frequency or severity. Three subclasses are recognized; A and B (below) are primarily useful under conditions of established endemicity as a means leading toward prompt control measures and to judge the effectiveness of control programs. The main purpose of C (below) is to stimulate control measures or to acquire essential epidemiological data.

A. Case report by telephone, telegraph, or other rapid means in specified areas where the disease ranks in importance with Class 2A; not reportable in many countries; examples—tularemia, scrub typhus.
B. Case report by most practicable means; forwarded to next superior jurisdiction as a collective report by mail weekly or monthly; not reportable in many countries; examples—bartonellosis, coccidioidomycosis.
C. Collective report weekly by mail to local health authority; forwarded to next superior jurisdicition by mail weekly, monthly, quarterly, or sometimes annually; examples—clonorchiasis, sandfly fever.

Class 4: Obligatory Report of Epidemics—No Case Report Required

Prompt report of outbreaks of particular public health importance by telephone, telegraph, or other rapid means; forwarded to next superior jurisdiction by telephone or telegraph. Pertinent data include number of cases, within what time, approximate population involved, and apparent mode of spread; examples—food poisoning, infectious keratoconjunctivitis.

Class 5: Official Report Not Ordinarily Justifiable

Diseases of this class are of two general kinds: those typically sporadic and uncommon, often not directly transmissible from man to man (chromoblastomycosis); or of such epidemiological nature as to offer no practical measures for control (common cold).

Diseases are often made reportable but the information gathered is put to no practical use. This frequently leads to deterioration in the general level of reporting, even for diseases of much importance. Better case reporting usually results when official reporting is restricted to those diseases for which control services are provided, or potential control procedures are under evaluation, or epidemiological information is needed for a definite purpose.

ACKNOWLEDGMENTS—Grateful acknowledgment is hereby made to all the experts, both within and without the American Public Health Association, who have prepared and critically reviewed sections in their area of expertise. The willing cooperation of the editorial committee, and of the individual members of the profession at large, has simplified the task of the chairman. The wise counsel of Dr. Gordon has helped to maintain continuity within the previous edition; his cooperation and encouragement were always forthcoming and have proved invaluable. The quarantine sign appears on the back cover of this edition by courtesy of Sylvan M. Fish, M.D., Communicable Disease Section, City of Philadelphia Department of Public Health, who made available to us his choice collection of otherwise unavailable medical antiques. Appreciation is also due the administrative staffs of the Jefferson Medical College of Philadelphia, and of the University of Kentucky Medical Center, for their assistance in coping with the many mundane tasks associated with this project, *Control of Communicable Diseases in Man*, eleventh edition.

ABRAM S. BENENSON, M.D.

TABLE OF CONTENTS

ACTINOMYCOSIS

1. Identification—A chronic suppurative or granulomatous disease most frequently localized in jaw, thorax or abdomen, rarely limited to skin and subcutaneous tissues. The lesions are firmly indurated granulomata; they spread slowly to contiguous tissues and break down focally to form multiple draining sinuses which penetrate to the surface. Discharges from sinus tracts contain "sulfur granules," which are colonies of the infectious agent.

Diagnosis is confirmed by culture.

2. Occurrence—An infrequent disease of man, occurring sporadically throughout the world. All races, both sexes, and all age groups may be affected; greatest frequency at 15 to 35 years of age and the ratio of males to females approximately two to one. Occurs also in cattle, swine, horses and other animals.

3. Infectious agent—*Actinomyces israelii* is the usual pathogen of man and *A. bovis* that of animals only. *A. naeslundii* and *Arachnia propionica* (*Actinomyces propionica*) have also been reported to cause disease in man. All species are gram-positive nonacid-fast anaerobic to microaerophilic organisms.

4. Reservoir—The natural reservoir of *A. israelii* is man. In the normal oral cavity *Actinomyces* grows as a saprophyte in and around carious teeth, in dental plaques, and in tonsillar crypts, without apparent penetration or cellular response of adjacent tissues. Sample surveys in U.S.A., Sweden and other regions have demonstrated *A. israelii* microscopically in granules from crypts of 40% of extirpated tonsils; and isolation in anaerobic culture from as many as 69% of specimens of saliva or material from carious teeth. No external environmental reservoir such as straw or soil has been demonstrated.

5. Mode of transmission—Presumably the agent passes by contact from man to man as a part of the normal oral flora. From the oral cavity the fungus may be swallowed, inhaled or introduced into jaw tissues by injury or at the site of a neglected or irritating dental defect. The source of clinical disease is endogenous. Transmission by human bite has been reported but is a rare event.

6. Incubation period—Irregular; probably many years after appearance in the normal oral flora, and days or months after precipitating trauma and actual penetration of tissues.

7. Period of communicability—Time and manner in which *A. israelii* becomes a part of the normal oral flora unknown and not pertinent. Except for the rare instances of human bite, not dependent upon exposure to an infected person or animal.

8. Susceptibility and resistance—Natural susceptibility is low. Immunity following attack has not been demonstrated.

1

9. **Methods of control—**

A. *Preventive measures:* None, except that maintenance of good dental hygiene will reduce risk of infection around teeth.

B. *Control of patient, contacts, and the immediate environment:*
1) *Report to local health authority:* Official report not ordinarily justifiable, Class 5 (see Preface).
2) *Isolation:* None.
3) *Concurrent disinfection:* None.
4) *Quarantine:* None.
5) *Immunization of contacts:* None.
6) *Investigation of contacts:* Not profitable.
7) *Specific treatment:* No spontaneous recovery. Prolonged administration of penicillin in high doses is usually effective. Tetracycline antibiotics are often effective and are the second choice.

C. *Epidemic measures:* Not applicable, a sporadic disease.

D. *International measures:* None.

AMEBIASIS

1. **Identification**—A disease of the large intestine due to invasion of the submucosa by pathogenic protozoa. Infection may be asymptomatic, or manifested by mild abdominal discomfort and diarrhea alternating with constipation; an acute dysentery with profuse blood and mucus, usually little pus (amebic dysentery); or a chronic dysentery with mucus and some blood. Infection may spread by the bloodstream or by direct extension to produce abscess of liver, lung or brain, or ulceration of skin. Amebiasis is an uncommon cause of death.

Diagnosis is by identifying trophozoites or cysts of *Entamoeba histolytica* in feces, or trophozoites in smears or sections from lesions; radiographic liver scan and serological data may be required for diagnosing liver abscess.

Differential diagnosis includes shigellosis, appendicitis, ulcerative colitis, balantidiasis and giardiasis. Other intestinal protozoa also are associated with diarrhea in man and may exist concomitantly with *E. histolytica*. Conversely, amebae often are present in diarrheas due to bacterial infections or other cause.

2. **Occurrence**—Infection is worldwide, to the extent of 50% or more of people in unsanitated areas, especially tropical countries and mental institutions; low (1 to 5%) in well-sanitated cities. The percent of infected persons who have clinical disease may be low. Clinical amebic dysentery is prevalent in warm and hot countries and relatively infrequent in temperate regions although infection rates may be high.

3. Infectious agent—*Entamoeba histolytica,* a protozoan.

4. Reservoir—Usually a chronic or asymptomatic patient. Acute cases are of little menace because of the fragility of trophozoites.

5. Mode of transmission—In epidemics, mainly by contaminated water containing cysts from feces of infected persons. Endemic spread is by water, by hand-to-mouth transfer of fresh feces and by contaminated vegetables, especially those served raw; by flies and by soiled hands of food handlers.

6. Incubation period—From 5 days to several months, commonly from 3 to 4 weeks.

7. Period of communicability—During intestinal infection, which may continue for years.

8. Susceptibility and resistance—Susceptibility to infection is general; relatively few persons harboring the organism develop recognizable symptoms; acute cases tend to become chronic. Immunity to reinfection has not been clearly demonstrated.

9. Methods of control—

A. *Preventive measures:*

1) Sanitary disposal of human feces.
2) Protect public water supplies against fecal contamination, and boil drinking water where necessary. Chlorination of water supplies as generally practiced does not destroy cysts; but filtration removes nearly all cysts, diatomaceous earth filters remove them completely. Avoid cross-connections between public and private auxiliary water supplies and back-flow connections in plumbing systems. Small quantities of water, as in Lyster bags and canteens, are best protected by relatively high concentrations of chlorine or iodine.
3) Health education of the general public in personal hygiene, particularly as to sanitary disposal of feces, hand washing after defecation and before preparing or eating food; also in the risks of eating moist foods raw.
4) Fly control and protection of foods against fly contamination by screening or other appropriate means.
5) Supervision by health agencies of the health and sanitary practices of persons preparing and serving food in public eating places; also general cleanliness of the premises. Routine examination of food handlers as a control measure is impractical.
6) Disinfectant dips for fruits and vegetables have no proved value.

B. *Control of patient, contacts, and the immediate environment:*

1) *Report to local health authority:* In selected endemic areas (U.S.A.); in many states and countries not reportable, Class 3C (see Preface).

2) *Isolation:* None. Exclusion of patient from preparation, processing and serving of food until treatment is completed.

3) *Concurrent disinfection:* Sanitary disposal of feces. Terminal cleaning.

4) *Quarantine:* None.

5) *Immunization of contacts:* Not applicable.

6) *Investigation of contacts and source of infection:* Microscopic examination of feces of household members and other suspected contacts, supplemented by search for direct contamination of water.

7) *Specific treatment:* Acute amebic dysentery : metronidazole (Flagyl), tetracycline, emetine hydrochloride or paromomycin (Humatin). Emetine hydrochloride will relieve symptoms but usually not eliminate the infection, and should be accompanied or followed by a standard amebicide, such as diiodohydroxyquin (Diodoquin), carbarsone, glycobiarsol (Milibis), iodochlorhydroxyquin (Entero-vioform), or emetine bismuth iodide to eliminate infection from lumen of the intestine. These amebicides are effective treatment for mild and asymptomatic infections. Extraintestinal amebiasis (liver abscess) is treated with metronidazole (Flagyl), chloroquine (Aralen) or emetine hydrochloride. If abscess requires aspiration, precede by chloroquine or emetine to limit infection.

Repeated fecal examinations at intervals up to 3 months are necessary to assure that amebae have been eliminated.

C. *Epidemic measures:* Any grouping of several cases from a single area or in an institution requires prompt epidemiologic investigation to determine source of infection and mode of transmission. If a common vehicle is indicated, such as water or food, take appropriate measures to correct the situation. If epidemiologic evidence points to person-to-person transmission, emphasis should be on personal cleanliness, sanitary disposal of feces, and fly control.

D. *International measures:* None.

ANCYLOSTOMIASIS (HOOKWORM DISEASE)

1. Identification—A chronic, debilitating disease with a variety of vague symptoms varying greatly according to extent of infection, nutritional state of the patient, and degree of anemia. The bloodsucking activity of the nematode, along with malnutrition, leads to hypochromic microcytic anemia, a major cause of disability. Heavily infected children may be retarded in mental and physical development. Death is infrequent either in acute or chronic stages, and then usually in association with other infections. Light hookworm infections generally produce few or no clinical effects. Synonym: Uncinariasis.

Infection is confirmed by finding hookworm eggs in feces; species recognition is through microscopic examination of adult worms.

2. Occurrence—Widely endemic in those tropical and subtropical countries where disposal of human feces is inadequate, and soil, moisture, and temperature favor development of infective larvae. *Necator americanus* is the prevailing species throughout tropical West Africa and southeastern U.S.A.; and *Ancylostoma duodenale* in Mediterranean countries, including the Nile Valley. Both forms occur in many parts of Asia, Central and South America, and the West Indies.

3. Infectious agents—*Necator americanus* and *Ancylostoma duodenale*.

4. Reservoir—Reservoir is an infected person discharging eggs in feces.

5. Mode of transmission—Eggs in feces are deposited on the ground and, under favorable conditions of moisture, temperature and type of soil, hatch, and larvae develop to the 3rd stage, becoming infective in 7 to 10 days. Infection of man occurs when the infective larvae penetrate the bare skin, usually of the foot; in so doing they characteristically produce a dermatitis (ground itch). Infection by ingestion is possible, but rare. The filariform larvae normally enter the skin and pass via lymphatics and blood stream to the lungs, enter the alveoli, migrate up the trachea to the pharynx, are swallowed, and reach the small intestine, where they attach to the intestinal wall, develop to maturity in about 5 weeks and produce eggs.

6. Incubation period—Symptoms may develop after a few weeks to many months or even years, depending on intensity of infection and nutrition of the host. Eggs appear in the feces about 6 weeks after infection (prepatent period).

7. Period of communicability—Infected persons are potential spreaders of infection for several years in the absence of treatment. Under favorable conditions, 3rd stage infective larvae remain alive in soil for several weeks.

8. Susceptibility and resistance—Susceptibility is universal. Some immunity develops with infection.

9. Methods of control—

    A. Preventive measures:

        1) Prevention of soil contamination by installation of sanitary disposal systems for human feces, especially sanitary privies in rural areas.

        2) Education of the public as to dangers of soil contamination, and in preventive measures, i.e., the practice of personal hygiene, especially the wearing of shoes.

B. Control of patient, contacts, and the immediate environment:

1) *Report to local health authority:* Official report ordinarily justifiable, Class 5 (see Preface).
2) *Isolation:* None.
3) *Concurrent disinfection:* Sanitary disposal of feces to prevent contamination of soil.
4) *Quarantine:* None.
5) *Immunization of contacts:* None.
6) *Investigation of contacts:* Each infected contact and carrier is a potential or actual spreader of the disease.
7) *Specific treatment:* Tetrachlorethylene or hexylresorcinol; toxic reactions are infrequent and therapy can be repeated if necessary; communicability is shortened. If present, ascariasis should be treated before tetrachlorethylene is administered. Bephenium hydroxynaphthoate is of value and is preferred for *A. duodenale* infections. Protein and iron supplementation of the diet is desirable.

C. Epidemic measures: Surveys for prevalence in highly endemic areas, public health education in sanitation of the environment and in personal hygiene, provision of facilities for excreta disposal and facilities for treatment of patients.

D. International measures: None.

ANGIOSTRONGYLIASIS

1. Identification—A disease of the central nervous system due to the nematode, *Angiostrongylus cantonensis;* meninges are predominantly involved. Invasion may be asymptomatic or mildly symptomatic; more commonly is characterized by severe headache, stiffness of neck and back, and various paresthesias. Temporary facial paralysis occurs in 5% of patients. Low-grade fever may be present. The worm has been found in the eye. Cerebrospinal fluid usually exhibits pleocytosis with 25–100% eosinophils; blood eosinophilia not always present. Illness may last a few days to several months; symptoms recur. Deaths have rarely been reported. Synonyms: Eosinophilic meningitis; Eosinophilic meningoencephalitis.

Diagnosis, especially in endemic areas, is suggested by eosinophils in the cerebrospinal fluid. A skin test with worm antigen is also useful in diagnosis. Differential diagnosis includes tuberculous meningitis, cerebral cysticercosis or hydatidosis.

2. Occurrence—The disease is endemic in Hawaii, Tahiti, Micronesia, Australia, Eastern Asia including Viet Nam, Thailand, Indonesia, Taiwan, and the Philippines. The nematode is also found in Ceylon, Mauritius and Madagascar.

3. Infectious agent—*Angiostrongylus cantonensis,* a nematode (lungworm of rats). The third-stage larva is infective.

4. Reservoir—The rat is the normal definitive host of this parasite.

5. Mode of transmission—Ingestion of raw or insufficiently cooked snails, slugs or land planarians, which are intermediate hosts harboring infective larvae. Prawns, fish and land crabs that have consumed snails or slugs transport the larvae, which remain infective. Lettuce and other similar vegetables contaminated by mollusks may serve as a source of infection. In some areas, other as yet unknown vectors may exist.

6. Incubation period—Usually 2–4 weeks, though it may be longer.

7. Period of communicability—Not transmitted from man to man.

8. Susceptibility and resistance—Susceptibility to infection is general. It is believed that in endemic areas repeated exposure to low-level infection has led to immunity among a fair number of the population. Malnutrition and other debilitating disease may contribute to an increase in severity and even a fatal outcome.

9. Methods of control—

A. Preventive measures:

1) Rat control.
2) Thorough cooking of all foods. Boiling snails, prawns, fish and crabs for 3–5 minutes or freezing at −15 C for 24 hours is effective in killing all larvae.
3) Thorough cleansing of lettuce and other greens to eliminate mollusks and their products.
4) Health education of the general public in preparation of seafoods and land snails.

B. Control of patient, contacts, and the immediate environment:

1) Report to local health authority: Official report not justifiable, Class 5 (see Preface).
2) Isolation: None.
3) Concurrent disinfection: Not necessary.
4) Quarantine: None.
5) Immunization of contacts: Not applicable.
6) Investigation of contacts and source of infection: The source of food involved and its preparation should be investigated.
7) Specific treatment: Thiabendazole (Mintezol) has been reported to be effective, especially in the early stages of the illness.

C. Epidemic measures: Any grouping of several cases from a single source or in an institution warrants prompt epidemiologic investigation.

D. International measures: None.

ANTHRAX

1. Identification—An acute bacterial disease, usually of the skin. Initial vesicle(s) at the site of inoculation develop into a depressed black eschar, at times surrounded by mild to moderate edema. Pain is unusual, and if present is related to edema or secondary infection. Untreated infections may spread to regional lymph nodes and bloodstream with overwhelming septicemia and death. Initial symptoms of inhalation anthrax are mild and nonspecific, resembling common upper respiratory infection, but acute symptoms of respiratory distress, fever and shock follow in from 3 to 5 days, with death commonly 7 to 24 hours thereafter. Untreated cutaneous anthrax has a fatality from 5 to 20%; with effective antibiotic therapy, essentially no deaths. The usual lesion evolves through the local changes even after the initiation of antibiotic therapy. Inhalation and gastrointestinal anthrax are highly fatal. Synonyms: Malignant pustule, Woolsorter's disease.

Laboratory confirmation is by direct demonstration of bacilli in lesions or discharges; by culture; by inoculation of mice, guinea pigs or rabbits with exudates from lesions, or blood or other tissues, or with pure cultures; also by use of *Bacillus anthracis* gamma bacteriophage. Fluorescent antibody techniques can be used for identification of the bacillus in vesicular fluid smears, cultures, or tissue sections.

2. Occurrence—Infrequent and sporadic in U.S.A. and most industrial countries; inhalation and gastrointestinal anthrax are rare. Primarily an occupational hazard of industrial workers who process hides, hair (especially from goats), bone and bone products, and wool, and of veterinarians and agricultural workers who handle infected animals. Endemic in numerous agricultural regions of the world where anthrax in animals is common. New areas of infection in livestock may develop through introduction of animal feed containing contaminated bone meal. Altered environmental conditions such as floods or droughts may provoke epizootics through germination and multiplication of anthrax spores dormant in soil.

3. Infectious agent—*Bacillus anthracis.*

4. Reservoir—Reservoir is any one of several animals: cattle, sheep, goats, horses, pigs and others. The spores of *B. anthracis,* which resist environmental and disinfection factors, remain viable in contaminated areas for many years after the source-animal infection has terminated.

5. Mode of transmission—Infection of skin is by contact with tissues of animals dying of the disease; or contaminated hair, wool, hides, and soil associated with infected animals. Inhalation anthrax results from inhalation of spores. Gastrointestinal anthrax arises from ingestion of contaminated undercooked meat; no evidence that milk from infected animals transmits anthrax. The disease spreads among omnivorous and carnivorous animals through contaminated meat, bone meal or other feed products. Biting flies and other insects have been reported to serve as mechanical vectors. Vultures have spread the organism from one area to another. Accidental infections occur among laboratory workers.

6. Incubation period—Within 7 days, usually 2 to 5.

7. Period of communicability—Never reported to have been transmitted from man to man. Articles and soil contaminated with spores may remain infective for years.

8. Susceptibility and resistance—Uncertain; some evidence of inapparent infection among persons in frequent contact with the infectious agent. No well-documented second attack has been reported.

9. Methods of control—

A. Preventive measures:

1) A cell-free vaccine, available in the U.S.A. from the National Communicable Disease Center for high-risk persons, is effective in preventing cutaneous and probably inhalation anthrax; recommended for veterinarians and for persons handling potentially contaminated industrial raw materials.
2) Education in personal cleanliness, in modes of transmission, and in care of skin abrasions for employees handling potentially contaminated articles.
3) Dust control and proper ventilation in hazardous industries. Continuing medical supervision of employees, with prompt medical care of all suspicious skin lesions. Adequate facilities for washing and changing clothes after work. Eating facilities separate from place of work.
4) Thorough washing, disinfection or sterilization, when possible, of hair, wool or hides, and bone meal or other feed of animal origin, prior to processing.
5) Hides of animals suspected of anthrax should not be sold, nor carcasses used as food or feed supplements.
6) Conduct postmortem examination of animals dying of suspected anthrax, with care not to contaminate soil or environment with blood or infected tissues. Burn carcasses or bury deeply with anhydrous calcium oxide (quicklime), preferably at site of death. Decontaminate soil seeded with bodily discharges.
7) Promptly isolate and treat animals suspected of anthrax. Milk from animals in herds with anthrax may be boiled and fed to swine or chickens.
8) Annual vaccination of animals in enzootic areas.
9) Control effluents and trade wastes of rendering plants handling potentially infected animals, and those from factories that manufacture products from hair, wool or hides likely to be contaminated.

B. Control of patient, contacts, and the immediate environment:

1) *Report to local health authority:* Case report obligatory in most states and countries, Class 2A (see Preface). Report also to appropriate livestock or agriculture authority.

2) *Isolation:* Wound isolation until lesions are bacteriologically free of anthrax bacilli. Inhalation anthrax should be under strict isolation.

3) *Concurrent disinfection:* Of discharges from lesions and articles soiled therewith. Spores require steam sterilization or burning. Terminal cleaning.

4) *Quarantine:* None.

5) *Immunization of contacts:* None.

6) *Investigation of contacts and source of infection:* Search for history of exposure to infected animals or contaminated animal products, and trace to place of origin. If in a manufacturing plant, inspect for adequacy of preventive measures outlined in 9A above.

7) *Specific treatment:* Penicillin is the drug of choice; tetracyclines or another broad-spectrum antibiotic may be used.

C. Epidemic measures: The occasional epidemics in man in U.S.A. are local industrial outbreaks among employees who work with animal products, especially goat hair; outbreaks may be related to butchering of infected cattle or may be an occupational hazard of animal husbandry.

D. International measures: Sterilization of imported bone meal before use as animal feed. Disinfection of wool, hair, hides and other products when indicated and practicable; formaldehyde has been used successfully; cobalt irradiation has also been used.

ARTHROPOD-BORNE VIRAL DISEASES
(Arboviral Diseases)

Summary

A large number of arboviruses are known to produce diseases in man, and the number is growing rapidly. These diseases present principally in three clinical syndromes: (1) an acute *central nervous system disease, usually with encephalitis* but ranging in severity from mild aseptic meningitis to coma, paralysis and death; (2) acute *benign fevers* of short duration—many resembling dengue, with and without an exanthem, although on occasion some of these may give rise to a more serious illness with central nervous system involvement or hemorrhages; (3) *hemorrhagic fevers,* which include acute febrile diseases with extensive hemorrhagic involvement, external or internal, frequently serious, and associated with shock and significant fatality. One of them, yellow fever, also causes severe liver damage and jaundice; milder clinical forms may resemble the second syndrome (benign fever) and a few patients may also have an encephalitic component.

Most of these diseases are zoonoses, accidentally acquired by man through an arthropod vector, with man an unimportant host in the cycle. In the presence of a suitable vector and viremia, a few may become epidemic, with man the principal source of vector infection. For still others the animal-arthropod cycle is not recognized to involve a nonhuman host. Most of the viruses are mosquito-borne, several are tick-borne, others *Phlebotomus*-borne. A few, producing disease in animals, are transmitted by *Culicoides* (midges, gnats). Laboratory infections occur, some by aerosols.

Many epidemiologic factors in the transmission cycle, chiefly relating to the vector, are common—a feature important in control. Consequently, the selected diseases under each clinical syndrome are arranged in four groups: Mosquito-borne, tick-borne, *Phlebotomus*-borne and unknown. Diseases of major importance are described individually or in groups where clinical and epidemiological similarities exist. Some of the less important or less well-studied diseases are presented only in the accompanying table.

Approximately 80 viruses presently classified as arboviruses produce disease in man. Most of these are further classified, by hemagglutination or complement fixation, into antigenic groups, of which A and B are the largest and best known. Both groups A and B contain agents predominantly causing encephalitis and agents predominantly causing other febrile illnesses. Group A contains only mosquito-borne viruses, group B both mosquito- and tick-borne agents and some agents without a recognized vector. Viruses of group C and several other groups produce principally febrile diseases with syndromes resembling more or less the dengue syndrome. Several human pathogens for which no common antigens have been demonstrated necessarily remain in a miscellaneous category.

Viruses believed associated with human disease are listed in the table by type of vector reasonably established or suspected, predominant character of recognized disease, and geographical area where found. In some instances, observed cases are too few to be certain of the usual clinical reaction. Some have been recognized only through laboratory-acquired exposure. None is included where evidence of human infection is based solely on serological survey; otherwise the number would be much greater.

DISEASES IN MAN CAUSED BY ARTHROPOD-BORNE VIRUSES

Virus Group	Name of Virus	Vector	Disease in Man	Where Found
Group A	*Bebaru	Mosquito	Fever, polyarthritis	Malaya, Australia
	*Chikungunya (TH-35)	Mosquito	Fever, hemorrhagic fever	Africa, Southeast Asia, Philippines
	*Eastern equine	Mosquito	Encephalitis	Americas
	*Mayaro (Uruma)	Mosquito	Fever	South America
	Mucambo	Mosquito	Fever	South America
	*Onyong-nyong (Gulu)	Mosquito	Fever	Africa
	*Pixuna	Mosquito	Fever	South America
	*Ross River	Mosquito	Fever	Australia
	Semliki Forest	Mosquito	Fever	Africa
	Sindbis	Mosquito	Fever	Africa, India, Southeast Asia, Philippines, Australia
	*Venezuelan equine	Mosquito	Fever, encephalitis	South America, Mexico, U.S.A.
	*Western equine	Mosquito	Encephalitis	Americas
Group B	Banzi	Mosquito	Fever	South Africa
	Bat salivary gland (Rio Bravo)	Unknown	Encephalitis, aseptic meningitis	U.S.A.
	Bussuquara	Mosquito	Fever	South America
	*Dengue 1, 2, 3, 4	Mosquito	Fever, hemorrhagic fever	See Dengue fever, p. 20.
	*Diphasic meningo-encephalitis	Tick	Encephalitis	U.S.S.R., Europe
	Ilheus	Mosquito	Fever, encephalitis	South America, Central America
	*Japanese (B)	Mosquito	Encephalitis	Asia, Pacific Islands
	*Kunjin	Mosquito	Fever	Australia
	*Kyasanur Forest	Tick	Hemorrhagic fever	India

Group	Virus	Disease	Vector	Location
Group B—cont'd	*Langat	Fever, encephalitis	Tick	Malaysia
	*Louping ill	Encephalitis	Tick	Great Britain
	*Murray Valley	Encephalitis	Mosquito	Australia, New Guinea
	Negishi	Encephalitis	Unknown	Japan
	*Omsk hemorrhagic	Hemorrhagic fever	Tick	U.S.S.R.
	*Powassan	Encephalitis	Tick	Canada, U.S.A.
	*Russian spring-summer (tick-borne encephalitis)	Encephalitis	Tick	Europe, Asia
	Spondweni	Fever	Mosquito	Africa
	*St. Louis	Encephalitis	Mosquito	Americas, Jamaica
	Uganda S	Fever	Mosquito	Africa
	Wesselsbron	Fever	Mosquito	Africa
	*West Nile	Fever, encephalitis	Mosquito	Africa, India, Middle East, Europe
	*Yellow fever	Hemorrhagic fever	Mosquito	Africa, South and Central America
Group C*	Zika	Fever	Mosquito	Africa, Southeast Asia
	Apeu	Fever	Mosquito	South America
	Caraparu	Fever	Mosquito	South America
	Itaqui	Fever	Mosquito	South America
	Madrid	Fever	Mosquito	South America
	Marituba	Fever	Mosquito	South America
	Murutucu	Fever	Mosquito	South America
	Oriboca	Fever	Mosquito	South America
	Ossa	Fever	Mosquito	South America
	Restan	Fever	Mosquito	South America
Bunyamwera group	Batai (Calovo)	Fever	Mosquito	Europe, Malaya, India
	*Bunyamwera	Fever	Mosquito	Africa
	Germiston	Fever	Mosquito	Africa
	Guaroa	Fever	Mosquito	South America, Panama
	Ilesha	Fever	Unknown	Africa
	Wyeomyia	Fever	Mosquito	South America, Panama
Bwamba group	*Bwamba	Fever	Mosquito	Africa

* Asterisked viruses and groups are discussed individually in text. See Index for page numbers.

DISEASES IN MAN CAUSED BY ARTHROPOD-BORNE VIRUSES (cont'd)

Virus Group	Name of Virus	Vector	Disease in Man	Where Found
California group	*California	Mosquito	Encephalitis	U.S.A., Canada
	*LaCrosse	Mosquito	Encephalitis	U.S.A., Canada
	Tahyna	Mosquito	Fever	Europe
Changuinola group	*Changuinola	Phlebotomus	Fever	Central America
Guama group	Catu	Mosquito	Fever	South America
	Guama	Mosquito	Fever	South America
Kemerovo group*	Kemerovo	Tick	Fever	Europe
	Tribec	Tick	Fever	Europe
Sandfly fever group* (Phlebotomus fever)	Candiru	Unknown	Fever	South America
	Chagres	Unknown	Fever	Central America
	Naples type	Phlebotomus	Fever	Europe, Africa, Asia
	Punta Toro	Unknown	Fever	Panama
	Sicilian type	Phlebotomus	Fever	Europe, Africa, Asia
Piry group	Chandipura	Mosquito	Fever	India
	Piry	Mosquito	Fever	South America
Simbu group	Manzanilla	Mosquito	Fever	South America
	*Oropouche	Mosquito	Fever	South America
Vesicular stomatitis group	*Vesicular stomatitis, Indiana	Phlebotomus	Fever	North and Central America
Miscellaneous and ungrouped*	Colorado tick fever	Tick	Fever	U.S.A.
	Congo	Tick	Hemorrhagic fever	Europe, Africa
	Ganjam	Tick	Fever	India
	Nairobi sheep disease	Tick	Fever	Africa
	Quaranfil	Tick	Fever	Africa
	Rift Valley	Mosquito	Fever	Africa

ARTHROPOD-BORNE VIRAL ENCEPHALITIDES

I. Mosquito-borne

EASTERN EQUINE, WESTERN EQUINE, CALIFORNIA, JAPANESE B, MURRAY VALLEY, AND ST. LOUIS ENCEPHALITIS

1. Identification—A group of acute inflammatory diseases of short duration, involving parts of the brain, spinal cord and meninges. Signs and symptoms are similar but vary in severity and rate of progress. Mild cases often occur as aseptic meningitis. Severe infections usually marked by acute onset, high fever, meningeal signs, stupor, disorientation, coma, spasticity, tremors, occasionally convulsions—especially in infants—and spastic but rarely flaccid paralysis. Case fatality ranges from 5 to 60%, that of Japanese B and Eastern equine types being highest. With most viruses, conspicuous sequelae are rare except in infants; more with Eastern equine and Japanese B than others; no parkinsonism. Mild leucocytosis is usual; leucocytes in spinal fluid from 50 to 200 per cu mm occasionally 1,000 or more in infants.

Specific identification is by demonstrated titer changes in antibody between early and late specimens of serum, by neutralization, complement fixation and hemagglutination inhibition; group reactions may occur. Virus may be isolated by inoculation of suckling mice or tissue culture with the brain of fatal cases, rarely with blood or cerebrospinal fluid; histopathological changes are not specific for individual viruses.

These diseases require differentiation from the tick-borne encephalitides, encephalitic and nonparalytic poliomyelitis, rabies, mumps meningoencephalitis, lymphocytic choriomeningitis, aseptic meningitis due to enteroviruses, herpes encephalitis, postvaccinal or postinfection encephalitides, bacterial, protozoal, leptospiral and mycotic meningitides or encephalitides; also the von Economo type of encephalitis (encephalitis lethargica), of unknown etiology and frequent occurrence just before and after 1920, but now rarely reported. Venezuelan equine virus, primarily producing an arthropod-borne viral fever (pp. 21–24), is increasingly responsible for cases of encephalitis.

2. Occurrence—Eastern equine encephalitis cases are recognized in eastern and North Central U.S.A. and adjacent Canada, in scattered areas of Central and South America and in the Caribbean Islands; Western equine cases in western U.S.A. and Canada, in scattered areas further east from Connecticut to Florida, and in South America; California type is scattered east and west; Japanese B, in western Pacific Islands from Japan to the Philippines, many eastern areas of Asia from Korea to Singapore, and India; Murray Valley, in parts of Australia and New Guinea; and St. Louis in most of U.S.A., also in Trinidad, Jamaica, Panama and Brazil. Cases occur in temperate latitudes in summer and early fall, commonly limited to areas and years of high temperature and many mosquitoes. Tend to persist endemically in hot, irrigated valley regions; irregularly noted in dry farming areas. May also be seasonal in tropical countries, depending on rainfall and vector population.

3. Infectious agents—Each disease is caused by a specific virus: Eastern equine and Western equine in Group A; Japanese B, Murray Valley and St. Louis in Group B viruses; LaCrosse and possibly others in the California group. Venezuelan equine (Group A) and West Nile (Group B) viruses may also cause encephalitis.

4. Reservoir—True reservoir or means of winter carry-over unknown—possibly bird, rodent, bat, reptile, amphibian or surviving adult mosquito, possibly differing for each virus.

5. Mode of transmission—By bite of infective mosquitoes. Most important vectors are: for Eastern equine in U.S.A., probably *Culiseta melanura,* from bird to bird and one or more *Aedes* species to man; for Western equine in western U.S.A., *Culex tarsalis;* for California, several species of *Aedes;* for Japanese B, *Culex tritaeniorhynchus* in temperate climates and *Culex gelidus* in tropics; for Murray Valley, probably *Culex annulirostris;* for St. Louis in U.S.A., *Culex tarsalis, Culex pipiens-quinquefasciatus* complex, and *Culex nigripalpus.* Mosquitoes usually acquire the infection from wild birds or rodents, but pigs are of some importance for Japanese B; for others, occasionally a mammal, such as the horse.

6. Incubation period—Usually 5 to 15 days.

7. Period of communicability—Not directly transmitted from man to man. Virus is not usually demonstrable in the blood of man after onset of disease. Mosquito remains infective for life. Viremia in birds usually lasts 2 to 5 days but may be prolonged in bats, reptiles and amphibia, particularly if interrupted by hibernation. Horses develop active disease with the two equine viruses and with Japanese B, but viremia is rarely present for long periods or in high titer; therefore, man and horses are uncommon sources of mosquito infection.

8. Susceptibility and resistance—Susceptibility to clinical disease usually highest in infancy and old age; inapparent or undiagnosed infection is more common at other ages. Varies with virus; thus, St. Louis tends to spare young children. Infection results in homologous immunity. In highly endemic areas, adults are largely immune to local strains by reason of mild and inapparent infections and susceptibles are mainly children.

9. Methods of control—

A. Preventive measures:

1) Destruction of larvae and elimination of breeding places of known or suspected vector mosquitoes.
2) Killing mosquitoes by space and residual spraying of human habitations. See Malaria 9A1, p. 141.
3) Screening of sleeping and living quarters; use of mosquito bed nets.
4) Avoid exposure to mosquitoes during hours of biting, or use repellents. See Malaria 9A4, p. 142.
5) Education of the public as to mode of spread and control.

6) Mouse brain-inactivated vaccine is used against Japanese B encephalitis for children in Japan and experimentally in a few other countries. Tissue culture vaccines are under development; no licensed vaccines for others.
7) Passive protection of accidentally exposed laboratory workers by human or animal immune serum.

B. Control of patient, contacts, and the immediate environment:

1) *Report to local health authority:* Case report obligatory in most states of U.S.A. and in some other countries, Class 2A (see Preface). Report under the appropriate disease; or as Encephalitis, other forms; or as Aseptic meningitis, with etiology or clinical type specified when known.
2) *Isolation:* None; virus not usually found in blood, secretions or discharges during clinical manifestations.
3) *Concurrent disinfection:* None.
4) *Quarantine:* None.
5) *Immunization of contacts:* None.
6) *Investigation of contacts and source of infection:* Search for missed cases and the presence of vector mosquitoes; primarily a community problem (see 9C).
7) *Specific treatment:* None.

C. Epidemic measures:

1) Identification of disease among horses or birds and recognition of human cases in the community have epidemiological value to indicate frequency of infection and areas involved. Immunization of horses probably does not limit spread of the virus in the community.
2) Fogging or airplane-spraying with suitable insecticide has shown promise for aborting urban epidemics of St. Louis encephalitis.

D. International measures: Insecticide spray of airplanes arriving from recognized areas of prevalence.
WHO Reference Centres (see Preface).

II. Tick-borne

**RUSSIAN SPRING-SUMMER ENCEPHALITIS,
DIPHASIC MENINGOENCEPHALITIS,
LOUPING ILL, POWASSAN ENCEPHALITIS**

1. Identification—A group of diseases clinically resembling mosquito-borne encephalitides except that Russian spring-summer type often is associated with flaccid paralysis, particularly of shoulder girdle, with residua. Diphasic meningoencephalitis (diphasic milk fever or

Central European tick-borne encephalitis) has a longer course, averaging 3 weeks; initial febrile stage is unassociated with symptoms referrable to central nervous system; a second phase of fever and meningoencephalitis follows 4 to 10 days after apparent recovery; fatality and severe residua are less frequent than for the Russian spring-summer disease. Louping ill in man also has a diphasic pattern and is relatively mild.

Specific identification is by serological tests or by isolation of virus from blood during acute illness by inoculation of suckling mice or tissue culture. More common serological tests cannot be expected to differentiate members of this group, but do distinguish the group from most other similar diseases.

2. Occurrence—CNS disease from this virus complex is distributed spottily over much of USSR, other parts of Eastern and Central Europe, Scandinavia and Britain. In general, the spring-summer type has a more eastern or Asian distribution; diphasic meningoencephalitis predominates in Europe, with louping ill present in Scotland, Northern England, and Ireland. Powassan virus is present in Canada and the U.S.A. Seasonal incidence depends on activity of the tick, with *Ixodes persulcatus* usually active in spring and early summer, while *Ixodes ricinus* continues into late summer or early autumn. Areas of highest incidence are those where man has intimate association with large numbers of infected ticks, generally in rural or forest areas but also in urban populations. Local epidemics of diphasic meningoencephalitis have occurred among persons consuming raw milk from goats or sheep—thus the name diphasic milk fever. Laboratory infections are common, a number with serious sequelae and some fatal.

3. Infectious agents—Minor antigenic differences exist, more with Powassan than others, but viruses in these diseases are closely related and form a complex within group B.

4. Reservoir—The tick or a combination of tick and mammal appears to be the true reservoir; transovarian tick passage of some USSR viruses has been demonstrated. Sheep and deer are the hosts most involved in louping ill. Rodents—sometimes other mammals and birds, rarely man—give rise to tick infections in Europe and Asia.

5. Mode of transmission—By the bite of infective ticks, or by consumption of milk from certain infected animals. *I. persulcatus* is the principal vector in eastern USSR and *I. ricinus* in western USSR and other parts of Europe; the latter is also the vector of louping ill of sheep in Scotland. *Ixodes cookei* is principal vector in eastern Canada and U.S.A. Larval ticks usually ingest virus by feeding on rodents, sometimes other mammals and birds. Adult ticks may acquire infection from man. Raw milk may be a vehicle for diphasic meningoencephalitis.

6. Incubation period—Usually 7 to 14 days.

7. Period of communicability—Not directly transmitted from man to man. A tick infected at any stage remains infective for life. Viremia in a variety of vertebrates may last for several days; in man up to a week or 10 days.

8. Susceptibility and resistance—Both sexes and all ages are susceptible, but age pattern varies widely in different regions as influenced by exposure to ticks, consumption of milk from an infected animal, or previously acquired immunity. Infection, whether inapparent or overt, leads to immunity.

9. Methods of control—

A. *Preventive measures:*
1) See Tick-borne Rickettsial Fevers 9A1 and 2, for measures against ticks (p. 207).
2) Formalinized virus vaccines have been used extensively in the USSR with reported safety and effectiveness.
3) Boil or pasteurize milk of animals of susceptible species in endemic areas of diphasic meningoencephalitis.

B. *Control of patient, contacts, and the immediate environment:*
1) *Report to local health authority:* In selected endemic areas; in most countries not a reportable disease, Class 3B (see Preface).
2) *Isolation:* None, if patient is tick-free.
3) *Concurrent disinfection:* None.
4) *Quarantine:* None.
5) *Immunization of contacts:* None.
6) *Investigation of contacts and source of infection:* Search for missed cases, presence of tick vectors, and animals excreting virus in milk.
7) *Specific treatment:* None.

C. *Epidemic measures:* See Tick-borne Rickettsial Fevers (p. 207).

D. *International measures:* WHO Reference Centres (see Preface).

ARTHROPOD-BORNE VIRAL FEVERS

I. Mosquito-borne

A. DENGUE FEVER

1. Identification—An acute febrile disease of sharp onset, occasionally with two periods of short duration; fever for about 5 days and rarely more than 7, intense headache, postorbital pains, joint and muscle pains, and rash. Early, general erythema in some cases; rash usually appears 3 to 4 days after onset of fever and is either maculopapular or scarlatiniform; petechiae may appear on feet, legs, axillae, or palate on last day of fever or shortly thereafter. Dark-skinned races frequently have no visible rash. Recovery is associated with prolonged fatigue and depression. Leucopenia and lymphadenopathy are usual. Epidemics are explosive, fatality exceedingly low. Synonym : Breakbone fever.

Differential diagnosis includes all diseases listed in Section B below, Colorado tick fever (p. 24), the sandfly fevers (p. 25), and others.

Hemagglutination, complement-fixation or neutralization tests are diagnostic aids. Virus is isolated from blood by inoculation of suckling mice or by tissue culture techniques.

2. Occurrence—Endemic areas are limited to parts of the world where mosquito vectors survive in adequate numbers throughout the year; also may depend on continued immigration of susceptibles. Islands of the Southwest Pacific, Southeast Asia, the Philippine Islands, Indonesia, India, and Pakistan are commonly involved. Epidemics can occur wherever vectors are present and virus is introduced, urban or rural; large outbreaks in several Caribbean islands and Venezuela in recent years.

3. Infectious agent—The viruses of dengue fever; at least four immunological types have been identified in dengue fever, Types 1, 2, 3 and 4. The same viruses or others closely related and not yet distinguishable are responsible for a different disease syndrome (see Arthropod-borne Viral Hemorrhagic Fevers, pp. 27–34).

4. Reservoir—Man, together with the mosquito, is one reservoir; the existence of an added animal-mosquito reservoir, the monkey, was recently demonstrated in Malaya.

5. Mode of transmission—By the bite of infective mosquitoes, *Aedes aegypti, Aedes albopictus,* or one of the *Aedes scutellaris* complex, infected by biting a human being or possibly a monkey.

6. Incubation period—3 to 15 days, commonly 5 to 6 days.

7. Period of communicability—Not directly transmitted from man to man. Patients are usually infective for mosquitoes from the day before onset to the 5th day of disease. The mosquito becomes infective 8 to 11 days after the blood meal and remains so for life.

8. Susceptibility and resistance—Susceptibility is apparently universal, but children usually have a milder disease than adults, and due to its mildness the disease may not resemble dengue. Homologous-type immunity is of long duration; heterologous immunity, though present, is very brief and may permit mild, undiagnosed febrile illness.

9. Methods of control—

A. Preventive measures:

1) Community survey to determine density of vector mosquitoes, to identify breeding places, and to promote plans for elimination.
2) Public health education on personal measures for protection against mosquitoes, including use of repellents (see Malaria 9A3 and 4, p. 142).

B. Control of patient, contacts, and the immediate environment:

1) Report to local health authority: Obligatory report of epidemics; no case report, Class 4 (see Preface).

2) Isolation: Patient should be kept in screened room for at least 5 days after onset, or in quarters treated with residual insecticide.

3) Concurrent disinfection: None.

4) Quarantine: None.

5) Immunization of contacts: None.

6) Investigation of contacts: Place of residence of patient during fortnight previous to onset. Search for unreported or undiagnosed cases.

7) Specific treatment: None.

C. Epidemic measures:

1) Search for and destruction of *Aedes* mosquitoes in places of human habitation.

2) Use of mosquito repellents by persons exposed through occupation or other necessity to bites of vector mosquitoes.

D. International measures: Enforcement of international agreements designed to prevent spread of the disease by man, and mosquito transfer via ships, airplanes and land transport from areas where an epidemic exists.

WHO Reference Centres (see Preface).

B. BUNYAMWERA, BWAMBA, CHIKUNGUNYA, MAYARO, O'NYONG-NYONG, RIFT VALLEY, VENEZUELAN EQUINE, WEST NILE, GROUP C VIRAL FEVERS, OROPOUCHE, AND OTHERS

1. Identification—A group of brief febrile illnesses of usually a week or less, many of which are dengue-like (see table for mosquito-borne viruses). Usual onset is with headache, malaise, arthralgia or myalgia and occasionally nausea and vomiting; generally some conjunctivitis and photophobia. Fever may or may not be diphasic (saddleback); rashes are common in West Nile, chikungunya and o'nyong-nyong disease, possibly hemorrhages in chikungunya fever in Southeast Asia and India; leucopenia common; convalescence frequently prolonged. Meningoencephalitis is an occasional feature of West Nile. Venezuelan equine virus in recent years has been responsible for an increase of encephalitic cases; it is still included under Viral fevers because most cases fulfill the requirements of this group. The several demonstrated related viruses within the Venezuelan equine complex make indefinite the proportion of fevers and encephalitides attributable to that specific virus. Several group C viruses are reported to produce weakness of lower limbs. Rarely fatal, except encephalitis from Venezuelan equine.

Serological tests differentiate other fevers of viral or unknown origin, but chikungunya, o'nyong-nyong, and others in group A are difficult to distinguish from one another. Specific diagnosis is possible by virus isolation from blood during febrile period by inoculation of suckling mice or tissue culture; Venezuelan equine also from nasopharyngeal washings. Laboratory infections occur with many of these viruses.

2. Occurrence—West Nile virus in Egypt, Israel, India, France and probably widespread in a number of parts of Africa and the northern Mediterranean; chikungunya in Africa, India, Southeast Asia and the Philippine Islands; Rift Valley, o'nyong-nyong, Bwamba and Bunyamwera fevers thus far identified only in Africa. Mayaro and group C fevers occur in tropical South America, Panama and Trinidad; Venezuelan equine or other closely related members of the complex (Mucambo, Pixuna) there and in Florida, Middle America and Mexico; Oropouche fever in Trinidad and Brazil. Ross River and Kunjin viruses produce disease in Australia. Seasonal incidence depends on vector prevalence. Recognized occurrence is primarily rural; occasionally chikungunya occurs in explosive urban outbreaks.

3. Infectious agents—Each disease is due to an independent virus of the same name as the disease. West Nile, Banzi, Kunjin, Spondweni, Uganda S and Zika viruses are in group B; the closely related chikungunya and o'nyong-nyong with Mayaro, Bebaru, Mucambo, Pixuna, Ross River and Venezuelan equine viruses in group A. Group C viruses are Apeu, Caraparu, Itaqui, Madrid, Marituba, Murutucu, Oriboca, Ossa and Restan. Others in smaller groups are listed in the table preceding.

4. Reservoir—Unknown for most viruses in the group. All appear to be tropics-dependent, with a continuous vertebrate-mosquito cycle essential. Horses are a source of mosquito infection with Venezuelan equine encephalitis; birds, with West Nile; and sheep, other domestic ruminants, game, monkeys and rodents, with Rift Valley; rodents, with group C.

5. Mode of transmission—In most instances by bite of an infective mosquito: for chikungunya, *A. aegypti* and possibly others; West Nile, *Culex univittatus* in Egypt, *C. pipiens molestus* in Israel; O'nyong-nyong, *Anopheles* species; Mayaro, *Mansonia venezuelensis;* Bunyamwera, *Aedes;* group C viruses, species of *Aedes, Mansonia, Psorophora* and *Sabethini.* Viruses of the Venezuelan equine complex isolated from many genera and species, many of them susceptible in the laboratory, including *Mansonia, Psorophora, Aedes, Culex, Haemagogus, Sabethini* and *Anopheles.* For Rift Valley in sheep, etc., *Aedes caballus, A. circumluteolus* and *A. theileri;* species of *Eretmapodites* probably important in forest cycles; however, most human infections are predominantly associated with handling of infective material of animal origin during necropsy and butchering.

6. Incubation period—Usually 3 to 12 days.

7. Period of communicability—Not directly transmitted from man to man except possibly Venezuelan equine virus in pharynx. Infective mosquitoes probably transmit virus throughout life. Viremia, essential to vector infection, is present for many of these viruses during early clinical illness in man.

8. Susceptibility and resistance—Susceptibility appears general, in both sexes and throughout life. Inapparent infections and mild undiagnosed disease are common. Infection leads to immunity, and susceptibles in highly endemic areas are mainly young children.

9. Methods of control—

A. Preventive measures:

1) The general measures applicable to mosquito-borne viral encephalitides (9A1 through 5 and 9A7, p. 16). For Rift Valley, precautions in care and handling of infected animals and their products.

2) An experimental attenuated virus vaccine for Venezuelan equine has been used effectively to protect laboratory workers and other adults at high risk. This vaccine is also effective in protecting horses. An experimental inactivated tissue culture vaccine is used similarly for Rift Valley.

B. Control of patient, contacts, and the immediate environment:

1) *Report to local health authority:* In selected endemic areas; in most countries not a reportable disease, Class 3B (see Preface).

2) *Isolation:* Keep patient in screened room for at least 5 days after onset, or in quarters treated with residual insecticide.

3) *Concurrent disinfection:* None.

4) *Quarantine:* None.

5) *Immunization of contacts:* None.

6) *Investigation of contacts:* Place of residence of patient during fortnight previous to onset. Search for unreported or undiagnosed cases.

7) *Specific treatment:* None.

C. Epidemic measures:

1) Community survey to determine density of vector mosquitoes, to identify their breeding places, and to promote plans for their elimination.

2) Use of mosquito repellents by persons exposed through occupation or other necessity to bites of vector mosquitoes.

3) Identification of the disease among horses (Venezuelan) or sheep and other animals (Rift Valley) and serological survey of birds (West Nile), or rodents (group C viruses) have epidemiological value to indicate frequency of infection and areas involved.

D. *International measures:* For Rift Valley fever, restrict movement of animals from enzootic areas to those free from disease; for others, none except enforcement of international agreements designed to prevent transfer of mosquitoes by ships, airplanes and land transport.

WHO Reference Centres (see Preface).

II. Tick-borne

COLORADO TICK FEVER AND OTHER TICK-BORNE FEVERS

1. Identification—The Colorado type is an acute febrile dengue-like disease, usually without rash; a brief remission is usual, followed by a second bout of fever, each lasting 2 or 3 days. Characteristically mild but may be severe in children, occasionally with encephalitis or tendency to bleed; deaths are uncommon.

Laboratory confirmation is by isolation of virus by inoculation of suckling mice; complement-fixing and neutralizing antibodies do not appear for 2 weeks or longer. Clinical manifestations of other types and diagnostic methods vary only slightly.

2. Occurrence—Known areas of occurrence of Colorado type are Western Canada and in Washington, Oregon, Idaho, Montana, California, Nevada, Utah, Wyoming, Colorado and South Dakota. Virus has been isolated from *Dermacentor andersoni* in British Columbia and New Mexico. The disease is most frequent in adult males, but also affects children and women; seasonal incidence parallels period of greatest tick activity, distribution is endemic, and the disease is common in much of the affected area. Geographic distribution of other types as shown in table preceding.

3. Infectious agents—The viruses of Colorado tick fever and Nairobi sheep disease and the Langat, Kemerovo, Tribec, Quaranfil, Ganjam and Congo viruses.

4. Reservoir—For Colorado type, small mammals; ground squirrels, porcupine, chipmunk and *Peromyscus* have been identified; also nymphal and larval ticks.

5. Mode of transmission—To man by bite of the infective adult vector tick. In Colorado type, immature ticks (*Dermacentor andersoni*) acquire infection by feeding on infected animals during viremia; they remain infected through the various moults and transmit virus to man by feeding as adult ticks.

6. Incubation period—Usually 4 to 5 days.

7. Period of communicability—Not directly transmitted from man to man; the wildlife cycle maintained by ticks is the important consideration. Ticks remain infective throughout life. Virus is present in man during course of the fever, from 1 to 10 days after onset.

8. Susceptibility and resistance—Susceptibility is apparently universal. Second attacks are unknown; experimental reinfection is unsuccessful.

9. Methods of control—

A. Preventive measures:

1) Control of ticks; see Rocky Mountain Spotted Fever, 9A1 and 9A2, p. 207.
2) No available vaccine.

B. Control of patient, contacts, and the immediate environment:

1) Report to local health authority: In endemic areas (U.S.A.); in most states and countries not a reportable disease, Class 3B (see Preface).

2) Isolation: None.

3) Concurrent disinfection: None; destroy ticks on patient.

4) Quarantine: None.

5) Immunization of contacts: None.

6) Investigation of contacts and source of infection: Identification of tick-infested areas.

7) Specific treatment: None.

C. Epidemic measures: Not applicable.

D. International measures: WHO Reference Centres (see Preface)

III. *Phlebotomus*-borne

SANDFLY FEVER

1. Identification—A 3- or 4-day fever clinically not unlike influenza except for absence of inflammation of the respiratory tract. Headache, fever of 38.3 to 39.5 C (101 to 104 F), retrobulbar pain on motion of the eyes, injected sclerae, malaise, nausea and pain in limbs and back are characteristic. Leucopenia is usual on 4th or 5th day after onset of fever. Temperature occasionally exceeds 104 F; may present alarming symptoms, but death is unknown. Diagnosis is clinical and by epidemiological means, through occurrence of multiple and similar cases. Synonyms: Pappataci fever, Phlebotomus fever, Three-day fever.

Diagnosis may be confirmed by neutralization test, using mouse-adapted viruses, or by isolation of virus from blood in newborn mice.

2. Occurrence—In those parts of Europe, Africa and Asia where the vector exists; recently recognized in Central and South America, where closely related viral agents are present. A disease of subtropical and tropical areas with long periods of hot, dry weather; in general, a belt extending around the Mediterranean and eastward into Burma and China. Seasonal, between April and October, and prone to appear as a disease of troops and travelers from nonendemic areas.

3. Infectious agents—The viruses of sandfly fever; at least five related immunological types (Naples, Sicilian, Candiru, Chagres and Punta Toro) have been isolated from man and differentiated. In addition, Changuinola virus and vesicular stomatitis virus of Indiana type have been isolated from *Phlebotomus,* and both produce febrile disease in man.

4. Reservoir—Principal reservoir is the man-sandfly complex; an animal reservoir is suspected but not demonstrated. Cattle, horses and swine are principal hosts of vesicular stomatitis virus.

5. Mode of transmission—By bite of infective sandfly. Vector of the classical viruses is a small hairy, blood-sucking midge, *Phlebotomus papatasii,* the common sandfly, which bites at night and has a limited flight range. Sandflies of the genus *Sergentomyia* have been found infected and may be vectors. Other types of *Phlebotomus* are involved in Central and South America.

6. Incubation period—Up to 6 days, usually 3 to 4 days, rarely less.

7. Period of communicability—Virus is present in the blood of an infected person at least 24 hours before and 24 hours after onset of fever. *Phlebotomus* becomes infective about 7 days after biting an infected person and remains so for life.

8. Susceptibility and resistance—Susceptibility is essentially universal; homologous acquired immunity is possibly lasting. Relative resistance of native populations in sandfly areas is probably attributable to infection early in life.

9. Methods of control—

A. *Preventive measures:* Control of sandflies is the important consideration. See Cutaneous Leishmaniasis 9A1, pp. 126–127.

B. *Control of patient, contacts, and the immediate environment:*

1) *Report to local health authority:* In selected endemic areas; in most countries not a reportable disease, Class 3C (see Preface).

2) *Isolation:* None; protect infected individual from bites of sandflies for the first few days of illness by very fine screening or mosquito bed nets (25–30 mesh to the inch, aperture size not more than 0.035 inches) impregnated with residual insecticide, or by spraying quarters with the insecticide.

3) *Concurrent disinfection:* None; destruction of sandflies in the dwelling.

4) *Quarantine:* None.

5) *Immunization of contacts:* No measures currently available.

6) *Investigation of contacts and source of infection:* Search for breeding areas of sandflies around dwellings, especially in rubble heaps, masonry cracks, and under stones.

7) *Specific treatment:* None.

C. *Epidemic measures:*
1) Community use of insecticide to destroy sandflies in and about human habitations.
2) Public health education on conditions leading to infection; and importance of preventing bites of sandflies by use of repellents while in infected areas, particularly after sundown.

D. *International measures:* WHO Reference Centres (see Preface).

ARTHROPOD-BORNE VIRAL HEMORRHAGIC FEVERS

I. Mosquito-borne

A. YELLOW FEVER

1. Identification—An acute infectious disease of short duration and varying severity. The mildest cases are clinically indeterminate; typical attacks are characterized by sudden onset, fever, headache, backache, prostration, nausea and vomiting. As the disease progresses, the pulse rate slows in relation to temperature, and albuminuria becomes pronounced; anuria may occur. Leucopenia appears early, most pronounced about the 5th day. Common hemorrhagic symptoms include epistaxis, buccal bleeding, hematemesis, and melena. Jaundice is moderate early in the disease, later is intensified; postmortem icterus may be pronounced. Case fatality among indigenous populations of endemic regions is less than 5%.

Laboratory diagnosis is by isolation of virus from blood by inoculation of suckling mice or monkeys, demonstration of a rising titer of antibodies in paired acute-phase and convalescent sera, and demonstration of typical lesions of the liver.

2. Occurrence—Except for a few cases in Trinidad, W.I., in 1954 no urban yellow fever outbreak has been transmitted by *Aedes aegypti* in the Americas since 1942. Urban yellow fever outbreaks are still reported from Africa in areas contiguous to rain forest regions, where jungle yellow fever is endemic. Urban yellow fever, when first introduced into a community in the Americas, tended to attack both sexes and all ages and races, whereas jungle yellow fever of tropical America occurs predominantly among adult males 20 to 40 years of age who are exposed in the jungle.

Jungle yellow fever is present from time to time in all mainland countries of the Americas, from Mexico to South America, with the exception of El Salvador, Uruguay and Chile. In Africa it extends from the West Coast south of the Sahara Desert through the Republic of the Congo (Leopoldville) into Zambia, Botswana, Malawi, Uganda, Tanzania, Kenya, Ethiopia, the Somali Republic and the Sudan. There is no evidence that yellow fever ever has been present in Asia.

3. Infectious agent—The virus of yellow fever.

4. Reservoir—In urban areas the reservoir of infection is man and *Aedes aegypti;* in forest areas, vertebrates other than man—mainly monkeys, marmosets, possibly marsupials and forest mosquitoes. Man has no essential role in transmission of jungle yellow fever, nor in maintaining the virus.

5. Mode of transmission—In urban and certain rural areas, by the bite of infective *Aedes aegypti* mosquitoes. In forests of South America, by the bite of several species of forest mosquitoes of the genus *Haemagogus* and by *A. leucocelaenus*. In tropical Africa, *Aedes africanus* is the vector in the monkey population, while *Aedes simpsoni,* a semidomestic mosquito, and probably other *Aedes* species transmit the virus from monkey to man. In recent large epidemics in Ethiopia, good epidemiological evidence incriminated *A. simpsoni* as a man-to-man vector.

6. Incubation period—3 to 6 days.

7. Period of communicability—Blood of patients is infective for mosquitoes shortly before onset of fever and for the first 3 days of illness. Highly communicable where many susceptible persons and abundant vector mosquitoes coexist. Not communicable by contact or common vehicles. The extrinsic period of incubation before *A. aegypti* becomes infective is commonly 9 to 12 days at the usual summer temperatures. *A. aegypti* mosquitoes, once infected, remain so for life, but transovarian passage does not occur.

8. Susceptibility and resistance—Recovery from yellow fever is followed by lasting immunity; second attacks are unknown. Mild inapparent infections are common in endemic areas. Transient passive immunity in infants born to immune mothers may persist up to 6 months. In natural infection, antibodies appear in the blood within the first week.

9. Methods of control—

A. *Preventive measures:*

1) Urban yellow fever, by eradication or control of *A. aegypti* mosquitoes.

2) Sylvan or jungle yellow fever, transmitted by *Haemagogus* and forest species of *Aedes,* cannot be controlled by any known method except vaccination, which is recommended for all persons living in rural areas whose occupation brings them into forests in yellow fever areas, and for persons who intend to visit those areas.

3) Active immunization of all persons necessarily exposed to infection because of residence, occupation or travel. A single subcutaneous injection of a vaccine containing viable 17D strain of virus cultivated in chick embryo is effective. Antibodies appear from 7 to 10 days after vaccination and persist for at least 17 years, probably much longer. This is the only vaccine used in the Americas. A second method

employs a living neurotropic yellow fever virus (Dakar strain prepared in mouse brain) administered by cutaneous scarification to persons 10 years of age and over. Reactions are more frequent, with fatal encephalitis an occasional complication.

B. Control of patient, contacts, and the immediate environment:

1) *Report to local health authority:* Case report universally required by International Sanitary and Health Regulations, Class 1 (see Preface).
2) *Isolation:* None; prevent access of mosquitoes to patient during first 3 days by screening sickroom or by spraying quarters with insecticide having residual effect, or by bed net.
3) *Concurrent disinfection:* None; home of patient and all houses in vicinity should be sprayed promptly with an effective residual insecticide.
4) *Quarantine:* None.
5) *Immunization of contacts:* Family and other contacts and neighbors not previously immunized should be vaccinated promptly.
6) *Investigation of contacts and source of infection:* Inquiry about all places, including forest areas, visited by patient 3 to 6 days before onset, to locate focus of yellow fever; observe all persons visiting that focus. Search of premises and place of work for mosquitoes capable of transmitting infection. Attention to mild febrile illnesses and unexplained deaths suggesting yellow fever.
7) *Specific treatment:* None.

C. Epidemic measures:

1) Urban or *aegypti*-transmitted yellow fever:
   a) Mass vaccination, beginning with persons most exposed and those living in *aegypti*-infested parts of the area.
   b) Spray all houses in community with residual insecticide.
   c) Apply larvicide to all actual and potential breeding places of *A. aegypti*.
2) Jungle or sylvan yellow fever:
   a) Immediate vaccination of all persons living in or near forested areas or entering such areas.
   b) Avoidance by unvaccinated individuals of those tracts of forest where infection has been localized, and similarly by vaccinated persons for the first week after vaccination.
3) In regions where yellow fever may occur, a viscerotomy service should be organized to collect for diagnostic purposes small specimens of liver from fatal febrile illnesses of 10 days' duration or less; many cases and outbreaks otherwise missed are thereby discovered.

4) In South and Central America, confirmed deaths of howler and spider monkeys in the forest are presumptive evidence of the presence of yellow fever. Confirmation by the histopathological examination of livers of moribund or recently dead monkeys or by virus isolation is highly desirable.

5) Immunity surveys by mouse neutralization tests of wild primates captured in forested areas are useful in defining enzootic areas. Serological surveys of human populations are practically useless where yellow fever vaccine has been widely used.

D. International measures:

1) Telegraphic notification by governments to WHO and to adjacent countries of the first imported, first transferred, or first nonimported case of yellow fever in an area previously free of the disease; and of newly discovered or reactivated foci of yellow fever infection among vertebrates other than man.

2) Measures applicable to ships, aircraft and land transport arriving from yellow fever areas are specified in the International Health Regulations,* WHO, Geneva.

3) *Animal quarantine:* Quarantine of monkeys, marmosets and other wild primates arriving from yellow fever areas may be required until 7 days have elapsed after leaving such areas.

4) *International travelers:* A valid international certificate of vaccination against yellow fever is required by many countries for entry of travelers coming from or through recognized yellow fever zones of Africa and South America; otherwise, quarantine measures are applicable. The international certificate of vaccination is valid from 10 days after date of vaccination and for 10 years; if revaccinated within that time, from date of that revaccination and for 10 years.

∾

B. HEMORRHAGIC FEVERS OF THE PHILIPPINES AND SOUTHEAST ASIA

1. Identification—A group of endemic acute hemorrhagic fevers recognized thus far principally in children under 7 years of age, although higher ages are affected in Singapore and Calcutta. Sudden onset, with high fever, prostration, headache, malaise and frequently nausea and vomiting. Conjunctivitis, epistaxis and abdominal pain

---

* These will come into force on January 1, 1971. Until that date, the *International Sanitary Regulations,* 3rd edition (Geneva: WHO, 1966) are applicable.

soon appear, along with an early petechial rash first noted on extremities and not infrequently involving face and trunk but not axillae or chest. Purpuric lesions may appear early and extensive ecchymoses later. Many patients have serious shock on the 3rd to 5th day; blood platelets reduced, bleeding time prolonged; hemoconcentration; usually no leucopenia or leucocytosis in severe cases. Hemorrhage into gastrointestinal or pulmonary tract may or may not be evident. Significant differences in clinical manifestations are observed in different countries; hepatomegaly is conspicuous in Thailand and absent in the Philippines; epistaxis more frequent in Philippines. Duration is usually 5 to 8 days, with prompt uncomplicated recovery. Fatality is about 5%, with death mainly during period of shock.

Serologic tests show a rise in titer with responsible viruses and others closely related; virus isolation from blood during acute febrile stage by inoculation of suckling mice or tissue culture. Isolation from organs at autopsy rare.

2. Occurrence—All recognized outbreaks have been in urban areas of the Philippine Islands, Thailand, Malaysia, South Vietnam, or semiurban India. Major outbreaks in Manila and Bangkok, but also smaller urban areas, observed almost exclusively among Oriental members of the population except in Calcutta. Occurrence is limited to rainy seasons and areas of high *Aedes aegypti* prevalence; not yet observed where only *A. albopictus* is present.

3. Infectious agents—Viruses presently classed as dengue virus, types 1, 2, 3 and 4, possibly others. Chikungunya virus may be responsible for some mild cases in Bangkok, for more severe cases in Calcutta. May be caused by combined infection of more than one virus or sensitization to previous dengue infection.

4. Reservoir—Unknown; probably man and *A. aegypti*.

5. Mode of transmission—By bite of an infective *A. aegypti* mosquito. Viruses have been isolated from this mosquito during epidemics. *A. albopictus* isolations are less common.

6. Incubation period—Unknown.

7. Period of communicability—No evidence of transmission from man to man.

8. Susceptibility and resistance—Modal age of attack in epidemics thus far recognized, except Singapore and Calcutta, is about 3 to 5 years, with the range from 4 months to the young adult years. Prevalence of dengue antibodies in the general population is high in older children and in adults. Many mild cases are recognized by serologic tests. Absence, in most areas, of hemorrhagic disease in Caucasians of European descent is not understood; classical dengue has been observed in Caucasians during epidemics of hemorrhagic disease in Orientals. A host factor involved in susceptibility is strongly suspected.

9. Methods of control—See Arthropod-borne viral fevers, Dengue fever, 9A to 9D, pp. 20–21.

II. Tick-borne

A. CRIMEAN HEMORRHAGIC FEVER AND CENTRAL ASIAN HEMORRHAGIC FEVER

1. Identification—Sudden onset with fever, malaise, weakness, irritability, headache, severe pain in limbs and loins, and marked anorexia. Vomiting, abdominal pain, and diarrhea occur occasionally. Early development of flush on face and chest, and injection of conjunctivae. Associated with hemorrhagic enanthem of soft palate, uvula and pharynx, and a fine petechial rash spreading from chest and abdomen to the body generally; occasionally large purpuric areas. Some bleeding from gums, nose, lungs, uterus and intestine; in large amount, only in serious or fatal cases. Hematuria and albuminuria slight or absent. Fever constantly elevated for 5 to 12 days, falling by lysis with prolonged convalescence. Leucopenia, with marked neutropenia; relative lymphocytosis but absolute lymphopenia and eosinophilia. Thrombocytopenia present, but bleeding time is normal. Reported case fatality ranges from 2% to 50%.

Virus of Crimean type has recently been isolated in suckling mice.

2. Occurrence—Crimean type recognized in the steppe regions of Western Crimea, and on the Kersch peninsula and in the Rostov-Don and Astrakhan regions; the Central Asian type in Kazakstan and Uzbekistan. Most patients are agricultural workers in fallow lands and dairy workers. Seasonal occurrence from June to September, the period of vector activity. Sporadic cases of similar disease have been observed in several areas of Central Africa.

3. Infectious agent—The Crimean virus, identified as the Congo virus originally isolated in Africa (Congo, Uganda, and Nigeria). Central Asia type not available in the laboratory.

4. Reservoir—In nature, believed to be hares, birds and *Hyalomma* ticks.

5. Mode of transmission—By bite of infective adult *Hyalomma marginatum* or *H. anatolicum*. Immature ticks are believed to acquire infection from the animal hosts.

6. Incubation period—7 to 12 days.

7. Period of communicability—Not directly transmitted from man to man. Infected tick probably remains so for life.

8. Susceptibility and resistance—Immunity for at least 1 year.

9. Methods of control—

A. *Preventive measures:* See Rocky Mountain Spotted Fever (p. 207) for preventive measures against ticks. No available vaccine.

B. *Control of patient, contacts, and the immediate environment:*

1) *Report to local health authority:* In selected endemic areas; in most countries not a reportable disease, Class 3B (see Preface).

2) Isolation: None if patient is tick-free.
3) Concurrent disinfection: None.
4) Quarantine: None.
5) Immunization: None.
6) Investigation of contacts and source of infection: Search for missed cases and the presence of hares and other possible vectors.
7) Specific treatment: Convalescent serum reported useful.

C. Epidemic measures: See Rocky Mountain Spotted Fever, p. 207.

D. International measures: WHO Reference Centres (see Preface).

B. OMSK HEMORRHAGIC FEVER AND KYASANUR FOREST DISEASE

1. Identification—These two diseases have marked similarities. Onset is sudden, with headache, fever, pain in lower back and limbs, and severe prostration; often associated with conjunctivitis, diarrhea and vomiting by the 3rd to 4th day. A papulovesicular eruption on the soft palate is an important diagnostic sign. Usually no involvement of central nervous system. Severe cases are associated with hemorrhages but with no cutaneous rash. Bleeding occurs from gums, nose, gastrointestinal tract, uterus and lungs (but rarely from the kidneys) sometimes for many days and, when serious, results in shock and death. However, shock may occur without manifest hemorrhage. Estimated fatality is from 1% to 10%. Leucopenia and thrombocytopenia are marked. Febrile period ranges from 5 days to 2 weeks, at times with a secondary rise in the 3rd week. Convalescence tends to be slow and prolonged.

Diagnosis is by isolation of virus from blood by inoculation of suckling mice or tissue cultures as long as 10 days following onset, or by serological tests.

2. Occurrence—In the Kyasanur Forest of the Shimoga District, Mysore State, India, principally in young adult males exposed in the forest during the dry season from January to June. Omsk type formerly occurred in rural workers and children exposed to infected ticks in the steppe regions of the Omsk Oblast in Siberia, recently only in the Novosibirsk region. Seasonal occurrence in each area coincides with vector activity. Laboratory infections are common with both viruses.

3. Infectious agents—Viruses of these two diseases are closely related. The agents belong to group B, are of the Russian spring-summer-louping ill complex, and are similar antigenically to other members.

4. Reservoir—In Kyasanur Forest disease, probably rodents and monkeys; in Omsk disease, rodents, muskrats, and possibly the tick, since transovarian passage has been reported for other viruses of this complex.

5. Mode of transmission—By bite of infective ticks (especially nymphal stages), probably *Haemaphysalis spinigera* in Kyasanur Forest disease; possibly *Dermacentor pictus* and *Dermacentor marginatus* in the Omsk type. Most recent data implicate direct transmission from muskrat to man and suggest ticks may not be vectors.

6. Incubation period—Usually 3 to 8 days.

7. Period of communicability—Not directly transmitted from man to man. Infected tick remains so for life.

8. Susceptibility and resistance—All ages and sexes are probably susceptible; previous infection leads to immunity.

9. Methods of control—See Tick-borne Encephalitis and Rocky Mountain Spotted Fever (pp. 19 and 207). A formalinized mouse brain virus vaccine has been reported effective for Omsk but as yet has been inadequately tested for Kyasanur Forest disease.

ASCARIASIS

1. Identification—A chronic nematode disease of the small intestine. Symptoms are variable, often vague or absent, and ordinarily mild; live worms passed in stools or vomited are frequently the first sign of infection. Heavy infection may cause digestive disturbances, abdominal pain, vomiting, restlessness, and disturbed sleep. Serious complications among children in tropical countries include bowel obstruction and occasional deaths, due to migration of adult worms into liver, peritoneal cavity and appendix. Deaths from other causes are often attributed to this more obvious infection.

Identification of eggs in feces is the usual method of diagnosis.

2. Occurrence—Common and worldwide, with greatest frequency in moist tropical countries, where prevalence may exceed 50% of a population. Children of preschool and early school age are more frequently and more heavily infected than older children and adults. In U.S.A. the disease is most prevalent in the South.

3. Infectious agent—*Ascaris lumbricoides,* the large intestinal round worm of man.

4. Reservoir—Reservoir is an infected person whose feces contain eggs.

5. Mode of transmission—By direct or indirect transmission of embryonated eggs to the mouth from soil in and about houses where facilities for sanitary disposal of human excreta are lacking or are not used. Embryonation requires 9 days to several weeks after passage of the egg. Salads and other foods eaten raw are the usual vehicles. Contaminated soil may be carried long distances on feet or footwear into houses and conveyances; transmission of infection by dust is also possible. Embryonated eggs are ingested, hatch in intestinal canal, and larvae penetrate the wall and reach liver and lungs by way of lymphatic and circulatory systems. Most larvae reaching the lungs pass into air passages, ascend bronchi, are swallowed, and eventually reach the small intestine, where they grow to maturity and mate. Eggs are passed from gravid females and are discharged in feces.

6. Incubation period—Worms reach maturity about 2 months after ingestion of embryonated eggs.

7. Period of communicability—As long as mature fertilized female worms live in intestine. Most adult worms live less than 6 months; maximum life under 1½ years. The female can produce about 200,000 eggs a day. Embryonated eggs, under favorable conditions, remain viable in soil for months and even years.

8. Susceptibility and resistance—Susceptibility is general.

9. Methods of control—

   A. Preventive measures:

     1) Provision of adequate facilities for proper disposal of feces and prevention of soil contamination in areas immediately adjacent to houses, particularly in play areas of children.

     2) In rural areas, construction of privies in such manner as to obviate dissemination of ascarid eggs through overflow, drainage, or similar circumstance. Composting is practiced to advantage where such facilities are lacking.

     3) Education of all persons, particularly children, to use toilet facilities and to wash hands after defecating. Encouragement of satisfactory hygienic habits on the part of children; in particular they should be trained to wash their hands before handling food, and not to eat food which has been dropped on the floor.

   B. Control of patient, contacts, and the immediate environment:

     1) Report to local health authority: Official report not ordinarily justifiable, Class 5 (see Preface).

     2) Isolation: None.

     3) Concurrent disinfection: Sanitary disposal of feces.

     4) Quarantine: None.

     5) Immunization of contacts: None.

     6) Investigation of contacts and source of infection: Individual and environmental sources of infection should be sought, particularly in persons and premises of family affected.

     7) Specific treatment: Piperazine hexahydrate or piperazine citrate (Antepar).

   C. Epidemic measures: Surveys for prevalence in highly endemic areas, education in sanitation of environment and in personal hygiene, and provision of treatment facilities.

   D. International measures: None.

ASPERGILLOSIS

1. Identification—A variety of clinical syndromes can be produced by *Aspergillus:* (1) Inhalation of the fungus may cause asthmatic attacks in hypersensitized persons. (2) Saprophytic endobronchial colonization in patients with bronchitis or bronchiectasis may cause bronchial plugs and atelectasis, or a large mass of hyphae may fill a previously existing cavity (fungus ball). In such patients, *Aspergillus* may appear in bacterial lung abscess or empyema. (3) *Aspergillus* pneumonia may occur, particularly in patients receiving cytotoxic or immunosuppressive therapy; it may disseminate to brain, kidneys and other organs and is usually fatal. Invasion of blood vessels with thrombosis and infarction is characteristic of pneumonic and disseminated infection. (4) Otomycosis is usually caused by *Aspergillus* species. (5) Rarely, the fungus may cause granulomas of the orbit or paranasal sinuses. (6) Growing on certain foods, many isolates of *Aspergillus flavus* and occasionally other species of *Aspergillus* will produce aflatoxins. These toxins are a possible cause of disease in animals and are carcinogenic for experimental animals, but no adverse effects on man have been recognized.

Among findings that suggest a diagnosis of allergic aspergillosis are (1) isolation of *Aspergillus* from sputum and (2) demonstration, by the use of *Aspergillus* antigens, of any or all of the following: bronchial constriction on inhalation, serum precipitins, and immediate cutaneous reactions after scratch test. Diagnosis of saprophytic endobronchial colonization is based on culture or microscopic demonstration of *Aspergillus* in sputum or in plugs of expectorated hyphae. Serum precipitins to *Aspergillus* antigens are usually present. Radiologic evidence of fungus ball is often obtainable. Diagnosis of invasive aspergillosis depends upon microscopic demonstration of the fungus in infected tissue. Cultural confirmation is desirable.

2. Occurrence—An uncommon sporadic disease. No distinctive differences in incidence by race or sex.

3. Infectious agent—*Aspergillus fumigatus* is the usual cause of aspergillosis. Isolation of other species has been chiefly confined to noninvasive disease.

4. Reservoir and source of infection—Compost piles undergoing fermentation and decay are prominent reservoirs and sources of infection. Fungi also are found in hay stored when damp, in decaying vegetation, and in cereal grains stored under conditions which permit the grain to heat up.

5. Mode of transmission—Inhalation of airborne spores.

6. Incubation period—Probably a few days to weeks.

7. Period of communicability—Not directly transmitted from man to man.

8. Susceptibility and resistance—The frequency of the fungus in the external environment and the usual occurrence of the disease as a secondary infection suggest a high degree of resistance by healthy persons.

9. **Methods of control—**

    A. Preventive measures: None.

    B. Control of patient, contacts, and the immediate environment:
        1) Report to local health authority: Official report ordinarily not justifiable; Class 5 (see Preface).
        2) Isolation: None.
        3) Concurrent disinfection: Ordinary cleanliness. Terminal cleaning.
        4) Quarantine: None.
        5) Immunization of contacts: None.
        6) Investigation of contacts: Ordinarily not profitable.
        7) Specific treatment: Amphotericin B should be tried in tissue-invasive forms. Solely endobronchial colonization should be treated by measures to improve bronchopulmonary drainage.

    C. Epidemic measures: Not applicable—a sporadic disease.

    D. International measures: None.

BALANTIDIASIS

1. **Identification**—A disease of the colon characteristically producing diarrhea or dysentery, accompanied by abdominal colic, tenesmus, nausea, and vomiting. Infection often asymptomatic. Occasionally the dysentery is of amebic type and stools may contain much blood, pus and mucus. In some individuals constipation prevails. Balantidiasis may also result in loss of appetite, headache, insomnia, colonic tenderness, muscular weakness, weight loss and anemia. Peritoneal and urogenital invasion is rare. Synonyms: Balantidiosis; Balantidial dysentery.

Diagnosis is by identifying the trophozoites or cysts of *Balantidium coli* in feces, or trophozoites in material obtained by sigmoidoscopy.

2. **Occurrence**—Worldwide in distribution, but the incidence of disease in man is low. Water-borne epidemics occasionally occur in areas of poor environmental sanitation. Association with hogs may result in a higher incidence.

3. **Infectious agent**—*Balantidium coli,* a ciliated protozoan.

4. **Reservoir**—Reservoir is swine and man.

5. **Mode of transmission**—Infection is by ingestion of cysts from feces of infected hosts; in epidemics, mainly by fecally contaminated

water. Sporadic transmission is by water, by hand-to-mouth transfer of feces, by contaminated raw vegetables, by flies and by soiled hands of food handlers.

6. Incubation period—Unknown; sometimes only a few days.

7. Period of communicability—During the whole period of intestinal infection.

8. Susceptibility and resistance—Man appears to have a high natural resistance. In otherwise debilitated individuals the infection may be serious and even fatal.

9. Methods of control—

A. Preventive measures:
1) Sanitary disposal of feces.
2) Avoidance of contact with hog feces.
3) Protection of public water supplies against fecal contamination. Diatomaceous earth filters remove all cysts. Usual chlorination of water does not destroy cysts. The efficacy of iodine is unproven. Small quantities of water are best purified by boiling.
4) Health education of the general public in personal hygiene.
5) Fly control and protection of foods against fly contamination.
6) Supervision by health agencies of food handlers.

B. Control of patient, contacts, and the immediate environment:
1) *Report to local health authority:* Official report not justifiable, Class 5 (see Preface).
2) *Isolation:* None.
3) *Concurrent disinfection:* Sanitary disposal of feces.
4) *Quarantine:* None.
5) *Immunization of contacts:* Not applicable.
6) *Investigation of contacts and source of infection:* Microscopic examination of feces of household members and suspected contacts. Also investigation of hogs. (These also harbor *Balantidium suis,* which is nonpathogenic to man.)
7) *Specific treatment:* Di-iodohydroxyquin (Diodoquin) and tetracyclines eliminate infection.

C. Epidemic measures: Any grouping of several cases in a single area or institution requires prompt epidemiological investigation.

D. International measures: None.

BARTONELLOSIS

1. Identification—An illness occurring in 2 stages, an interval of weeks to months usually separating an initial acute febrile period and an eruptive period. The febrile Oroya fever stage is characterized by irregular fever, severe anemia, pain in bones and joints, and lymphadenopathy. The eruptive Verruga Peruana stage may merge with the febrile stage; an intervening quiescent period is usual. The eruption is in crops of papules or nodules resembling hemangiomas, sometimes with many small lesions, sometimes with a few tumor-like subepithelial nodules. Fatality of untreated Oroya fever ranges from 10 to 40%, usually associated with Salmonella septicemia; Verruga Peruana has a prolonged course but few deaths. Synonyms: Oroya fever, Verruga Peruana, Carrión's disease.

Diagnosis is by demonstration of the infectious agent within red blood cells during the acute stage, in sections of skin lesions during the eruptive stage, or by blood culture during either stage.

2. Occurrence—Limited to certain altitudes in mountain valleys of Peru, Ecuador and southwest Colombia, where vector is present. No special predilection for age, race or sex.

3. Infectious agent—*Bartonella bacilliformis.*

4. Reservoir—Reservoir is an infected person with the agent present in the blood. In endemic areas the asymptomatic carrier rate may reach 5%.

5. Mode of transmission—By bite of sandflies of the genus *Phlebotomus;* species not identified for all areas; *Phlebotomus verrucarum* is important in Peru.

6. Incubation period—Usually 16 to 22 days, but occasionally 3 to 4 months.

7. Period of communicability—Not directly transmitted from man to man. Infectivity of man for the sandfly is long; the infectious agent may be present in blood weeks before and up to several years after actual illness. Duration of infectivity of sandfly, unknown.

8. Susceptibility and resistance—Susceptibility is general but the disease is milder in children than adults. Inapparent infections and carriers are known. Recovery from untreated Oroya fever almost invariably gives permanent immunity to this form. The verruga stage may recur.

9. Methods of control—

A. *Preventive measures:*
1) Control sandflies. See Cutaneous Leishmaniasis, pp. 126–127.
2) Avoid known endemic areas after sundown; otherwise apply insect repellent to exposed parts of the body.

B. *Control of patient, contacts, and the immediate environment:*
1) *Report to local health authority:* In selected endemic areas;

in most countries not a reportable disease, Class 3B (see Preface).

2) Isolation: None. The infected individual should be protected from bites of *Phlebotomus* (see 9A).

3) Concurrent disinfection: None.

4) Quarantine: None.

5) Immunization of contacts: None.

6) Investigation of contacts and source of infection: Identification of sandflies, particularly in localities where the infected person was exposed after sundown during preceding 3 to 8 weeks.

7) Specific treatment: Penicillin, streptomycin, chloramphenicol and tetracyclines are all effective in reducing fever and bacteremia. Chloramphenicol is drug of choice; believed to work directly against *Bartonella,* but more importantly it is best drug for the frequent secondary salmonellosis.

C. Epidemic measures: Intensification of case finding and systematic spraying of houses with a residual insecticide.

D. International measures: None.

BLASTOMYCOSIS, NORTH AMERICAN

1. Identification—Systemic blastomycosis is a chronic granulomatous mycosis, primarily of the lungs. Begins with a fever and symptoms of respiratory infection resembling influenza; progresses gradually with fever, loss of weight, cachexia with cough and purulent sputum. Dissemination results in abscesses in subcutaneous tissues, bones, central nervous system, reproductive and other visceral organs and is frequently fatal if untreated.

Cutaneous blastomycosis is characterized by a papule which ulcerates and spreads slowly and peripherally for months or years, leaving an irregular crusted ulcer with a granulomatous base and an elevated papilliform to verrucous border containing minute abscesses. The center of the ulcer heals with a thin scar. The lesions are usually on exposed parts of the body such as face, hands, wrists, feet and ankles. Cutaneous blastomycosis ordinarily is a local manifestation of existing systemic disease.

Direct microscopic examination of unstained smears of sputum and materials from lesions shows characteristic budding forms of the fungus which can be cultured. The complement-fixation test titer is of questionable value. Blastomycin skin test is often negative and misleading.

2. Occurrence—Uncommon, occurring sporadically in central and southeastern U.S.A., Central America, Canada and Africa. Rare in children; much more frequent in males than in females. Infection of dogs and horses occurs.

3. Infectious agent—*Blastomyces dermatitidis,* a dimorphic fungus which grows as a yeast in the tissues and in enriched culture media at 37 C, and as a mold at 30 C on simple media.

4. Reservoir—Reservoir is probably soil.

5. Mode of transmission—Resistant spores typical of the mold or saprophytic growth form probably are inhaled in spore-laden dust.

6. Incubation period—Probably a few weeks or less, to months.

7. Period of communicability—Not transmitted directly from man or animals to man. Contamination of the environment with resultant conversion of the fungus from the parasitic to the saprophytic disseminative mold form is potentially possible for duration of the disease.

8. Susceptibility and resistance—Unknown. Inapparent pulmonary infections are probable but of undetermined frequency. No information on immunity; rarity of the disease and of laboratory infections suggests man is relatively resistant.

9. Methods of control—

   A. Preventive measures: Unknown.

   B. Control of patient, contacts, and the immediate environment:
      1) Report to local health authority: Official report not ordinarily justifiable, Class 5 (see Preface).
      2) Isolation: None.
      3) Concurrent disinfection: Sputum, discharges and all contaminated articles. Terminal cleaning.
      4) Quarantine: None.
      5) Immunization of contacts: None.
      6) Investigation of contacts: Not profitable.
      7) Specific treatment: Amphotericin B (Fungizone) is the present drug of choice. Hydroxystilbamidine isethionate is an effective alternative.

   C. Epidemic measures: Not applicable—a sporadic disease.

   D. International measures: None.

BLASTOMYCOSIS, SOUTH AMERICAN

1. Identification—A serious, at times fatal, chronic mycosis characterized by lung involvement and/or ulcerative lesions of the mucosa (oral, nasal, rectal) and of the skin. Lymphadenopathy is frequent. In disseminated cases all viscera may be affected, especially the adrenal. Synonyms: Paracoccidioidal granuloma, Paracoccidioidomycosis.

Diagnosis confirmed histologically or by cultivation of the parasite. Serological techniques at present of questionable value.

Keloidal blastomycosis, a disease formerly confused with South American blastomycosis, is caused by *Loboa loboi.*

2. Occurrence—Endemic in South America, particularly rural Brazil. Highest incidence in adults aged 20 to 50 years; 10 times as common in males as in females.

3. Infectious agent—*Paracoccidioides brasiliensis (Blastomyces brasiliensis),* a dimorphic fungus.

4. Reservoir—Probably soil or spore-laden dust.

5. Mode of transmission—Presumably but not proven to be acquired through inhalation of contaminated soil or dust.

6. Incubation period—Highly variable, from 1 month to 30 years.

7. Period of communicability—Not known to be transmitted directly from man to man.

8. Susceptibility and resistance—Unknown.

9. Methods of control—

   A. *Preventive measures:* None.

   B. *Control of patient, contacts, and the immediate environment:*
   1) *Report to local health authority:* Official report not ordinarily justifiable, Class 5 (see Preface).
   2) *Isolation:* None.
   3) *Concurrent disinfection:* Of discharges and contaminated articles. Terminal cleaning.
   4) *Quarantine:* None.
   5) *Immunization of contacts:* None.
   6) *Investigation of contacts:* Not profitable.
   7) *Specific treatment:* Amphotericin B (Fungizone) given intravenously promptly arrests spread of lesions and is drug of choice. Sulfadiazine, sulfamerazine, and combinations of sulfonamides control the disease but treatment must be continued indefinitely to prevent relapse. Amphotericin B probably should be followed by treatment with sulfonamides.

   C. *Epidemic measures:* Not applicable; a sporadic disease.

   D. *International measures:* None.

BRUCELLOSIS

1. Identification—A systemic disease with acute or insidious onset, characterized by continued, intermittent or irregular fever of variable duration, headache, weakness, profuse sweating, chills or chilliness, arthralgia and generalized aching. The disease may last for several days, many months, or occasionally several years. Recovery is usual but disability is often pronounced. Fatality is 2% or less; higher for *Brucella melitensis* infections than for other biotypes. Clinical diagnosis is often difficult and uncertain. Death is rare in persons without complications. Synonyms: Undulant fever, Malta fever, Mediterranean fever, Bang's disease.

Laboratory diagnosis is by isolation of the infectious agent from blood, bone marrow or other tissues, or from discharges of the patient. The agglutination test is valuable, especially with paired sera to show rise in antibody. Tests for specific gamma-G antibody also useful, particularly in chronic cases.

2. Occurrence—Worldwide, especially in Mediterranean countries of Europe and North Africa, USSR, Mexico and South America. Males affected more often than females because of occupational risks. Sporadic cases and outbreaks occur among consumers of unpasteurized milk or milk products from cows, sheep and goats. Reported incidence in U.S.A. is less than 300 cases annually and declining, but many occupational cases are not diagnosed, which results in incomplete reporting.

3. Infectious agents—*Brucella abortus*, biotypes I–IX; *Brucella canis; Brucella melitensis*, biotypes I–III; and *Brucella suis*, biotypes I–IV.

4. Reservoir—Reservoirs of human infection are cattle, swine, sheep, goats, horses and reindeer; in U.S.A., mainly swine, cattle and Alaskan caribou. *B. canis*, which can infect laboratory workers, is a problem in laboratory dog colonies.

5. Mode of transmission—By contact with tissues, blood, urine, vaginal discharges, aborted fetuses, and especially placentas, and by ingestion of milk or dairy products (cheese) from infected animals. Airborne infection may occur among animals in pens and stables, and also in laboratories and abattoirs.

6. Incubation period—Highly variable and difficult to ascertain; usually 5 to 21 days, occasionally several months.

7. Period of communicability—No evidence of communicability from man to man.

8. Susceptibility and resistance—Severity and duration of clinical illness are subject to wide differences. Children are less likely to have manifest disease than are adults. Mild and inapparent infections are frequent. Duration of acquired immunity is uncertain.

9. Methods of control—Ultimate control of brucellosis in man rests in the elimination of the disease among domestic animals.

A. Preventive measures:

    1) Education of farmers and workers in slaughter houses, packing plants and butcher shops as to the nature of the

disease and the danger of handling carcasses or products of infected animals.

2) Search for infection among livestock by the agglutination reaction; eliminate infected animals by segregation or slaughter. Infection among swine usually requires slaughter of the drove. Calf immunization is recommended in enzootic areas.

3) Pasteurization of milk and dairy products from cows, sheep or goats. Boiling of milk is practical when pasteurization is impossible.

4) Care in handling and disposal of discharges and fetus from an aborted animal. Disinfection of contaminated areas.

5) Meat inspection and condemning of carcasses of diseased swine; not a useful procedure for cattle or goats.

B. *Control of patient, contacts, and the immediate environment:*

1) *Report to local health authority:* Case report obligatory in most states and countries, Class 2B (see Preface).

2) *Isolation:* None.

3) *Concurrent disinfection:* Of purulent discharges.

4) *Quarantine:* None.

5) *Immunization of contacts:* None.

6) *Investigation of contacts and source of infection:* Trace infection to the common or individual source, usually infected domestic goats, swine or cattle, or unpasteurized milk or dairy products from cows and goats. Test suspected animals, remove reactors.

7) *Specific treatment:* Tetracycline alone adequate for moderately ill cases. In severe cases the best results are with a combination of chlortetracycline (Aureomycin) and streptomycin. Steroids useful as antitoxemic agents. Treatment should be continued for at least 3 weeks. The relapse rate is high.

C. *Epidemic measures:* Search for common vehicle of infection, usually unpasteurized milk or milk products from an infected herd. Stop distribution or provide pasteurization.

D. *International measures:* Control of domestic animals and animal products in international trade and transport. WHO Reference Centres (see Preface).

CANDIDIASIS

1. **Identification**—A mycosis characterized by pseudomembranes on mucosal surfaces, eczematoid skin lesions and rarely granulomata

in various tissues. Common but ordinarily benign clinical manifesta-tions are oral thrush, vaginitis or vulvovaginitis, and intertriginous skin lesions of various kinds, onychomycosis and paronychia. Uncom-mon but grave manifestations include pneumonitis, meningitis, endo-carditis, and ulcers of the gastrointestinal tract. The kidney is very susceptible to blood-borne infection. Synonyms: Moniliasis, Thrush, Candidosis.

Laboratory confirmation is by repeated microscopic demonstration of budding and mycelial forms in direct smears of sputum or material from lesions. Fresh sputum is essential; the fungus multiplies rapidly at room temperature and 24-hour specimens are useless. The fungus is cultured easily.

2. Occurrence—Worldwide and sporadic. More common in fe-males than males. Infection of fingers is associated with maceration through long exposure to water (bartenders, housewives). Skin lesions are common in obese persons with excessive perspiration in frictional folds; in diabetics, and in lactating women. Oral and dermal thrush occur in newborn, premature and debilitated infants and oral thrush in older persons with ill-fitting dentures, or receiving broad-spectrum antibiotic therapy. The fungus also is found in fowl and other animals.

3. Infectious agents—*Candida albicans (Monilia albicans)*, a fungus, and occasionally other species of *Candida*.

4. Reservoir—Reservoir is man.

5. Mode of transmission—By contact with excretions of mouth, skin, vagina, and especially feces from patients or carriers. From mother to infant during childbirth, and by endogenous spread. Sites which may originate disseminated candidiasis include mucosal lesions, unsterile narcotic injections, percutaneous intravenous catheters and retention catheters of the bladder.

6. Incubation period—Variable, 2 to 5 days in thrush of infants.

7. Period of communicability—Presumably for duration of lesions.

8. Susceptibility and resistance—The frequency of isolating *Can-dida* from sputum, throat, stool or voided urine in the absence of clini-cal evidence of infection suggests widespread immunity. Many adults have dermal delayed hypersensitivity to the fungus and possess humoral antibodies. Second attacks are common; clinical manifestations are likely to follow general or locally lowered resistance. Susceptibility is enhanced by diabetes mellitus or therapy with broad-spectrum an-tibiotics, cytotoxic agents or adrenal corticosteroids.

9. Methods of control—

> **A. Preventive measures:** Detection and treatment of vaginal thrush during third trimester of pregnancy to prevent neonatal thrush. Early detection and local treatment of thrush in mouth, esoph-agus or urinary bladder of debilitated patients, especially those receiving antibiotics or adrenal corticosteroids, to prevent sys-temic spread.

B. Control of patient, contacts, and the immediate environment:

1) *Report to local health authority:* Official report ordinarily not justifiable, Class 5 (see Preface).
2) *Isolation:* In nurseries, segregation of patients with oral thrush.
3) *Concurrent disinfection:* Of secretions and contaminated articles.
4) *Quarantine:* None.
5) *Immunization of contacts:* None.
6) *Investigation of contacts:* Not profitable in sporadic cases.
7) *Specific treatment:* Infections developing during antibiotic therapy sometimes disappear when medication is discontinued. Nystatin (Mycostatin) is useful in gastrointestinal infections, amphotericin B (Fungizone) in generalized disease. Topical application of nystatin or gentian violet to lesions of skin and mucous membrane.

C. Epidemic measures: Epidemics are largely limited to thrush in nurseries for the newborn. Cultures should be taken from the mouths of infants during the first 2 days of life. If *Candida albicans* is demonstrated, clinical thrush can be confidently predicted. Such infants and those with oral thrush should be segregated with emphasis on general cleanliness increased. Concurrent disinfection and terminal cleaning are to be practiced; compare epidemic diarrhea in hospital nurseries, p. 73.

D. International measures: None.

CAPILLARIASIS, INTESTINAL

1. **Identification**—A helminthic disease of the small bowel, first described in 1968. Clinical manifestations include recurrent vague abdominal pain, borborygmi, malaise, anorexia, copious vomiting and frequent voluminous, watery stools. The tremendous protein loss in stools causes weight loss and edema. Death is common in untreated cases.

Diagnosis is by identifying eggs of the parasite in the feces.

2. **Occurrence**—Described only in the northern portion of Luzon in the Philippines.

3. **Infectious agent**—*Capillaria philippinensis,* a roundworm.

4. **Reservoir**—Unknown.

5. **Mode of Transmission**—Unknown. Fish may be an intermediate host. Autoinfection apparently is an important part of the life cycle.

6. **Incubation period**—Unknown.

7. **Period of communicability**—Unknown.

8. **Susceptibility and resistance**—Unknown aside from occurrence of the disease only in Filipinos.

9. **Methods of control**—

A. *Preventive measures:* Specific measures not known but probably should include sanitary disposal of human excreta, attention to hygienic habits, and the cooking of all foods of animal origin.

B. *Control of patient, contacts and the immediate environment:*
1) *Report to local health authority:* Class 3B, Preface.
2) *Isolation:* None.
3) *Concurrent disinfection:* Sanitary disposal of excreta.
4) *Quarantine:* None.
5) *Immunization of contacts:* None.
6) *Investigation of contacts:* Family members and associates for evidence of infection.
7) *Specific treatment:* Thiabendazole (Mintezol) combined with appropriate initial fluid and electrolyte replacement.

C. *Epidemic measures:* Probably not applicable.

D. *International measures:* None.

CARDITIS, VIRAL

1. **Identification**—An acute or subacute myocarditis or pericarditis, which may occasionally complicate various virus infections and which also occurs as a primary disease. The main identified causes are enteroviruses of the Coxsackie B group. The following description is based on Coxsackie carditis:

The myocardium is particularly affected in young children, in whom fever and lethargy may be followed rapidly by heart failure, with pallor, cyanosis, dyspnea, tachycardia and enlargement of heart and liver. Heart failure may be progressive and fatal, or recovery may take place over a few weeks; some cases run a relapsing course over months and may show residual heart damage. In adults, pericarditis is the commonest manifestation, with acute chest pain, disturbance of heart rate and rhythm, and often dyspnea. The disease may complicate Pleurodynia (see pp. 174–175).

Specific diagnosis is made by isolation of the infectious agent (e.g., coxsackievirus from feces, pericardial fluid or postmortem heart tissue) or, less reliably, by demonstrating a rise in specific antibody in convalescent- as compared with acute-phase sera.

2. Occurrence—An uncommon disease, mainly sporadic but commoner during epidemics of Coxsackie B virus infection. Institutional outbreaks with high fatality in the newborn have been described in maternity units.

3. Infectious agents—Various Coxsackie B viruses (types 1, 2, 3, 4, 5) ; occasionally Coxsackie A viruses (types 1, 4, 9, 16, 23) ; also severe poliovirus infections. Influenza, mumps, measles, rubella, varicella-zoster, vaccinia, smallpox, arboviruses, and echovirus 6 (see Index for page location herein) have been reported in association with carditis.

Reservoir, Mode of transmission, Incubation period, Period of communicability, Susceptibility and resistance and Methods of control—(numbered paragraphs 4, 5, 6, 7, 8 and 9, respectively) depend on the specific infectious agent.

CAT-SCRATCH DISEASE

1. Identification—A subacute, self-limited infectious disease characterized by malaise, granulomatous lymphadenitis, and variable degrees and patterns of fever. Usually preceded by a cat scratch in which a primary lesion often develops, followed by regional lymph node involvement. Suppuration occurs in about $\frac{1}{4}$ of patients; pus obtained from lymph nodes is sterile and may be used to prepare a skin test antigen of varying sensitivity and specificity. Recurrent and chronic forms are rare; rashes, erythema nodosum, thrombocytopenia, Parinaud's oculoglandular syndrome (conjunctivitis with enlargement of homolateral preauricular node), and encephalitis are reported rarely. Synonyms : Cat-scratch fever, Benign inoculation lymphoreticulosis.

Diagnosis is based on a consistent clinical picture and histopathological characteristics of involved lymph nodes; some observers insist on a positive skin test for diagnosis. Pasteurellosis, a bacterial infection with *Pasteurella multocida,* acquired by animal bite, may cause a similar clinical picture.

2. Occurrence—Worldwide, uncommon. It occurs in all seasons. Striking increase in cases in some winters has been reported in northern U.S. and Canada. Sexes equally affected; more frequent in children and young people. Familial clustering occurs.

3. Infectious agent—Unknown.

4. Reservoir—Probably one of several animals, usually with inapparent infection, most frequently the cat.

5. Mode of transmission—Infected animals suspected of transmitting infection to man by scratching, biting, licking, or other means. Minor trauma after insect bites, or contact with splinters or thorns is advanced as the mode of transmission in the absence of known direct contact with animals.

6. **Incubation period**—Usually 7 to 14 days from inoculation to primary lesion; possibly as short as 2 days.

7. **Period of communicability**—Unknown for reservoir hosts. Not directly transmitted from man to man.

8. **Susceptibility and resistance**—Unknown.

9. **Methods of control**—

A. Preventive measures: Unknown.

B. Control of patient, contacts, and the immediate environment:

1) *Report to local health authority:* Official report not ordinarily justifiable, Class 5 (see Preface).
2) *Isolation:* None.
3) *Concurrent disinfection:* Of discharges from purulent lesions.
4) *Quarantine:* None.
5) *Immunization of contacts:* None.
6) *Investigation of contacts:* Examination of family contacts for similar illness.
7) *Specific treatment:* None.

C. Epidemic measures: Not applicable.

D. International measures: None.

CHANCROID

1. **Identification**—An acute, localized, self-limiting autoinoculable genital infection characterized clinically by necrotizing ulcerations at site of inoculation, frequently accompanied by painful inflammatory swelling and suppuration of regional lymph nodes. Extragenital lesions are on record. Synonyms: Ulcus molle, Soft chancre.

Diagnostic aids: Microscopic examination of stained exudate from edges of lesions, culture of pus from buboes, intradermal skin test (Ito-Reenstierna test), and biopsy.

2. **Occurrence**—No particular differences in incidence according to age, race or sex except as determined by sexual habits. Geographically widespread; most common in tropical and subtropical countries and in seaports. Incidence sometimes higher than that of syphilis.

3. **Infectious agent**—*Haemophilus ducreyi,* the Ducrey bacillus.

4. **Reservoir**—Reservoir is man.

5. **Mode of transmission**—Direct sexual contact with discharges from open lesions and pus from buboes; suggestive evidence of asymptomatic infection in women. Rare instances of professionally acquired

lesions on hands of physicians and nurses; accidental inoculation of children is known. Indirect transmission rare. Prostitution, indiscriminate sexual promiscuity and uncleanliness favor transmission.

6. Incubation period—From 3 to 5 days, occasionally longer; if abrasions of mucous membranes are present, as short as 24 hours.

7. Period of communicability—As long as infectious agent persists in original lesion or discharging regional lymph nodes; usually parallels healing; in most instances a matter of weeks.

8. Susceptibility and resistance—Susceptibility general; no evidence of natural or acquired resistance.

9. Methods of control—

    A. *Preventive measures:* Except for measures specific for chancroid, preventive measures are those of syphilis (p. 245). Thorough washing of genitalia with soap and water promptly after intercourse very effective.

    B. *Control of patient, contacts, and the immediate environment:*
        1) Report to local health authority: Case report obligatory in many states and countries, Class 2B (see Preface).
        2) Isolation: None; avoid sexual contact until all lesions are healed.
        3) Concurrent disinfection: None; stress personal cleanliness.
        4) Quarantine: None.
        5) Immunization of contacts: Not applicable; prompt treatment on recognition of disease or clinical suspicion.
        6) Investigation of contacts: Search for sexual contacts of 2 weeks before and after onset.
        7) Specific treatment: Sulfonamides. Streptomycin or tetracyclines only if infectious agent is sulfonamide resistant; may mask syphilis.

    C. *Epidemic measures:* Persisting levels of occurrence or an increased incidence are indications for more rigid application of measures outlined in 9A and 9B.

    D. *International measures:* (See Syphilis 9D, p. 247).

CHICKENPOX

1. Identification—An acute generalized viral disease of sudden onset with slight fever, mild constitutional symptoms and an eruption of the skin which is maculopapular for a few hours, vesicular for 3 to 4 days, and leaves a granular scab. Lesions tend to be more abundant on covered than on exposed parts of the body; may appear on scalp, and mucous membranes of upper respiratory tract; commonly occur in sucessive crops, with several stages of maturity present at the same time; may be so few as to escape observation. Mild, atypical and inapparent infections occur. Rarely fatal; a primary viral pneumonia is the commonest cause of death in adults and septic complications and encephalitis in children. Synonym: Varicella.

HERPES ZOSTER is a local manifestation of recurrent or recrudescent infection with the same virus. Vesicles with an erythematous base are restricted to skin areas supplied by sensory nerves of a single or associated group of dorsal root ganglia. Lesions may appear in crops in irregular fashion along nerve pathways, are deeper seated and more closely aggregated than chickenpox; histologically they are identical. Severe pain and paresthesia are common. Occurs mainly in older adults. Occasionally a varicelliform eruption follows some days after zoster, and rarely a secondary eruption of zoster type after chickenpox.

Laboratory tests, such as visualization of the virus by electron micros-copy, isolation of virus in tissue culture, or the demonstration of a rise in complement-fixing serum antibody, are useful but not readily available. Multinucleate giant epithelial cells may be detected in Giemsa-stained scrapings of the base of a lesion; these are not found in vaccinia or variola lesions.

2. Occurrence—Worldwide. Infection with varicella-zoster virus is nearly universal. In metropolitan communities, roughly ¾ of the population have had chickenpox by age 15. Zoster occurs in older people. In temperate zones chickenpox occurs most frequently in winter and early spring.

3. Infectious agent—The varicella-zoster virus.

4. Reservoir—Reservoir is the infected person.

5. Mode of transmission—From person to person by direct con-tact, droplet, or airborne spread of secretions of respiratory tract of infected persons. Indirectly through articles freshly soiled by dis-charges from vesicles and mucous membranes of infected persons. In contrast to vaccinia and variola, scabs from varicella lesions are not infective. One of the most readily communicable of diseases, espe-cially in the early stages of the eruption. Susceptibles may contract chickenpox from patients with herpes zoster.

6. Incubation period—From 2 to 3 weeks; commonly 13 to 17 days.

7. Period of communicability—As long as 5 days before the erup-tion of chickenpox, not more than 6 days after the first crop of vesicles.

8. Susceptibility and resistance—Susceptibility to chickenpox is universal among those not previously infected; ordinarily a more severe disease of adults than of children. One infection confers long immunity; second attacks are rare. Infection apparently remains latent and recurs years later as herpes zoster in a proportion of older adults, sometimes in children.

Patients on steroid therapy and leukemic children on steroid or antimetabolite therapy may suffer severe, prolonged and fatal chickenpox. Adults with cancer, especially of lymphoid tissue with or without steroid therapy, may have an increased frequency of zoster.

9. Methods of control—

A. *Preventive measures:*
1) Cases reported as chickenpox in persons over 15 years, or at any age during an epidemic of smallpox, should be investigated to eliminate possibility of smallpox.
2) Protect susceptible patients receiving steroid therapy against exposure; and if exposed, reduce the dose of steroid to physiologic levels. Gamma globulin from zoster convalescent patients is effective in preventing disease.

B. *Control of patient, contacts, and the immediate environment:*
1) *Report to local health authority:* Official report is not ordinarily justifiable. Case report of chickenpox in adults (Class 3B, Preface) may be required where smallpox is endemic.
2) *Isolation:* None; exclusion from school for 1 week after eruption first appears and avoidance of contact with susceptibles.
3) *Concurrent disinfection:* Articles soiled by discharges from the nose and throat and from lesions.
4) *Quarantine:* None.
5) *Protection of contacts:* Immune serum globulin, while it may not prevent disease, may produce a milder attack, whereas gamma globulin from zoster convalescent patients can prevent disease.
6) *Investigation of contacts:* Of no practical importance except where there is suspicion of smallpox.
7) *Specific treatment:* None.

C. *Epidemic measures:* None.

D. *International measures:* None.

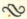

CHOLERA

1. Identification—A serious acute intestinal disease characterized by sudden onset, profuse watery stools, vomiting, rapid dehydration, acidosis and circulatory collapse. Death may occur within a few hours of onset. Case fatality in untreated cases may exceed 50%. Mild cases with only diarrhea also occur, especially in children. Inapparent and wholly asymptomatic infections are many times more frequent than clinically recognized cases.

The diagnosis is confirmed by culturing cholera vibrios from feces or vomitus, or by demonstrating a significant rise in titer of vibriocidal or bacterial agglutinating antibodies in acute and convalescent sera.

2. Occurrence—During the 19th century pandemics, cholera repeatedly spread from its traditional home in Bengal and other parts of India to most parts of the world. During the 20th century the disease has been largely confined to Asia although a severe epidemic occurred in Egypt in 1947.

Since 1960 the disease has been recognized as an increasingly serious endemic and epidemic problem in many countries of South Asia and the Western Pacific. In 1965 and 1966 epidemics and outbreaks occurred in Afghanistan, Iran, Southern USSR, and Iraq.

Except for 2 laboratory-acquired cases in 1966, there have been no reports of naturally occurring cholera in the U.S.A. since 1911.

3. Infectious agent—*Vibrio cholerae,* comma vibrio, including the classical and El Tor biotypes and the Inaba and Ogawa serotypes. The diseases caused by these variants are clinically indistinguishable. In any single epidemic one particular variant tends to be dominant.

4. Reservoir—Reservoir is man.

5. Mode of transmission—Transmission occurs through ingestion of water contaminated with feces and vomitus of patients, to a lesser extent feces of carriers; or of food contaminated by water, soiled hands or flies. Spread from person to person by direct contact is of relatively minor importance.

6. Incubation period—From a few hours to 5 days, usually 2 to 3 days.

7. Period of communicability—Unknown, but presumably for the duration of the stool-positive carrier state, which usually lasts for only a few days after recovery. However, carriers of several months' duration are not unusual. A rare chronic biliary infection lasting for years has been observed, associated with intermittent shedding of vibrios in the stool.

8. Susceptibility and resistance—Susceptibility is variable and poorly understood. Clinical cholera is usually confined to the lowest socioeconomic groups. Even in severe epidemics attack rates rarely exceed 1 or 2%, although inapparent infection rates are much higher. Infection results in significant serological response in agglutinating, vibriocidal and antitoxic antibodies. Resistance to clinical disease correlates with the level of circulating vibriocidal antibody. In endemic areas, most persons acquire immunity by early adulthood. Partial acquired immunity (about 50% protection) to overt disease is induced by antibacterial vaccines, but the duration is short-lived (a few months) and does not prevent asymptomatic infection.

9. Methods of Control—

A. *Preventive measures:*

1) Sanitary disposal of human feces.
2) Protection and purification of water supplies (see Typhoid Fever 9A1, p. 270).
3) Boiling of milk or pasteurization of milk and dairy products (see Typhoid Fever 9A4, p. 270).
4) Sanitary supervision of processing, preparation, and serving of foods, especially those eaten moist and raw; special attention to provision and use of hand-washing facilities.
5) Destruction of flies, control of fly breeding, and screening to protect foods against fly contamination (see Typhoid Fever 9A3, p. 270).
6) Education of the public in personal hygiene, especially washing hands before eating and after defecation.
7) Active immunization with cholera vaccine of persons subject to unusual or continued risk. Vaccines prepared from classical strains have proven effective against El Tor disease (see 8 above).

B. *Control of patient, contacts, and the immediate environment:*

1) *Report to local health authority:* Case report universally required by International Sanitary Regulations, Class 1 (see Preface).
2) *Isolation:* Desirable in hospital during presence of acute symptoms, but strict isolation is not called for if it inhibits provision of prompt and adequate rehydration of acutely ill patients. Crowded cholera wards can be operated without hazard to staff and visitors if attendants will practice scrupulous cleanliness.
3) *Concurrent disinfection:* Of feces and vomitus, and of articles used by patient; disinfection of hands each time after handling articles contaminated by feces. Terminal cleaning.
4) *Quarantine:* Surveillance of contacts for 5 days from last exposure and longer if feces contain cholera vibrios.
5) *Management of contacts:* No passive immunization. Inoculation of contacts with cholera vaccine can be expected to do no more than protect against subsequent or continued exposure. Chemoprophylaxis of family contacts with tetracycline is justifiable.
6) *Investigation of contacts and source of infection:* Search for unreported cases. Investigate possibilities of infection from polluted drinking water or from contaminated foods.
7) *Specific treatment:* Prompt parenteral therapy using adequate volumes of isotonic balanced electrolyte solutions to correct dehydration, acidosis and hypokalemia can lower the case fatality ratio to less than 1%. Liquids containing

glucose and saline are partially absorbed and are helpful when given by mouth. Tetracycline and other antimicrobial agents reduce the volume of intravenous fluids required by limiting the duration of the diarrhea and reducing the fluid loss; they shorten the period of excretion of vibrios.

C. Epidemic measures:

1) Adopt emergency measures to assure a safe water supply; boiling of water used for drinking, cooking, or washing dishes or food containers, unless water supply is treated adequately, as by chlorination, and protected from contamination thereafter. An accessible and sufficient water supply for hygienic purposes is important.
2) Provide inspection service for early detection of infected persons; provision of temporary facilities, by requisition or otherwise, for isolation and adequate treatment of patients and for screening suspects; identification and isolation of carriers may be desirable, but is usually impractical. The culturing of prospective travelers and their detention in isolation camps prior to departure are impractical measures of questionable value.
3) Institute immediate administration of cholera vaccine to exposed population groups, despite its limited value.
4) Assure careful supervision of food and drink. After cooking or boiling, protect against contamination as by flies and human handling.
5) Control flies by limiting fly breeding, by use of appropriate insecticides, and by screening kitchens and eating places. See Typhoid Fever 9A3, p. 272.
6) Promulgate temporary regulations to assure proper execution of the above control measures.

D. International measures:

1) Telegraphic notification by governments to WHO and to adjacent countries of the first imported, first transferred or first nonimported case of cholera in an area previously free of the disease.
2) Measures applicable to ships, aircraft and land transport arriving from cholera areas are specified in International Health Regulations,* WHO, Geneva.
3) International travelers: Under international health regulations, cholera patients or suspects (see Definition 43, Suspect) are not permitted to leave the country. Many countries require that travelers from an area where cholera is present possess a valid international cholera vaccination

* These will come into force on January 1, 1971. Until this date the *International Sanitary Regulations,* 3rd edition (Geneva: WHO, 1966) are applicable.

certificate for entry. Validity of the certificate shall extend for a period of 6 months beginning 6 days after an injection of cholera vaccine, or in the event of revaccination within 6 months, from the date of the revaccination.

4) WHO Reference Centres (see Preface).

CHROMOBLASTOMYCOSIS

1. Identification—A chronic spreading mycosis of the skin and subcutaneous tissues, usually of a lower extremity. Hematogenous spread to the brain has been reported. Progression to contiguous tissues is slow, over a period of years, with eventual large verrucous or even cauliflower-like masses, and lymph stasis. Rarely a cause of death. Synonyms: Chromomycosis, Dermatitis verrucosa.

Microscopic examination of scrapings or biopsies from lesions reveals characteristic brown hyphae or thick-walled, rounded brown cells. Confirmation of the diagnosis by culture of the fungus is desirable but not mandatory.

2. Occurrence—Worldwide distribution as sporadic cases in widely scattered areas but mainly Central America, Caribbean Islands, South America, Australia, Madagascar and South Africa. Primarily a disease of rural tropical regions, probably because of more frequent penetrating wounds of feet not protected by shoes. The disease is commonest in men aged 30 to 50 years; females are rarely infected.

3. Infectious agents—*Phialophora verrucosa, Phialophora pedrosoi, Phialophora compactum, Phialophora dermatitidis,* and *Cladosporium carrionii.*

4. Reservoir—Presumably wood, soil, or vegetation.

5. Mode of transmission—Traumatic contact with contaminated wood or other materials.

6. Incubation period—Unknown; probably months.

7. Period of communicability—Not directly transmitted from man to man.

8. Susceptibility and resistance—Unknown, but rarity of disease and absence of laboratory infections suggest man is relatively resistant.

9. Methods of control—

A. *Preventive measures:* Protection against small puncture wounds, as by wearing shoes or protective clothing.

B. *Control of patient, contacts, and the immediate environment:*

1) *Report to local health authority:* Official report not ordinarily justifiable, Class 5 (see Preface).

2) *Isolation:* None.

3) *Concurrent disinfection:* Of discharges from lesions and articles soiled therewith.
4) *Quarantine:* None.
5) *Immunization of contacts:* Not applicable.
6) *Investigation of contacts:* Not profitable.
7) *Specific treatment:* None. Calciferol or local injections of amphotericin B may be tried.

C. Epidemic measures: Not applicable, a sporadic disease.

D. International measures: None.

CLONORCHIASIS

1. Identification—A trematode disease of the bile ducts. Clinical reaction may be slight or absent in light infections. Symptoms result from local irritation of bile ducts by the flukes, from toxemia, and possibly from secondary bacterial invaders. Loss of appetite, diarrhea, and a sensation of abdominal pressure are common early symptoms. Bile duct obstruction, rarely producing jaundice, may be followed by cirrhosis, enlargement and tenderness of liver, and progressive ascites and edema. Eosinophilia (5 to 40%) is frequent. A chronic disease, sometimes of 30 years or longer in duration, but not often a direct or contributing cause of death. Synonym: Chinese liver fluke disease.

Direct diagnosis is by finding the characteristic fluke eggs in feces or by duodenal drainage; to be differentiated from heterophydiasis and opisthorchiasis in man in Southeast Asia (Thailand), Egypt, USSR and other countries.

2. Occurrence—Highly endemic in Southeast China, present throughout the country except in the northwest; Japan, widespread; Taiwan; South Korea and Vietnam, principally the Red River delta. In other parts of the world imported cases occur in immigrants.

3. Infectious agent—*Clonorchis sinensis,* Asiatic liver fluke.

4. Reservoir—Man, cat, dog, hog, and other animals are reservoir hosts of adult flukes.

5. Mode of transmission—Man (or other definitive host) is infected by freshwater fish eaten raw (fresh, dried, salted, or pickled) or partly cooked. During digestion, larvae are set free from cysts, and migrate via the common bile duct to biliary radicles. Eggs deposited in the bile passages are evacuated in feces. Eggs in feces contain a fully developed miracidium; ingested by a susceptible snail of the family *Amnicolidae,* they hatch in its intestine and penetrate vascular spaces. Cercariae develop and emerge into water; on contact with second intermediate host (40 species of freshwater fishes—*Cyprinidae*), cercariae penetrate the host and encyst, usually in muscle, occasionally on underside of scales. The complete life cycle, from man to man, requires at least 3 months.

6. Incubation period—Undetermined; flukes reach maturity within 16 to 25 days after encysted larvae are ingested.

7. Period of communicability—Infected individuals may pass viable eggs for as long as 30 years. Not directly transmitted from man to man.

8. Susceptibility and resistance—Susceptibility is universal. No resistance with age; in endemic areas, highest prevalence at age 55 to 60 years.

9. Methods of control—

A. *Preventive measures:*
1) In endemic areas, education regarding life cycle of the parasite.
2) Thorough cooking of all freshwater fish.
3) Treatment or storage of night soil before use as a fertilizer in fish ponds; 1 part of 0.7% solution of ammonium sulfate to 10 parts of feces will kill the miracidia in the eggs within 30 minutes.

B. *Control of patient, contacts, and the immediate environment:*
1) *Report to local health authority:* Official report not ordinarily justifiable, Class 5 (see Preface).
2) *Isolation:* None.
3) *Concurrent disinfection:* Sanitary disposal of feces.
4) *Quarantine:* None.
5) *Immunization of contacts:* Not applicable.
6) *Investigation of contacts and source of infection:* Of the individual case, unprofitable. A community problem (see 9C below).
7) *Specific treatment:* None; chloroquine hydrochloride (Aralen), trichloromethylbenzol and gentian violet, medicinal, are of some value.

C. *Epidemic measures:* Locate source of infected fish parasitized through use of night soil as fertilizer in fish ponds, or through fecal contamination of streams. Shipments of dried or pickled fish are the likely source in nonendemic areas.

D. *International measures:* Control of fish or fish products imported from endemic areas.

COCCIDIOIDOMYCOSIS

1. Identification—A deep mycosis beginning as a respiratory infection.

A. *Primary Infection:* May be entirely asymptomatic or resemble an acute influenzal illness with fever, chills, cough and pleural pain. About one-fifth of clinically recognized cases (an estimated 5% of all primary infections) develop erythema nodosum, a complication most frequent in white females and rarest in Negro males. Primary infection may (1) heal completely without detectable residuals, (2) leave fibrosis or calcification of pulmonary lesions, (3) leave a persistent thin-walled cavity, or (4) and most rarely, progress to the disseminated form of the disease comparable to progressive primary tuberculosis. Synonym: Valley fever.

The fungus may be demonstrated by microscopic examination of sputum or by culture. Reaction to skin test with coccidioidin appears usually within 2 to 3 days after onset of symptoms but may not become positive for up to 3 weeks; precipitin and complement-fixation tests are usually positive within the first 3 months of clinical disease. Serial skin and serological tests may be necessary to confirm a recent infection.

B. *Progressive Primary Coccidioidomycosis (Coccidioidal granuloma):* A progressive highly fatal and uncommon granulomatous disease characterized by lung lesions and single or aggregated abscesses throughout the body, especially in subcutaneous tissues, skin, bone, peritoneum, testes, thyroid and central nervous system. Coccidioidal meningitis resembles tuberculous meningitis.

A granulomatous disease, "paracoccidioidal granuloma" (see pp. 41–42), has no relation to coccidioidomycosis.

2. **Occurrence**—Primary infections are extremely common in scattered highly endemic arid and semiarid areas; in U.S.A. from southern California to west Texas; in northern Argentina and Mexico; occasionally in Central America. Dusty fomites from endemic areas can transmit infections elsewhere and infections occur in persons who have traveled through endemic areas. Affects all ages, both sexes and all races. Infection most frequent in summer, especially after wind and dust storms. An important disease among migrant workers and military recruits in endemic areas. Coccidioidal granuloma has the geographic distribution of Valley fever.

3. **Infectious agent**—*Coccidioides immitis,* a dimorphic fungus growing in soil and in culture media as a mold which reproduces by arthrospores; and in tissue and under special conditions of culture as spherical cells which become sporangia and produce sporangiospores (endospores).

4. **Reservoir**—Reservoir is soil; fungus apparently propagates in soil, especially in and around rodent burrows, in regions where temperature and moisture requirements are satisfactory, and infects man, cattle, dogs, horses, burros, sheep, swine and wild rodents.

5. Mode of transmission—Inhalation of spores from dust, soil and dry vegetation, and in laboratories from culture media. Infection through open wounds is possible but infrequent. Draining lesions and possibly expectorated sputum in rare instances may contaminate articles and permit indirect transmission following conversion of the fungus from parasitic to saprophytic form.

6. Incubation period—Eight days to 3 weeks in primary infection. Coccidioidal granuloma develops insidiously, not necessarily preceded by recognized symptoms of primary pulmonary infection.

7. Period of communicability—Not directly transmitted from animal or man to man. After 7 to 10 days *C. immitis* on casts or dressings may change from the parasitic to the disseminative saprophytic form.

8. Susceptibility and resistance—Susceptibility to primary infection is general as indicated by high incidence of positive coccidioidin reactors in endemic areas; recovery apparently is followed by solid immunity. More than half of patients with symptomatic infection are between 15 and 25 years of age; males are affected 5 times more frequently than females; Negroes and Filipinos 10 times oftener than others.

9. Methods of control—

A. Preventive measures: In endemic areas, planting of grass, oiling of air fields and other dust control measures. Individuals from nonendemic areas should not be recruited to dusty occupations, such as road building and picking cotton.

B. Control of patient, contacts, and the immediate environment:

1) *Report to local health authority:* Case report of recognized coccidioidal disease in selected endemic areas (U.S.A.); in many countries not a reportable disease, Class 3B (see Preface).

2) *Isolation:* None.

3) *Concurrent disinfection:* Of discharges and soiled articles. Terminal cleaning.

4) *Quarantine:* None.

5) *Immunization of contacts:* None.

6) *Investigation of contacts:* Not profitable except in cases appearing in nonendemic areas, where residence and travel history should be obtained.

7) *Specific treatment:* Amphotericin B (Fungizone) appears to be of benefit in disseminated infections but must be given near the toxic level.

C. Epidemic measures: Epidemics occur only when groups of susceptibles are infected by airborne spores. Dust control measures should be instituted where practicable (see 9A above).

D. International measures: None.

CONJUNCTIVITIS, ACUTE BACTERIAL

1. Identification—A clinical syndrome beginning with lacrimation, irritation, and vascular injection of the palpebral and bulbar conjunctivae of one or both eyes, followed by edema of lids, photophobia, and mucopurulent exudate; in severe cases, ecchymoses of bulbar conjunctiva and marginal infiltration in the cornea. Not fatal, with a usual clinical course of 2 to 3 weeks; many patients have no more than vascular injection of the conjunctivae and slight exudate for a few days. Synonyms: Sore eye, Pink eye.

Confirmation of clinical diagnosis is by bacteriologic culture or microscopic examination of smear of exudate; required to differentiate from viral conjunctivitis (trachoma and adenoviruses), and idiopathic conjunctivitis (Reiter's syndrome, etc.).

2. Occurrence—Widespread and common throughout the world, particularly in warmer climates; frequently epidemic. In U.S.A., infection with *Haemophilus aegyptius* is largely confined to southern rural areas, Georgia to California, primarily during summer and early autumn; in those areas it is an important cause of absence from school. Infection with other organisms occurs throughout U.S.A., often in association with acute viral respiratory disease during cold seasons.

3. Infectious agents—*Haemophilus aegyptius* (Koch-Weeks bacillus) and pneumococci appear to be the most important; *Haemophilus influenzae, Moraxella lacunata,* staphylococci, streptococci, and *Corynebacterium diphtheriae* produce the disease. A gram-negative diplococcus resembling the gonococcus is responsible for epidemics with much loss of sight among young children in North Africa and the Middle East.

4. Reservoir—Reservoir is man. Carriers of *H. aegyptius* are common in many areas during intervals between epidemics of the acute illness.

5. Mode of transmission—Contact with discharges from the conjunctiva or upper respiratory tract of infected persons, through contaminated fingers, clothing, or other articles. In some areas may be mechanically transmitted by eye gnats or flies, but their importance as vectors is undetermined and probably differs from area to area.

6. Incubation period—Usually 24 to 72 hours.

7. Period of communicability—During the course of active infection.

8. Susceptibility and resistance—Children under 5 years are most often affected and incidence decreases with age. The debilitated and aged are particularly susceptible to staphylococcal infections. Immunity after attack is low-grade and variable, according to the infectious agent.

9. Methods of control—

    A. *Preventive measures:* Personal hygiene, hygienic care and treatment of affected eyes.

B. *Control of patient, contacts, and the immediate environment:*

1) *Report to local health authority:* Obligatory report of epidemics; no case report, Class 4 (see Preface).

2) *Isolation:* None. Children should not attend school during the acute stage.

3) *Concurrent disinfection:* Of discharges and soiled articles. Terminal cleaning.

4) *Quarantine:* None.

5) *Immunization of contacts:* None.

6) *Investigation of contacts:* Usually not profitable.

7) *Specific treatment:* Local application of an ointment containing a tetracycline antibiotic, chloramphenicol or a sulfonamide such as sodium sulfacetamide.

C. *Epidemic measures:*

1) Adequate and intensive treatment of patients and their associates.

2) In areas where insects are suspected of mechanically transmitting infection, measures to prevent access of eye gnats or flies to eyes of sick and well persons.

3) Insect control, according to the suspected vector.

D. *International measures:* None.

CONJUNCTIVITIS, INCLUSION

1. Identification—An acute papillary conjunctivitis of the newborn with abundant mucopurulent exudate; in children and adults, an acute follicular conjunctivitis with preauricular adenopathy but no corneal changes. If untreated, the acute stage ends spontaneously in 10 days to a few weeks in the newborn, in 6 weeks to a few months in children and adults; the chronic phase with minimal exudate persists at least 3 months in infants and somewhat longer in adults. Genitourinary tract infection is usually asymptomatic or limited to a mild urethritis or cervicitis. Specific treatment results in rapid recovery. Synonyms: Neonatal inclusion blennorrhea, Paratrachoma, Swimming pool conjunctivitis.

Laboratory confirmation is through demonstration of basophilic intracytoplasmic inclusion bodies in epithelial scrapings or by isolation of the agent in chick embryo yolk sac. Isolation of the infectious agent is more difficult than for the closely related agent of trachoma.

Neonatal inclusion conjunctivitis is distinguished clinically from the more serious gonococcal ophthalmia neonatorum (see p. 100) by differences in incubation period: long (at least 5 days) for inclusion conjunctivitis, and short (less than 3 days) for gonococcal disease.

2. Occurrence—Probably worldwide as sporadic cases; small epidemics reported in North America, Europe and Japan.

3. Infectious agent—The agent of inclusion conjunctivitis, a bedsonia (chlamydia).

4. Reservoir—Reservoir is man.

5. Mode of transmission—Discharges of the genital tract of infected persons are infectious. Genital infections are transmitted during intercourse. Eye infection in the newborn is by direct contact with the infected birth passage. Most child and adult cases arise from non-chlorinated swimming pools, presumably contaminated with genitourinary exudates. Eye-to-eye transmission in series has not been reported.

6. Incubation period—5 to 7 days, occasionally 10 to 12 days.

7. Period of communicability—While genital infection persists; probably not longer than 10 months in the female.

8. Susceptibility and resistance—Inclusion conjunctivitis usually is rare in areas and in communities where trachoma is common but with no evidence of differences in racial susceptibility. Natural or acquired immunity has not been demonstrated.

9. Methods of control—

A. *Preventive measures:* Difficult to apply in view of the inapparent nature of genital infections; general preventive measures are those for the venereal diseases (Syphilis 9A, p. 245). Instillation of silver nitrate or penicillin into the eye soon after birth does not prevent neonatal infection.

B. *Control of patient, contacts, and the immediate environment:*

1) *Report to local health authority:* Case report of neonatal cases obligatory in most states and many countries, Class 2B (see Preface).

2) *Isolation:* For the first 48 hours after commencing treatment.

3) *Concurrent disinfection:* Aseptic techniques and hand washing by personnel appear to be adequate to prevent nursery transmission.

4) *Quarantine:* None.

5) *Immunization of contacts:* Not applicable.

6) *Investigation of contacts:* In neonatal infections, examination and treatment of mother and her consort. Prompt treatment on recognition or suspicion of infection.

7) *Specific treatment:* For ocular infections, local application of sulfonamides, tetracycline antibiotics or chloramphenicol in oil or in ointment form, 4 to 6 times daily, usually for 1 week. For genital infections, sulfonamides by mouth.

C. *Epidemic measures:* Sanitary control of swimming pools; ordinary chlorination suffices. Individuals contaminating swimming pools are difficult to trace.

D. *International measures:* WHO Reference Centres (see Preface).

CRYPTOCOCCOSIS

1. Identification—A mycosis usually presenting as a subacute or chronic meningoencephalitis. Infection of lung, kidney, prostate, bone or liver occurs, often with few local symptoms. Skin may show acneiform lesions, ulcers or subcutaneous tumor-like masses. Occasionally, *Cryptococcus neoformans* seems to be an endobronchial saprophyte in patients with lung disease of other origin. Synonyms: Torulosis, European blastomycosis.

Diagnosis of cryptococcal meningitis is aided by microscopic examination of spinal fluid mixed with India ink. Urine or pus may also contain encapsulated budding forms. Serologic tests for antigen or antibody are sometimes helpful. Diagnosis is confirmed by culture, ability of the isolate to grow at 37 C and its pathogenicity for mice. Media containing cycloheximide inhibit *Cryptococcus* and should not be used.

2. Occurrence—Sporadic cases occur in all parts of the world. All races are susceptible; males infected twice as frequently as females, mainly adults. Infection also occurs in cats, dogs, horses, monkeys and other animals.

3. Infectious agent—*Cryptococcus neoformans* (*Torula histolytica*), a fungus.

4. Reservoir—Saprophytic growth in the external environment. The infectious agent can be isolated consistently from old pigeon nests and pigeon droppings and sometimes from soil in many parts of the world.

5. Mode of transmission—Presumably by inhalation of *Cryptococcus*-laden dust.

6. Incubation period—Unknown. Pulmonary disease may precede brain infection by months or years.

7. Period of communicability—Not directly transmitted from man to man.

8. Susceptibility and resistance—The frequency of *Cryptococcus* in the external environment and the infrequency of disease suggest that man has an appreciable resistance. Susceptibility increased during adrenal corticosteroid therapy and in disorders of the reticuloendothelial system, particularly Hodgkin's disease.

9. Methods of control—

A. Preventive measures: Control of pigeons.

B. Control of patient, contacts, and the immediate environment:

1) *Report to local health authority:* Official report ordinarily not justifiable, Class 5 (see Preface).
2) *Isolation:* None.
3) *Concurrent disinfection:* Of discharges and contaminated dressings. Terminal cleaning.
4) *Quarantine:* None.
5) *Immunization of contacts:* None.

6) Investigation of contacts and source of infection: Investigate exposure to accumulations of pigeon droppings, especially on window ledges, in aviaries, roosts and nests.

7) Specific treatment: Amphotericin B (Fungizone) given intravenously is effective in many cases.

C. Epidemic measures: None.

D. International measures: None.

CYTOMEGALIC INCLUSION DISEASE

1. Identification—An incompletely defined disease. Its most severe form occurs in the perinatal period following transplacental or congenital infection. The neonate may exhibit signs and symptoms of severe generalized infection especially involving the central nervous system and liver; lethargy, convulsions, jaundice, petechiae and purpura, hepatosplenomegaly, chorioretinitis, intracerebral calcifications, and pulmonary infiltrates occur in varying degree. Survivors may exhibit mental retardation, microcephaly, motor disabilities, and evidence of chronic liver disease. Death *in utero* occurs; neonatal case fatality rate is high.

Infection acquired later in life is generally inapparent. In debilitated patients or those on immunosuppressive drugs, dissemination of latent infection may occur; in such cases, or after primary infection, abnormalities of liver function and structure or severe pulmonary disease may be seen. A disease resembling infectious mononucleosis may follow transfusion of contaminated blood.

Presence of infection is established by isolation of the virus in human cell cultures of the fibroblast type from urine, saliva, or tissue; by demonstration of typical "cytomegalic" cells in sediments of body fluids or in organs; and by demonstration of significant rise in titer of serum antibody. When infection is proven, its role in the patient's disease is a matter of clinical judgment.

2. Occurrence—Virus has been recovered and disease has been reported from many parts of the world. Serologic evidence of infection is present in a high proportion (80%) of persons after age 35.

3. Infectious agent—A cytomegalovirus, one of a group of antigenically related agents.

4. Reservoir—Man is the only known reservoir. Cytomegaloviruses not infectious for man are found in many animals.

5. Mode of transmission—Not precisely known. Virus is excreted in urine and saliva. Fetus may acquire infection *in utero;* indirect evidence suggests that this occurs only if mother's primary infection occurs during pregnancy. Viremia may be present in asymptomatic persons; virus may be transmitted by blood transfusion.

6. Incubation period—Little information is available. Transplacental transmission of the virus may result in acute disease from before birth to soon after. The illness following transfusion of blood containing the infectious agent begins typically several weeks after transfusion.

7. Period of communicability—Virus is excreted in urine or saliva for many months and perhaps longer but it should be recalled that mode of transmission is not precisely known.

8. Susceptibility and resistance—Inapparent infection is nearly universal. Fetuses, infants, and patients with debilitating diseases or those on immunosuppressive drugs show lowered resistance to disease.

9. Methods of control—

A. Preventive measures: Unknown.

B. Control of patient, contacts, and the immediate environment:

1) *Report to local health authority:* Official report not ordinarily justifiable, Class 5 (see Preface).
2) *Isolation:* None.
3) *Concurrent disinfection:* Discharges from hospitalized patients and articles soiled therewith.
4) *Quarantine:* None.
5) *Immunization of contacts:* None available.
6) *Investigation of contacts and source of infection:* None.
7) *Specific treatment:* None.

C. Epidemic measures: None.

D. International measures: None.

DERMATOPHYTOSIS (RINGWORM)

Ringworm is a general term applied to mycotic disease of keratinized areas of the body (hair, skin and nails). Various genera and species of fungi known collectively as the dermatophytes are causative agents. The dermatomycoses are subdivided according to sites of infection. Synonyms: Dermatomycosis, Tinea (including Favus, Athlete's foot and Jockey itch).

A. RINGWORM OF THE SCALP (TINEA CAPITIS)

1. Identification—Begins as a small papule and spreads peripherally, leaving scaly patches of baldness. Infected hairs become brittle and break off easily. Occasionally boggy, raised and suppurative lesions develop, called kerions. Examination of the scalp under Wood's light (ultraviolet) for yellow-green fluorescence is helpful in tinea capitis caused by *Microsporum canis* and *Microsporum audouinii.*

Favus of the scalp is a variety of tinea capitis caused by *Trichophyton schoenleinii* and characterized by a mousy odor and by formation of small, yellowish cup-like crusts or scutulae giving the appearance of being stuck on the scalp. Affected hairs do not break off but become gray and lusterless, eventually fall out and leave baldness which may be permanent.

Microscopic examination of scales and hair in 10% potassium hydroxide reveals characteristic arthrospores. The fungus should be cultured for confirmation of the diagnosis.

Tinea capitis is distinguished easily from Piedra, a fungus infection of the hair occurring in South America and some countries of Southeast Asia, an infection characterized by black, hard "gritty" or white, soft "pasty" nodules on the hair shafts, caused by *Piedraia hortai* and *Trichosporon beigelii,* respectively.

2. Occurrence—Tinea capitis caused by *Microsporum audouinii* is widespread in U.S.A., particularly in urban areas. *M. canis* infection occurs in both rural and urban areas wherever infected cats and dogs are present. *Trichophyton mentagrophytes* and *Trichophyton verrucosum* infections occur in rural areas where the disease exists in cattle, horses, rodents and wild animals. *Trichophyton tonsurans* infections are epidemic in urban areas in southern and eastern U.S.A., Puerto Rico and Mexico.

3. Infectious agents—Various species of *Microsporum* and *Trichophyton.* Identification of genus and species is important epidemiologically and to determine prognosis.

4. Reservoir—Principal reservoir of *M. audouinii, T. schoenleinii* and *T. tonsurans* is man; animals, especially dogs, cats and cattle, harbor the other organisms mentioned.

5. Mode of transmission—Direct or indirect contact, especially with backs of theater seats, barber clippers, toilet articles or clothing contaminated with hair from infected animals or man.

6. Incubation period—10 to 14 days.

7. Period of communicability—As long as lesions are present, and viable spores persist on contaminated materials.

8. Susceptibility and resistance—Children before the age of puberty are notoriously susceptible to *Microsporum audouinii.* All ages are subject to *M. canis* and *Trichophyton* infections. No permanent resistance follows infection.

9. Methods of Control—

A. Preventive measures:

1) In the presence of epidemics or in hyperendemic areas, young children should be surveyed by Wood's light before entering school. Spotty alopecia and well-circumscribed lesions should be searched for.

2) Education of the public, especially parents, of the danger of acquiring infection from infected children as well as from dogs, cats and other animals.

B. Control of patient, contacts, and the immediate environment:

1) *Report to local health authority:* Obligatory report of epidemics; no individual case report, Class 4 (see Preface). School outbreaks should be reported to school authorities.
2) *Isolation:* Impractical. Daily washing of the scalp in mild cases removes loose hair. In severe cases cover hair with a cap and wash daily.
3) *Concurrent disinfection:* Contaminated caps should be boiled after use.
4) *Quarantine:* Not practical.
5) *Immunization of contacts:* None.
6) *Investigation of contacts and source of infection:* Study household contacts, and pets and farm animals for evidence of infection and treat.
7) *Specific treatment:* Griseofulvin is treatment of choice; a 6 weeks' course is adequate in most cases. Topical antibacterial agents are useful in the treatment of secondarily infected lesions (kerions). Examine weekly and take cultures to assure complete recovery.

C. Epidemic measures: Epidemics in a school or institution require special measures such as education of children and parents, and enlistment of services of physicians and nurses for diagnosis. Follow-up surveys are important.

D. International measures: None.

B. RINGWORM OF THE BODY (TINEA CORPORIS)

1. Identification—An infectious disease of the skin other than of the scalp, bearded areas, and feet, characteristically appearing as flat, spreading ring-shaped lesions. The periphery is reddish, vesicular or pustular, and may be dry and scaly or moist and crusted. As the lesion progresses peripherally, the central area often clears, leaving apparently normal skin. Differentiation from inguinal candidiasis is necessary, since treatment differs.

Diagnosis is made by taking scrapings from the advancing margins, clearing in 10% potassium hydroxide and examining microscopically. This shows segmented branching filaments of fungus. Final identification is by culture.

2. Occurrence—Worldwide and relatively frequent. Males are infected more often than females. All ages are susceptible and racial differences are immaterial.

3. Infectious agents—*Epidermophyton floccosum* and various species of *Microsporum* and *Trichophyton*.

4. Reservoir—Reservoir is man and animals.

5. Mode of transmission—Direct or indirect contact with skin and scalp lesions of infected persons, lesions of animals, contaminated floors, shower stalls, benches and similar articles.

6. Incubation period—10 to 14 days.

7. Period of communicability—As long as lesions are present and viable spores persist on contaminated materials.

8. Susceptibility and resistance—Susceptibility is general. Clinical manifestations are commonly exaggerated under conditions of friction and excessive perspiration, as in axillary and inguinal regions.

9. Methods of Control—

A. *Preventive measures:* Proper laundering (with sterilization) of towels and general cleanliness in showers and dressing rooms of gymnasiums, especially repeated washing of benches. A fungicidal agent such as cresol should be used for disinfecting floors and benches.

B. *Control of patient, contacts, and the immediate environment:*

1) *Report to local health authority:* Obligatory report of epidemics; no individual case report, Class 4 (see Preface). Case report to school authority of infections of children.

2) *Isolation:* Infected children should be excluded from gymnasiums, swimming pools and activities likely to lead to exposure of others.

3) *Concurrent disinfection:* Effective frequent laundering of clothing.

4) *Quarantine:* None.

5) *Immunization of contacts:* None.

6) *Investigation of contacts and source of infection:* Examination of school and household contacts, and of household pets and farm animals and treatment of infections.

7) *Specific treatment:* Thorough bathing with soap and water, removal of scabs and crusts, and application of any of a number of topical agents: tolnaftate (Tinactin), salicylic acid or one of the higher fatty acids (propionic acid, undecylenic acid). Griseofulvin by mouth also useful.

C. *Epidemic measures:* Education of children and of parents concerning the nature of the infection, its mode of spread and necessity of maintaining good personal hygiene.

D. *International measures:* None.

C. RINGWORM OF THE FOOT (TINEA PEDIS)

1. Identification—Scaling or cracking of the skin, especially between the toes, or blisters containing a thin watery fluid are so characteristic that most laymen recognize "athlete's foot." In severe cases, vesicular lesions appear on various parts of the body, especially the hands. These dermatophytids do not contain the fungus and constitute an allergic reaction to fungus products.

Microscopic examination of potassium hydroxide-treated scrapings from lesions between the toes reveals segmented branching filaments. This examination is necessary to verify diagnosis; clinical appearances are not diagnostic.

2. Occurrence—Worldwide and a common disease. Adults more often affected than children; males more than females. No differences in racial susceptibility. Infections are more frequent in hot weather.

3. Infectious agents—Various species of *Trichophyton* and rarely *Epidermophyton floccosum.*

4. Reservoir—Reservoir is man.

5. Mode of transmission—Direct or indirect contact with skin lesions of infected persons or contaminated floors, shower stalls and other articles used by infected persons.

6. Incubation period—Unknown.

7. Period of communicability—As long as lesions are present and viable spores persist on contaminated materials.

8. Susceptibility and resistance—Susceptibility is variable and infection may be inapparent. Second attacks are frequent.

9. Methods of control—

A. *Preventive measures:* Those for tinea corporis above. Education of the public on maintenance of strict personal hygiene, with special care in drying areas between toes after bathing.

B. *Control of patient, contacts, and the immediate environment:*
   1) *Report to local health authority:* Official report not ordinarily justifiable, Class 5 (see Preface). Report school outbreaks to school authorities.
   2) *Isolation:* None.
   3) *Concurrent disinfection:* Boil socks of heavily infected individuals to prevent reinfection. Place shoes in a box and subject to formaldehyde for several hours; follow by airing to prevent irritation of skin from residual formalin.
   4) *Quarantine:* None.
   5) *Immunization of contacts:* None.
   6) *Investigation of contacts and source of infection:* None.
   7) *Specific treatment:* Topical agents as recommended for tinea corporis. Expose feet to air through wearing sandals, and use dusting powders. Griseofulvin may be useful.

C. *Epidemic measures:* Thorough cleaning and washing down of gymnasiums, showers and similar sources of infection. Education of the public concerning the mode of spread.

D. *International measures:* None.

D. RINGWORM OF THE NAILS (TINEA UNGUIUM)

1. Identification—A chronic infectious disease involving one or more nails of the hand or foot. The nail gradually thickens, becomes discolored and brittle, and an accumulation of caseous-appearing material forms beneath the nail, or the nail becomes chalky and disintegrates.

Diagnosis by microscopic examination of potassium hydroxide preparations of the nail and of detritus beneath the nail should be confirmed by culture.

2. Occurrence—Common.

3. Infectious agents—Various species of *Trichophyton*.

4. Reservoir—Reservoir is man.

5. Mode of transmission—Presumably by direct extension from skin or nail lesions of infected persons, possibly contaminated floors and shower stalls. Usually no transmission even to close family associates.

6. Incubation period—Unknown.

7. Period of communicability—As long as an infected lesion is present.

8. Susceptibility and resistance—Injury to nail predisposes to infection. Reinfection is frequent.

9. Methods of Control—

A. Preventive measures: Those for tinea corporis.

B. Control of patient, contacts, and the immediate environment:
  1) Report to local health authority: Official report not ordinarily justifiable, Class 5 (see Preface).
  2–6) See Section C, above (Tinea Pedis).
  7) Specific treatment: Griseofulvin is the treatment of choice; although improvement is usual, cure is infrequent.

C. Epidemic measures: Not applicable.

D. International measures: None.

DIARRHEA, ENTEROPATHOGENIC *ESCHERICHIA COLI*

1. Identification—An entity characterized in its most severe form by profuse watery diarrhea, with little mucus and no blood, acidosis, prostration, dehydration and cardiovascular collapse. Fever is often absent. This is a frequent cause of epidemic diarrhea in nurseries for the newborn, although older children and even adults may be affected.

Case fatality rate may be high (up to 40%), especially in the very young. There are no specific findings at autopsy.

Specific diagnosis is by isolation of *Escherichia coli* from stools on nonselective media (blood agar, Endo, MacConkey or eosin-methylene blue) and by serologic identification of the isolate as an enteropathogenic serogroup.

2. Occurrence—Epidemic outbreaks occur in nurseries and institutions, less often in food poisoning outbreaks in the community; a cause of endemic diarrhea in poorly sanitated areas, occurring most frequently in persons under 2 years of age.

3. Infectious agents—Several serogroups are more commonly encountered, e.g., $O26:B6$, $O55:B5$, $O86:B7$, $O111:B4$, $O112:B11$, $O119:B14$, $O124:B17$, $O125:B15$, $O126:B16$, $O127:B8$ and $O128:B12$. Other serogroups may be involved in disease of both children and adults. A variety of other unrelated infectious organisms cause a clinically similar illness.

4. Reservoir—Infected adults, who are often asymptomatic.

5. Mode of transmission—Fecal contamination during delivery from mother to infant, or by fecal-oral spread, possibly by fomites such as weighing scales or tables, and occasionally (among adults) food. Infants with diarrhea are particularly infectious, as they excrete extraordinarily large numbers of organisms. Faulty personal toilet hygiene of adult carriers and/or poor environmental sanitation contribute to perpetuation of an epidemic. Airborne (dust) transmission may be important.

6. Incubation period—One day or more.

7. Period of communicability—Readily communicable among newborn infants. Epidemics may persist for months.

8. Susceptibility and resistance—Infants are most susceptible, particularly prematures. Role of immunity unknown.

9. Methods of control—

A. Preventive measures:

1) For general measures for prevention of disease by fecal-oral spread, see Typhoid Fever 9A (p. 270).
2) Prevention of hospital nursery outbreaks depends primarily on maintenance of a clean nursery with adequate hand-washing facilities.
   a) Provide a nursery for the newborn and premature infants not connecting directly with other nurseries, and having separate isolation facilities for those ill or suspect. Provide each infant with individual equipment kept at his bassinet; no common bathing or dressing tables and no bassinet stands for holding or transporting more than one infant at a time.
   b) Prepare feeding formulas aseptically, bottle, apply nipple, cover with a cap, sterilize, and refrigerate, with

nipple and caps on bottles until feeding time. Control by periodic bacteriological sampling of heated stored formulas.

c) Keep no normal newborn infant in the same nursery with sick infants or older children. Admit to the nursery no infant born outside the hospital or to a mother with diarrheal or respiratory illness until after quarantine for at least 6 days, preferably after bacteriological examination of stools. Nurses caring for other patients should have no association with nurseries for healthy newborn infants; nurses engaged in the milk kitchen should not attend infants' toilet. Control of visitors to minimize spread of infection; and of laundry procedures to assure absence of pathogens from the finished product as returned to the nursery.

d) Systematic daily record for each infant of number and consistency of stools.

B. Control of patient, contacts and the immediate environment:

1) *Report to local health authority:* Obligatory report of epidemics; no individual case report, Class 4 (see Preface). Two or more concurrent cases in a nursery are to be interpreted as an epidemic.

2) *Isolation:* Of infected infants, also suspects.

3) *Concurrent disinfection:* Of all discharges and articles soiled therewith. Thorough terminal cleaning.

4) *Quarantine:* Complete quarantine of all newborn contacts.

5) *Immunization of contacts:* None.

6) *Investigation of contacts and source of infection:* See 9C2 below.

7) *Specific treatment:* Neomycin, tetracycline antibiotics, and chloramphenicol in illnesses due to enteropathogenic *E. coli;* colistin (Coly-Mycin S) if strains are resistant.

C. Epidemic measures: For nursery epidemics, the following—

1) Admit no more babies to the contaminated nursery; suspend maternity service unless a clean nursery is available with separate personnel and facilities. For babies exposed in the contaminated nursery, provide separate medical and nursing personnel skilled in the care of communicable disease. Observe contacts for at least 2 weeks after last case leaves the nursery; promptly remove each new case to isolation. Maternity service may be resumed after discharge of all contact babies and mothers and thorough cleaning. Put into practice recommendations of 9A above so far as is feasible in the emergency.

2) *Epidemiologic investigation:* (a) Assure adequate treatment of missed cases by follow-up examination of all infants discharged from hospital during the 2 weeks pre-

ceding first recognized case; (b) examine mothers and maternity service personnel for early signs of illness; (c) conduct laboratory examination of feces of all sick and exposed babies, mothers and maternity service personnel to detect missed cases and carriers; (d) survey hospital for sanitary hazards; (e) investigate preparation of feeding formulas; (f) inquire into techniques of aseptic nursing of infants, of changing diapers and other clothing. Chemoprophylaxis for contacts should be approached with caution but may have some value.

D. International measures: WHO Reference Centres (see Preface).

DIARRHEAL DISEASE, ACUTE UNDIFFERENTIATED

Acute diarrheal disease is a clinical syndrome of varied etiology with diarrhea and often fever as the common manifestations. It includes specific infectious diseases such as cholera, shigellosis, salmonellosis, and amebiasis, as well as infections with enteropathogenic *Escherichia coli*, viruses, other protozoa or helminths. A variety of organisms of low pathogenicity may be etiologically associated when present in large numbers. On the other hand, abnormal frequency and liquidity of fecal discharges, usually appearing in isolated cases, can have psychogenic, metabolic, nutritional or chemical etiology.

More often than not, no definable infectious agent can be identified in an outbreak of diarrhea. In some situations, salmonellae or shigellae can be recovered from asymptomatic members of the community in a frequency comparable to their occurrence among persons with diarrhea. The decline in overall incidence of diarrhea with increasing age, the appearance of epidemics when sanitary facilities fail, and the high incidence when a new population group is exposed suggest that most cases have an infectious origin and are disseminated by fecal-oral spread.

The specific diarrheas are usually recognized by laboratory identification of the infectious agent. Although these specific diseases have distinctive epidemiological characteristics, many features are shared. Patterns of distribution and frequency, modes of transmission and communicability, and incubation periods are, in general, similar to each other and to the diarrheas whose specific causes have not been identified by techniques presently available.

Although diarrheal disease is a symptom of infection by many agents and can even be the result of noninfectious factors, acute diarrheal disease is presented as an entity because facilities for clinical and laboratory differentiation are limited, especially in the undeveloped areas where diarrheal disease is most prevalent. It must be understood that the term "acute undifferentiated diarrheal disease" often includes a varying proportion of specific disease entities, as well as those diarrheas whose etiological agent is not known.

A. DIARRHEA OF EARLY CHILDHOOD (WEANLING DIARRHEA OF LESS DEVELOPED COUNTRIES)

This is a clinical syndrome, apparently of infectious origin and sometimes associated with specific pathogens, occurring particularly frequently during and around the weaning period of early childhood (4–30 months), and usually concerned with malnutrition and poor sanitation. The onset is acute and the course may be rapidly progressive with frequent liquid or semiliquid stools, varying from three to as many as 20 daily. Approximately one-third of cases have blood or mucus in the stools; pus is frequently present. Fever may be absent but often is at a low level, along with malaise, toxemia, intestinal cramps and tenesmus. The usual clinical course lasts four to five days, but low-grade indisposition may continue for one to three months with irregularly occurring loose stools, a progressively depleted nutritional state and occasional recurrent acute episode. Dehydration and electrolyte imbalance are common and difficult to correct. Protein-calorie malnutrition is commonly associated; acute diarrheal disease may precipitate Kwashiorkor. The overall case fatalities for infants in their first and second years of life range from 1 to 5% for the general population but are as high as 30–40% among hospitalized infants; fatality is far lower in older age groups. In economically advanced countries, illnesses may be relatively mild, are much less frequent and fatality is low; fifty years ago, however, case incidence and mortality rates were those of the developing regions today.

The condition is universally present and common in areas of poor sanitation and prevailing malnutrition. Incidence has been reported in some areas as 115 cases per 100 children per year for breast-fed infants under 5 months of age, reaching 275 attacks per year at the weaning age with mortality rates of over 50 per 1,000 preschool children per year. Highest prevalence tends to parallel hot, dry periods. In most cases no pathogenic agent can be demonstrated. In some localities, *Shigella,* enteropathogenic *E. coli, Salmonella, Entamoeba histolytica, Giardia lamblia* or other parasites as well as enteroviruses and adenoviruses may be found in as many as 10–40% of cases, either alone or as mixed infections. However, these are not necessarily the cause of the diarrhea.

Epidemiological observations suggest an infectious agent, with man as an important reservoir, spread by direct or indirect contact through fecal-oral transfer with a usually short 1–4 day incubation period. It is apparently readily communicable to other children in the family. Control is based on improved sanitation and nutrition, including the promotion of breast feeding and appropriate supplementation. Cases are treated by correction of fluid and electrolyte abnormalities and nutritional deficiencies; antibiotics are rarely justified.

B. ACUTE ENDEMIC GASTROENTERITIS OF GENERAL POPULATIONS

The entity of diarrheal diseases of early childhood is closely related to the diarrheas of the general population. In less developed regions, diarrheal disease is frequently listed as the first cause of death for populations as a whole, with death rates often above 100 per 100,000 population per year and sometimes reaching 500. Attack rates are high, and all ages are affected although incidence declines progressively with age. Environmental factors determine the modes of the spread. In U.S.A., the death rate is low, presently about 4 per 100,000 population per year. The disease is sporadic but family outbreaks occur and neighborhood epidemics are identified. Fecal-oral spread by indirect contact accounts for a large proportion of cases; food is a usual vehicle, water less so. In developed areas specific pathogens are rarely recovered.

Primary emphasis in the control of diarrhea among older children and adults rests on sanitary disposal of feces, the maintenance of a pure water supply, and other environmental measures. It is clear that long-term and ultimate community control depends on community-wide environmental sanitation.

Another large group of mild illnesses of unknown but presumable viral etiology is widespread. These infections tend to be associated more with vomiting and are variously termed epidemic vomiting and diarrhea, viral gastroenteritis, winter vomiting disease, and even intestinal influenza. They may be grouped in the general category of acute viral diarrheas, but evidence for viral etiology is largely inferential. Epidemiological evidence of contact spread through respiratory secretions is strong.

C. TRAVELER'S DIARRHEA

A clinical syndrome with worldwide distribution characterized by precipitous onset of watery stools, with variable upper and lower gastrointestinal symptoms and malaise. The disease is self-limited and lasts 1 to 3 days, although mild symptoms may persist longer. It affects travelers usually within a few days of their arrival in a new area. The syndrome is thought to be usually infectious but transmission probably involves multiple factors, including dietary change and excess. The disease primarily affects adults as sporadic cases, but families or groups of travelers of all ages may be affected in apparent common-source outbreaks. Control measures are based on probable fecal-oral transmission. In the absence of a specific diagnosis, symptomatic treatment is usually adequate for most cases.

D. EPIDEMIC DIARRHEA IN HOSPITAL NURSERIES

This clinical syndrome of infectious origin affecting infants under 1 month of age, characterized by severe diarrhea, dehydration, and acidosis so severe as to set it apart from the usual infantile diarrhea, occurs as epidemics in hospital nurseries caring for newborn infants. Recognition of the disease is thus restricted to economically advanced countries where hospital nurseries exist. Feces are watery, yellow, later green, with little mucus and no blood. Fever is absent or slight except when dehydration or pyogenic complications occur. Fatality was ordinarily high, with a range from 0 to 40% before effective antibiotics became available.

Epidemics have occurred in hospital nurseries in North America and Europe, and have continued as long as 4 to 5 months. Premature infants are most susceptible and have the highest fatality; most patients are 8–9 days old. The pathogen most commonly recovered on stool studies is enteropathogenic *E. coli* of one of 10 or more serotypes. Less frequently enteroviruses are recovered; *Salmonella* is occasionally involved and *Shigella* rarely. Often, no known pathogen is recovered.

Infection is spread from other cases or from carriers (including the hospital staff and attendants) when hospital routines permit fecal-oral transmission. Infection can be acquired from a mother with a contaminated birth canal. The incubation period is most frequently two to four days. Control depends on the high level of nursery sanitation and rapid identification of the infecting organism with appropriate antibiotic therapy, when pertinent. (See Diarrhea, Enteropathogenic *Escherichia coli,* pp. 72–73.)

DIPHTHERIA

1. **Identification**—An acute infectious disease of tonsils, pharynx, larynx or nose, occasionally of other mucous membranes or skin. Lesion is marked by a patch or patches of grayish membrane with surrounding dull red inflammatory zone. The throat is moderately sore in pharyngeal diphtheria, with cervical lymph nodes somewhat enlarged and tender; in severe cases, there is marked swelling and edema of neck. Laryngeal diphtheria is serious in infants and young children. Nasal diphtheria is mild, often chronic and marked by one-sided nasal discharge and excoriations. Inapparent infections outnumber recognized cases. Cutaneous diphtheria usually appears as a localized punched-out ulcer. Late effects of absorption of toxin include cranial and peripheral motor and sensory nerve palsies and myocarditis, often severe. Case fatality of 5 to 10% has changed little in 50 years.

Diagnosis is confirmed by bacteriologic examination of lesions. Failure to demonstrate the bacillus in suspected diphtheria is not a valid reason for withholding specific treatment.

Physicians should suspect diphtheria in differential diagnosis of bacterial and viral pharyngitis, Vincent's angina, infectious mononucleosis, syphilis, and candidial disease, especially following antibiotics. The tendency to prescribe antibiotics automatically for all sore throats, on the assumption that most are streptococcal, delays definitive diagnosis and therapy of diphtheria and has been responsible for deaths.

2. Occurrence—Endemic and epidemic; a disease of late autumn, winter and spring. Primarily a disease of unimmunized children under 15 years of age; in U.S.A., cases are seen in migrant labor camps and among vagrants and homeless men. Relatively, the tropics have more inapparent infection, less faucial and more cutaneous diphtheria than temperate zones.

3. Infectious agent—Toxicogenic *Corynebacterium diphtheriae,* the Klebs-Loeffler bacillus.

4. Reservoir—Reservoir is man.

5. Mode of transmisison—Contact with a patient or carrier or with articles soiled with discharges from mucous membranes of nose and nasopharynx, and from skin and other lesions of infected persons. Raw milk has served as a vehicle.

6. Incubation period—Usually 2 to 5 days, occasionally longer.

7. Period of communicability—Variable, until virulent bacilli have disappeared from discharges and lesions; usually 2 weeks or less, seldom more than 4 weeks.

8. Susceptibility and resistance—Infants born of immune mothers are relatively immune, a passive protection usually lost before the 6th month. Recovery from clinical attack is usually but not always followed by persisting immunity. Immunity is often acquired through unrecognized infection. Passive temporary immunity of from 15 days to 3 weeks and active immunity of prolonged duration can be induced artificially.

9. Methods of control—

A. *Preventive measures:*

1) The only effective control of diphtheria is through active immunization with diphtheria toxoid on a population basis including an adequate program to maintain immunity. Where protection has been neglected in infancy, immunization should be started as soon as the opportunity arises. Alternative procedures are: (a) *Multiple antigen*—At 2 or 3 months of age, diphtheria alum toxoid combined with tetanus toxoid and pertussis vaccine (DTP); 3 intramuscular injections of 0.5 ml each at 4 to 6 week intervals and a reinforcing dose approximately one year after the 3rd injection. A booster dose of DTP should be given to children 3 through 6 years of age at the time of school entrance, kindergarten or elementary. DTP may be given through 6 years of age; thereafter use tetanus and diphtheria toxoids, combined, alum precipitated (for adult use) (Td) which contains only 2 Lf of diphtheria toxoid. This is given on two occasions 4–6 weeks apart, followed by a reinforcing dose 1 year later. Booster doses of Td

should be given every 10 years. (b) *Single antigens*—Only used when there is a definite contraindication to the other components in the combined antigen; diphtheria alum toxoid, at 2 to 3 months of age and until 7 years, 2 intramuscular injections of 0.5 ml each at 4 to 6 week intervals. Give a reinforcing dose within one year following the 2nd dose. For primary immunization of children more than 6 years old and for adults, use 0.5 ml of a purified adult-type diphtheria toxoid (2 Lf of antigen), 2 doses at 4 to 6 week intervals and a 3rd dose within the next year. Booster dose schedule as above.

2) Adults subject to unusual risk, such as physicians, teachers, nurses, nursemaids, orderlies, and other hospital personnel, should be immunized and should receive booster doses every 10 years.

3) Educational measures to inform the public and particularly the parents of young children of the hazards of diphtheria and the necessity and advantages of active immunization.

B. Control of patient, contacts, and the immediate environment:

1) *Report to local health authority:* Case report obligatory in most states and countries, Class 2A (see Preface).

2) *Isolation:* Until 2 cultures each from throat and nose fail to show diphtheria bacilli; to be taken not less than 24 hours apart and after cessation of antimicrobial therapy. Where practicable, a virulence test should be made if throat cultures continue positive 3 weeks after onset. If the result is negative, isolation may be ended; if positive, repeat a course of antibiotic therapy. Where termination of isolation by culture is impractical, isolation may end with a fair degree of safety 14 days after onset.

3) *Concurrent disinfection:* Of all articles in contact with patient, and all articles soiled by discharges of patient. Terminal cleaning.

4) *Quarantine:* All intimate contacts should be placed under modified quarantine until nose and throat cultures are negative. All carriers should be treated (9B7 below). Adult contacts whose occupation involves handling of food or close association with children should be excluded from those occupations until bacteriological examination proves them not to be carriers.

5) *Immunization of contacts:* Child contacts less than 10 years old, intimately exposed and not previously immunized with toxoid, may be given a prophylactic dose of antitoxin, 10,000 units, and at the same time a first dose of toxoid. Daily examination by a physician is advised for older children and adults, with such further active immunization as may be indicated; persons previously immunized

should have a reinforcing dose of toxoid. Groups of older persons, as in institutions, barracks, or other congested quarters, may be given routine immunization with Td, or they may be screened for susceptibility with a Schick test, with immunization restricted to Schick-positives.

6) *Investigation of contacts:* Search for carriers and unreported and atypical cases; restrict and treat. These control measures are of little importance in well-immunized communities.

7) *Specific treatment:* If diphtheria is suspected, antitoxin should be given *without awaiting bacteriological confirmation,* 20,000 to 80,000 units depending upon the duration of symptoms, area of involvement and severity of the disease, and in a single dose after completion of sensitivity tests. Intramuscular administration usually suffices; in severe infections antitoxin both intravenously and intramuscularly is indicated. Sulfonamides are of no value. Penicillin or erythromycin should be used in conjunction with antitoxin but an antibiotic is not a substitute. Neither an antibiotic nor diphtheria antitoxin can be relied upon to shorten materially the period of communicability. Penicillin-soaked compresses (500 units per ml) are of value in cutaneous diphtheria; also erythromycin and bacitracin.

A virulence test may eliminate necessity for treatment of carriers. Otherwise, give 600,000 to 2,000,000 units of aqueous procaine penicillin intramuscularly daily for 7 days. If this fails, penicillin may be repeated after a virulence test, or erythromycin substituted. If antibiotic treatment fails, tonsillectomy may be performed but not before 3 months after onset of disease.

C. Epidemic measures:

1) Immediate intensification of efforts to immunize the largest possible number of the affected population, with emphasis on protection of infants and preschool children. Sample immunization surveys define levels of immunity and set priorities for selected area immunization.

2) In areas with good health facilities, prompt field investigation of reported cases to verify diagnosis, determine subtype of *C. diphtheriae,* identify contacts, trace sources of infection and define population groups at special risk.

D. International measures:
Active immunization of susceptible infants and young children traveling to or through countries where diphtheria is a common disease; a booster dose of toxoid for those previously inoculated.

DIPHYLLOBOTHRIASIS

1. Identification—A nonfatal intestinal tapeworm disease of long duration. Symptoms commonly are trivial or absent. A few patients develop vitamin B-12 deficiency anemia; massive infections may be associated with toxic symptoms. Synonym: Broad or Fish tapeworm disease.

Diagnosis is confirmed by identification in feces of eggs or proglottids (segments) of the worm.

2. Occurrence—Endemic worldwide in temperate zones. Where raw or only partly cooked fish is popular, 10 to 30% of some populations are infected, prevalence increasing with age. Persons in U.S.A. become infected through eating uncooked, infected fish from midwest· ern or Canadian lakes.

3. Infectious agent—*Diphyllobothrium latum,* a cestode; and also several other species.

4. Reservoir—The main reservoir is an infected person discharging eggs in feces; other reservoir hosts include dog, bear and other fish-eating mammals.

5. Mode of transmission—Man acquires the infection by eating raw or inadequately cooked fish. Larvae developing in flesh of freshwater fish infect definitive hosts, man or animals. Eggs from segments of worm are discharged into bodies of fresh water in which they mature, hatch, and produce infection in first intermediate host (copepods). Susceptible freshwater species of fish ingest infected copepods and become second intermediate hosts in which the worms transform into the stage infective for man.

6. Incubation period—From 3 to 6 weeks.

7. Period of communicability—Not directly transmitted from man to man. Man and other definitive hosts continue to disseminate eggs in the environment as long as worms remain in the intestine, sometimes for several years.

8. Susceptibility and resistance—Man is universally susceptible. No apparent resistance follows infection.

9. Methods of control—

A. Preventive measures:

1) Prevention of stream and lake pollution by installing disposal systems for human feces in cities and villages, by treatment of sewage effluents, by the use of sanitary privies in rural areas, and by education of the public in the life cycle of the parasite.

2) Thorough cooking of freshwater fish or freezing for 24 hours at −10 C insures protection. Inspection of fish is not practical.

B. Control of patient, contacts, and the immediate environment:

1) Report to local health authority: Official report not ordinarily justifiable, Class 5 (see Preface).

2) Isolation: None.

3) Concurrent disinfection: None; sanitary disposal of feces.

4) Quarantine: None.

5) Immunization of contacts: None.

6) Investigation of contacts: Not usually justified.

7) Specific treatment: Niclosamide (Yomesan), available from the NCDC, Atlanta, Ga., or quinacrine hydrochloride (Atabrine) are the drugs of choice. Oleoresin of aspidium, not available in the U.S.A., is an alternative choice.

C. Epidemic measures: None.

D. International measures: None.

DRACONTIASIS

1. Identification—An infection of the subcutaneous and deeper tissues with a large nematode. Blister appears, usually on a lower extremity, especially the foot. This vesicle forms as the gravid, meter-long female prepares to discharge her larvae. Burning and itching of the skin in the area of the lesion and frequently fever, nausea, vomiting, diarrhea, dyspnea, generalized urticaria and eosinophilia may precede vesicle formation. On rupture of the vesicle the worm discharges her larvae into water encountered by the infected leg. The prognosis is good unless there are multiple worms and unless a bacterial infection occurs which may produce severe crippling sequelae. Synonyms: Guinea worm disease, Dracunculiasis.

Diagnosis is by microscopic identification of larvae or recognition of the adult worm after removal.

2. Occurrence—In India, Africa, Middle East, West Indies, and northeastern South America. Local prevalence varies greatly; in some localities nearly all inhabitants are infected, in others few and mainly young adults. In North America, worms morphologically identical to *Dracunculus medinensis* occur in dogs, foxes, mink and raccoons; no authentic indigenous case reported in man.

3. Infectious agent—*Dracunculus medinensis,* a nematode worm.

4. Reservoir—Reservoir is an infected person.

5. Mode of transmission—Larvae discharged into fresh water are swallowed by crustacea of genus *Cyclops,* penetrate into body cavity and in about 2 weeks develop to the infective stage. Man swallows the infected copepods in drinking water from contaminated step-wells and ponds, larvae are liberated in stomach or duodenum, migrate through the viscera, become adults, and reach the subcutaneous tissues.

6. Incubation period—About 8 to 14 months.

7. Period of communicability—Until larvae have been completely evacuated from the uterus of the gravid worm, usually 15 to 20 days. Larvae may survive in water up to 3 weeks. Not directly transmitted from man to man.

8. Susceptibility and resistance—Susceptibility is universal. No acquired immunity; multiple and repeated infections occur in the same person.

9. Methods of control—

A. *Preventive measures:*
1) Provision of potable water. Abolition of step-wells and other measures to prevent contamination of drinking water by infected persons through immersion of affected parts.
2) Boiling of drinking water, or filtration through muslin cloth to remove copepods.
3) Control of copepods is by appropriate treatment of water.
4) Education of the public to drink only boiled or filtered water. Instruction of infected persons in mode of spread of the infection and the danger in contaminating wells or other water supplies.

B. *Control of patient, contacts, and the immediate environment:*
1) *Report to local health authority:* Official report not ordinarily justifiable, Class 5 (see Preface).
2) *Isolation:* None.
3) *Concurrent disinfection:* None.
4) *Quarantine:* None.
5) *Immunization of contacts:* None.
6) *Investigation of contacts and source of infection:* Obtain information as to source of drinking water at probable time of infection. Search for other cases, and examine drinking water microscopically for infected copepods.
7) *Specific treatment:* Niridazole.

C. *Epidemic measures:* In hyperendemic situations, field survey to determine prevalence, to discover sources of infection, and to guide control measures as described in 9A.

D. *International measures:* None.

ENTEROBIASIS

1. Identification—Generally a benign intestinal disease with mild or nonspecific symptoms. If severe, may cause pruritus ani with disturbed sleep and irritability, and local irritation from scratching. A variety of severe manifestations including appendicitis and salpingitis have been described, but the relationship to enterobiasis is indefinite. Synonyms: Pinworm disease, Oxyuriasis.

Diagnosis is by applying a cellulose tape applicator to the perianal region and examining it microscopically for eggs; the material is best obtained in the morning before bathing or defecation.

2. Occurrence—Distribution is worldwide and exceedingly common. An estimated 10% of the general population of the United States is infected. Prevalence is highest in children of school age, next highest in those of preschool age, and lowest in adults except for mothers of infected children. Infection is characteristically familial. Crowding is an important factor; incidence is often high in institutions.

3. Infectious agent—*Enterobius vermicularis,* an intestinal round worm infecting only man.

4. Reservoir—Infected persons, particularly children. Pinworms of animal hosts are not transmissible to man.

5. Mode of transmission—Direct transfer of infective eggs by hand from anus to mouth of the same host, or indirectly to same host or new hosts through clothing, bedding, food, or other articles contaminated with eggs of the parasite. Dustborne infection by inhalation is possible in heavily contaminated households. Eggs are infective within a few hours after leaving the gastrointestinal tract. After ingestion, eggs hatch in the stomach and small intestine; young worms mature in the lower small intestine, cecum, and upper portions of colon. Gravid worms migrate to the rectum to discharge eggs on perianal skin; may migrate up the genital tract of females and enter peritoneal cavity.

6. Incubation period—The life cycle requires 3 to 6 weeks. Infections ordinarily build up from successive reinfections and may not be recognized for several months.

7. Period of communicability—In the absence of treatment, for 2 to 8 weeks unless reinfected from self.

8. Susceptibility and resistance—Susceptibility is universal. Differences in frequency and intensity of infection are due to differences in exposure. No apparent resistance to repeated infections.

9. Methods of control—

A. Preventive measures:

1) Frequent bathing, with showers preferred to tub baths; use of clean underclothing, night clothes, and bed sheets at frequent intervals.
2) Public health education in personal hygiene of the toilet, particularly the washing of hands after defecation, and always before eating or preparing food; also to discourage habits of nail-biting and scratching bare anal area.
3) Reduction of overcrowding in living accommodations.

4) Adequate provision of toilets and privies with hand-washing facilities; and maintenance of clean facilities for defecation.

B. Control of patient, contacts, and the immediate environment:

1) Report to local health authority: Official report not ordinarily justifiable, Class 5 (see Preface). Advise school authorities of school outbreaks.

2) Isolation: None.

3) Concurrent disinfection: Sanitary disposal of feces. Change bed linen and underwear of infected person daily. Eggs on discarded linen are killed by exposure to temperatures of 55 C (132 F) for a few seconds, either by boiling or by the usual household washing machine.

4) Quarantine: None.

5) Immunization of contacts: None.

6) Investigation of contacts: Examine all members of an affected family or institution.

7) Specific treatment: Piperazine citrate (Antepar), pyrvinium pamoate (Povan). All infected members of a household or institution should be treated simultaneously.

C. Epidemic measures: Outbreaks in schools and institutions require strict hygienic measures and cleanliness. Toilet seats should be washed daily with disinfectants. Provide adequate treatment facilities.

D. International measures: None.

FASCIOLOPSIASIS

1. Identification—A trematode disease of the small intestine, particularly the duodenum. Diarrhea of a nondysenteric type usually alternates with constipation; vomiting and anorexia are frequent. Large numbers of worms may produce acute intestinal obstruction. Patients may show edema of face within 20 days after massive infection, also of abdominal wall and legs; ascites is common; eosinophilia is usual, secondary anemia occasional. Death is rare.

Diagnosis is by finding flukes (which measure 20–75 mm long, 8 to 20 mm wide and 0.5 to 3 mm thick) or characteristic eggs in feces; worms are occasionally vomited.

2. Occurrence—Widely distributed in the Orient, especially central and south China. Prevalence is often extremely high.

3. Infectious agent—*Fasciolopsis buski,* a large trematode or fluke.

4. Reservoir—Man, pig and dog are definitive reservoir hosts of adult flukes.

5. Mode of transmission—Eggs passed in feces develop in water within 3 to 7 weeks under favorable conditions; miracidia hatch, penetrate snails (*Segmentininae* of the *Planorbidae*) as intermediate hosts; cercariae develop, are liberated and encyst on aquatic plants. Man becomes infected by eating these plants uncooked. In China the chief sources of infection are the nuts of the red water-caltrop grown in enclosed ponds, and tubers of the so-called "water chestnut," as the hull or skin is peeled off with teeth and lips. Period of development from infection of snail to development of encysted infective metacercariae is 7 to 8 weeks.

6. Incubation period—About 6–8 weeks, from ingestion of infective larvae. Eggs appear in the stool a month after infection (prepatent period).

7. Period of communicability—As long as viable eggs are discharged by patient; without treatment, probably for many years. Not directly transmitted from man to man.

8. Susceptibility and resistance—Susceptibility is universal. In malnourished individuals the ill effects are pronounced; the number of worms also influences severity.

9. Methods of control—

A. Preventive measures:

1) Public health education of people in endemic areas on life cycle of parasite and mode of transmission.
2) Treat nightsoil before use as fertilizer; chemical treatment: anhydrous calcium oxide (unslaked lime, 1 part to 1,000 parts of water) destroys eggs, as does drying, freezing or heating.
3) Dry the suspected plants, or if eaten fresh, dip into boiling water for a few seconds; both methods kill metacercariae.
4) Destroy snail intermediate hosts and infected animals.

B. Control of patient, contacts, and the immediate environment:

1) *Report to local health authority:* In selected endemic areas; in most countries not a reportable disease, Class 3C (see Preface).
2) *Isolation:* None.
3) *Concurrent disinfection:* Sanitary disposal of feces.
4) *Quarantine:* None.
5) *Immunization of contacts:* None.
6) *Investigation of contacts and source of infection:* In the individual case, of little value. A community problem (see 9C below).
7) *Specific treatment:* Tetrachloroethylene and hexylresorcinol crystoids are reasonably effective.

C. Epidemic measures: Identify aquatic plants which are eaten fresh and bear encysted metacercariae; identify infected snail species living in water with plants and prevent access of human feces to the water.

D. International measures: None.

FASCIOLIASIS is an infection with *Fasciola hepatica,* the fluke commonly infecting the bile ducts of sheep, cattle and other ruminants throughout the world. The disease, fascioliasis, is reported in man in South America, the Caribbean, Europe and parts of the U.S.A.

FILARIASIS

1. Identification—An infection with a nematode parasite whose early acute manifestations include fever, lymphadenitis, retrograde lymphangitis of extremities, orchitis, epididymitis, funiculitis, and abscess. These are primarily allergic reactions, but secondary bacterial infection may occasionally cause death. Prolonged and repeated infection with obstruction to lymph flow often leads to hydrocele and elephantiasis of limbs, genitalia or breasts, or to chyluria. Many infected persons show no clinical manifestations. Female worms give rise to larvae (microfilariae), which, in the absence of lymphatic obstruction, reach the bloodstream. A nocturnal periodicity of microfilariae in the peripheral blood (10 p.m.–2 a.m.) occurs in all endemic areas except those Pacific Islands where the vector is an *Aedes* mosquito (day biter). Many persons with clinical manifestations do not have circulating microfilariae (occult filariasis) ; in some cases, infection is manifested by marked eosinophilia associated with pulmonary infiltrates (tropical eosinophilia or tropical pulmonary eosinophilia). Synonyms : Wucheriasis, Brugiasis.

Microfilariae are best detected in blood at optimum daily periodicity, examined in thick-film preparation or stained sediment of laked blood. Skin test is nonspecific, but of value in absence of microfilaremia.

Filariasis due to *Wuchereria bancrofti* and *Brugia malayi* requires differentiation from other filarial diseases, loiasis, onchocerciasis, and others (see pp. 135, 162, etc.).

2. Occurrence—*Wuchereria bancrofti* is endemic in most of the warm regions of the world, including Latin America, Asia, and Pacific Islands. *Brugia malayi* is endemic only in Southeast Asia, India, Central China, South Korea, and a few islands of Indonesia. Local foci of high prevalence are often surrounded by nonendemic areas. High prevalence depends upon a large reservoir of infection and abundant vector breeding; commonly a disease of heavily populated areas.

3. Infectious agents—*Wuchereria bancrofti,* and *Brugia malayi,* nematode worms.

4. Reservoir—Reservoir is man with microfilariae in the blood.

5. Mode of transmission—By bite of a mosquito harboring infective larvae. *W. bancrofti* is transmitted in nature by many species, the most important being *Culex fatigans, Culex pipiens, Aedes polynesiensis (pseudoscutellaris),* and several species of *Anopheles. B. malayi* is transmitted by various species of *Mansonia, Anopheles,* and *Aedes.* Microfilariae penetrate stomach wall of the mosquito, lodge in thoracic muscles, develop into infective larvae, migrate to the proboscis, and are transmitted to the new host as the mosquito bites.

6. Incubation period—Allergic hypersensitivity manifestations may appear as early as 3 months after infection. Microfilariae do not appear in the blood until at least 9 months after bite of infective mosquitoes.

7. Period of communicability—Not directly transmitted from man to man. Man remains infective for mosquitoes as long as microfilariae are present in the blood, which may be years. Communicability in the mosquito is from about 10 days after blood meal until all infective larvae are discharged.

8. Susceptibility and resistance—Universal susceptibility. Repeated infections apparently occur in endemic regions.

9. Methods of control—

A. Preventive measures:

1) Determine, by dissection, the vector or vectors; study times and places of feeding and locate breeding places. If vector is a night biter, attack adult mosquitoes by spraying building with an acceptable effective residual insecticide, screening of houses, use of bed nets, and insect repellents. Attack mosquito larvae by eliminating small breeding places and treating others with larvicides. Each local situation requires individual study.

2) Education of the public concerning mode of transmission, and methods of mosquito control.

B. Control of patient, contacts, and the immediate environment:

1) Report to local health authority: In selected endemic regions; in most countries not a reportable disease, Class 3C (see Preface). Reporting of cases with demonstrated microfilariae provides data on potential transmission. Cases of elephantiasis without microfilariae in the blood should not be reported as filariasis, but are usefully recorded in estimating prevalence or in planning control programs.

2) Isolation: Not practicable. So far as possible, patients with microfilariae in blood should be protected from mosquitoes to reduce transmission.

3) Concurrent disinfection: None.

4) Quarantine: None.

5) Immunization of contacts: None.

6) Investigation of contacts and source of infection: Only as a part of a general community effort (see 9A and 9C herein).

7) *Specific treatment:* Diethylcarbamazine (Hetrazan) results in rapid disappearance of most or all microfilariae from the blood, but may not destroy the adult female worm; microfilariae may again appear after several months. Sodium thiacetarsamide (Caparsolate sodium) causes slow disappearance of microfilariae during treatment without subsequent increase over a 2 year period. Action of this compound apparently is against adult worms rather than microfilariae.

C. *Epidemic measures:* In areas of high endemicity it is essential that the local situation be correctly appraised, particularly the bionomics of mosquito vectors, prevalence and incidence of disease, and environmental factors responsible for transmission. Vector control is the fundamental approach. Even partial control by antimosquito measures may reduce incidence and restrict the endemic focus. Measurable results are slow because of the long incubation period. Mass treatment of known infected persons with diethylcarbamazine (Hetrazan) contributes materially.

D. *International measures:*

1) Coordinated programs by neighboring countries where the disease is endemic, with the purpose of limiting migration of infected persons across international boundaries, and instituting treatment and control measures near such boundaries.

2) WHO Reference Centres (see Preface).

FOOD POISONING

Food poisoning is a generic term applied to certain illnesses of abrupt evolution, usually enteric in nature and acquired through consumption of food or water. The term applies to intoxications caused by chemical contaminants (heavy metals, fluorides and others); toxins elaborated by bacterial growth (staphylococcal toxins, botulinus toxins); and a variety of organic substances that may be present in natural foods such as certain mushrooms, mussels, eels and other seafood.

Acute salmonellosis is often classed with food poisoning; but, since it is more an acute enteric infection than an intoxication, it is presented herein as a separate entity (pp. 213–216). Food also may spread many other infectious diseases; these include typhoid and paratyphoid fever, shigellosis, streptococcal pharyngitis (septic sore throat), diphtheria, brucellosis, infectious hepatitis, amebiasis, trichinosis and other helminthic infections. These, however, are not usually classified as forms of food poisoning. Epidemic nausea and vomiting of presumed viral origin can be confused with food poisoning and also with the various forms of water-borne diarrhea.

Food-poisoning outbreaks are usually recognized by the sudden occurrence of a group of illnesses within a short period of time among individuals who have consumed one or more foods in common. The diagnosis is generally indicated by epidemiological findings. While single cases of food poisoning are undoubtedly common, they are difficult to identify unless, as in botulism, there is a distinctive clinical syndrome.

A. STAPHYLOCOCCAL FOOD POISONING

1. Identification—An intoxication (not an infection) of abrupt and sometimes violent onset, with severe nausea, cramps, vomiting, usually diarrhea, and prostration; often with subnormal temperature and sometimes markedly lowered blood pressure. Deaths are exceedingly rare; duration of illness is commonly not more than a day or two, but its intensity may result in surgical exploration in sporadic cases. Diagnosis is usually through recognition of a group of cases with the characteristic acute, predominantly upper gastrointestinal symptoms and the short interval between eating a common food item and the onset of symptoms.

Recovery of large numbers of enterotoxin-producing staphylococci on routine culture media from stomach contents or a suspected food item supports the diagnosis. Phage typing greatly aids epidemiologic investigation.

Differential diagnosis considers other recognized forms of food poisoning, and epidemic nausea, vomiting and diarrhea (winter vomiting disease).

2. Occurrence—Widespread and relatively frequent; one of the principal acute food poisonings in U.S.A.

3. Toxic agent—Several enterotoxins of staphylococci stable at boiling temperature. Staphylococci multiply in food, producing the toxin which causes poisoning.

4. Reservoir—In most instances man; occasionally cows.

5. Mode of transmission—By ingestion of any of a wide variety of contaminated food products: pastries, custards, salads and salad dressings, sandwiches, sliced meats and meat products in which toxin-producing staphylococci of human origin (from purulent discharges of an infected finger, abscesses, nasal secretions, or the apparently normal skin of hands and forearms) or of bovine origin (contaminated milk or milk products) had multiplied in food allowed to stand for several hours before serving. Ham and bacon, pressed meat, milk from cows with infected udders, occasionally dried milk, have sometimes been implicated in extensive outbreaks.

6. Incubation period—Interval between eating food and onset of symptoms is 1 to 6 hours, usually 2 to 4 hours.

7. Period of communicability—Not applicable.

8. Susceptibility and resistance—Most persons are susceptible, although individual reactions are variable.

9. Methods of control—

A. Preventive measures:

1) Prompt refrigeration of food (especially of sliced and chopped meats, custards and cream fillings) to avoid multiplication of staphylococci accidentally introduced. Fill pastries with custard just prior to sale, or subject the finished product to pasteurizing heat treatment. Immediate disposal or prompt refrigeration of left-over foods.

2) Temporary exclusion from food handling of persons suffering from pyogenic skin infections. Use of face masks for food handlers with respiratory infections and of disposable gloves for salad mixers.

3) Education of food handlers in strict attention to sanitation and cleanliness of kitchens, including proper refrigeration, hand washing, attention to fingernails; and to the danger of working while having a skin infection.

B. Control of patient, contacts, and the immediate environment:

1) Report to local health authority: Report promptly. Obligatory report of epidemics of suspected or confirmed cases Class 4 (see Preface).

2, 3, 4, 5, 6, 7: Not pertinent. Control is of epidemics; single cases are rarely identified.

C. Epidemic measures:

1) By quick review of reported cases, determine time and place of exposure and the population at risk. A study of the prominent clinical features of the disease, coupled with an estimate of the incubation period, provides useful leads to the most probable etiological agent. Collect appropriate specimens of feces and vomitus for laboratory examination. Obtain a complete listing of the foods served. Interview an appropriate sample of the patients, and of those remaining well, for specific foods eaten. Determine attack rates for each item of food. The rate for those eating the contaminated food will be higher, and the rate for those not eating the food will be lower, than the overall rate for the population group studied, thus incriminating the vehicle of infection.

2) Conduct a meticulous inquiry into the origin of the incriminated food, manner of preparation and storage before serving, particularly looking for possible sources of con-

tamination and periods of inadequate refrigeration that would permit incubation of the etiological agent. Submit any remainder of the incriminated food for laboratory examination. Failure to isolate staphylococci does not exclude the presence of the heat-resistant enterotoxin.

3) Search for food handlers with skin infections, particularly of the hands. Culture all purulent lesions; culture nasal swabs of all food handlers. Phage-typing of strains of enterotoxin-producing staphylococci isolated from foods and food handlers and from vomitus of patients is recommended.

D. *International measures:* WHO Reference Centres (see Preface).

B. *CLOSTRIDIUM PERFRINGENS (C. WELCHII)* FOOD POISONING

1. Identification—An intestinal disorder characterized by sudden onset of abdominal colic followed by diarrhea; nausea is common but vomiting is usually absent. Generally a mild disease of short duration, 1 day or less, and rarely fatal in healthy persons.

Diagnosis is supported by semiquantitative bacteriological examination of food and patients' stools, using anaerobic techniques, with demonstration of the same serotype in both.

2. Occurrence—Widespread and relatively frequent in countries with cooking practices that favor multiplication of the *Clostridium.*

3. Infectious agent—Type A strains of *Clostridium perfringens* (*C. welchii*), both heat-resistant and heat-sensitive.

4. Reservoir—Reservoir is the gastrointestinal tract of man and animals (cattle, pigs and vermin) and soil.

5. Mode of transmission—Ingestion of food contaminated by feces or soil in which conditions had permitted multiplication of the organism. Almost all outbreaks are associated with meat—sometimes with fresh meat not thoroughly cooked, but usually stews, meat pies, reheated meats, or gravies made of beef, turkey or chicken. Outbreaks are traced to food service industries such as catering firms, restaurants and cafeterias.

6. Incubation period—From 8 to 22 hours, usually 10 to 12 hours.

7. Period of communicability—Unknown.

8. Susceptibility and resistance—Most persons are probably susceptible. In volunteer studies, no resistance to repeated infection has been observed.

9. Methods of control—

A. *Preventive measures:*

1) Serve meat dishes hot, as soon as they are cooked, or cool rapidly and refrigerate until serving time; reheating, if necessary, should be rapid. Large cuts of meat should be adequately cooked; divide stews and similar dishes prepared in bulk into small lots for cooking and refrigeration.

2) Educate food handlers in the risks inherent in large-scale cooking, especially of meat dishes.

B. Control of patient, contacts, and the immediate environment: See Staphylococcal Food Poisoning 9B, p. 91.

C. Epidemic measures: Identify contaminated food (see A. Staphylococcal Food Poisoning 9C, pp. 91–92).

D. International measures: None.

C. BOTULISM

1. Identification—A serious intoxication (not an infection) characterized by weakness, dizziness, headache and constipation, soon followed by oculomotor or other symmetrical motor cranial-nerve paralyses. Clinical manifestations relate primarily to the nervous system. Change in voice, such as hoarseness, is often the first sign noted. Vomiting and diarrhea occasionally initiate illness. About two-thirds of patients die within 3 to 7 days, usually from respiratory or cardiac failure or from infectious complications.

Diagnosis is established by demonstration of the specific toxin in blood, or of its presence in a suspected food item. Isolation of the organism from the suspected food and feces is helpful but is not diagnostic.

2. Occurrence—Sporadic and family-grouped cases occur in most countries, always in relation to a food product so prepared or preserved as to permit toxin formation. A relatively rare disease.

3. Toxic agent—Toxins produced by *Clostridium botulinum* (botulinus bacillus) or *Clostridium parabotulinum*. Most outbreaks are due to type A, B, or E toxins of *C. botulinum*, a few to types F and C. Type E outbreaks are usually related to fish. Toxin is produced in improperly processed foods, only under anaerobic conditions, and especially in nonacid foods. Toxin is destroyed by boiling; inactivation of spores requires higher temperatures. Ordinary refrigeration does not necessarily prevent toxin production.

4. Reservoir—Soil, water, and the intestinal tract of animals, including fish.

5. Mode of transmission—By ingestion of contaminated food from jars or cans inadequately processed during canning and eaten without subsequent adequate cooking. Most poisonings in U.S.A. are due to home-canned vegetables and fruits or to fish; meats are infrequent vehicles. In Europe, most cases are due to sausages and to smoked or preserved meats or fish.

6. Incubation period—Symptoms usually appear within 12 to 36 hours, sometimes several days after eating contaminated food. In general, the shorter the incubation period the more severe the disease and the higher the fatality.

7. Period of communicability—Not applicable.

8. **Susceptibility and resistance**—Susceptibility is general.
9. **Methods of control**—

A. *Preventive measures:*

1) Governmental control by regulation and inspection of commercial processing of canned and preserved foods.
2) Health education of housewives and others concerned with home canning and other processing of foods in safe procedures (time, pressure and temperature required to destroy spores), and especially the need to boil home-canned vegetables 3 minutes with thorough stirring before serving.

B. *Control of patient, contacts, and the immediate environment:*

1) *Report to local health authority:* Case report of suspect and confirmed cases obligatory in most states and countries, Class 2A (see Preface).
2) *Isolation:* None.
3) *Concurrent disinfection:* None.
4) *Quarantine:* None.
5) *Immunization of contacts:* None for simple direct contacts. Those who are known to have eaten the specifically incriminated food within 36 hours may be given polyvalent botulism antitoxin, or monovalent antitoxin of the appropriate type if available.
6) *Investigation of contacts and source of infection:* Search for contaminated food. Study the food habits and recent food history of persons attacked.
7) *Specific treatment:* Intravenous and intramuscular administration of botulism antitoxin. Trivalent antitoxin (types A, B and E) and monovalent type E antitoxin may be obtained from the National Communicable Disease Center, Atlanta, Ga. Antitoxin types A and B can also be obtained from commercial sources.

C. *Epidemic measures:* Suspicion or recognition of a case of botulism should immediately raise the question of a group outbreak involving a commercially produced widely distributed food. Immediate search for persons who shared the suspected food and for any remaining food from the same source that may be similarly contaminated; such food, if found, to be submitted for laboratory examination. Blood from patients and others exposed but not ill should be obtained before administration of antitoxin and forwarded immediately to a reference laboratory.

D. *International measures:* None.

GIARDIASIS

1. Identification—A protozoal infection of the small bowel, often asymptomatic, but which has been associated with a variety of intestinal symptoms, most notably chronic diarrhea and steatorrhea. Heavy infections may be associated with abdominal cramps and bloating, frequent loose and pale, greasy, or malodorous stools, anemia, fatigue and weight loss. Malabsorption of fats and of fat-soluble vitamins has been demonstrated. Large numbers of organisms (*Giardia lamblia*) have been found in symptomatic patients, in whom improvement occurred upon removal of the parasite by appropriate chemotherapy. There is no invasion beyond the bowel lumen, but damage and inflammatory changes of duodenal and jejunal mucosal cells have been shown in severe giardiasis. Synonyms: *Giardia* enteritis, Lambliasis.

Diagnosis is by identification of cysts or trophozoites in feces or of trophozoites in duodenal drainage. The latter method is more reliable. The presence of *G. lamblia* (in either stools or duodenal drainage) is not necessarily indicative of a causal relationship to the symptoms, so that other intestinal pathogens or other causes of malabsorption should be considered.

2. Occurrence—*G. lamblia* has a worldwide distribution. Children are infected more frequently than adults. Prevalence is higher in areas of poor sanitation and in institutions. The carrier rate in different areas of the United States may range between 1.5 and 20%, depending on the community and age group surveyed.

3. Infectious Agent—*Giardia lamblia,* a flagellated protozoan.

4. Reservoir—Man.

5. Mode of transmission—Not clear, but probably by fecal contamination of water and by hand-to-mouth transfer of cysts from the feces of an infected individual. One epidemic of giardiasis reported in the United States presumably resulted from contamination of a public water supply by sewage.

Cyst passers are probably more important in transmission than those with active disease due to fragility of the trophozoite form. Resistance of *Giardia* cysts to chlorination is unknown but is probably similar to that of *Entamoeba histolytica* cysts, which are not killed by standard concentrations.

6. Incubation period—Variable. In experimental infections, prepatent periods have ranged from 6 to 22 days. In the waterborne epidemic in the United States, clinical illnesses occurred from approximately 1 week to 4 weeks after exposure.

7. Period of communicability—For the entire period of infection.

8. Susceptibility and resistance—Despite the high proportion of asymptomatic carriers, clinical studies have indicated that *G. lamblia* is pathogenic, but the mechanism of pathogenicity is not clear.

9. Methods of control—

A. Preventive measures:

1) Health education of families and institutions in personal hygiene.
2) Sanitary disposal of feces.
3) Protection of public water supplies against fecal contamination.

B. Control of patient, contacts, and the immediate environment:

1) Report to local health authority: Obligatory report of epidemics, Class 4 (see Preface).

2) Isolation: None.

3) Concurrent disinfection: Sanitary disposal of feces.

4) Quarantine: None.

5) Investigation of contacts and source of infection: Microscopic examination of feces of household members and other suspected contacts, supplemented by search for environmental contamination.

6) Specific treatment: Quinacrine hydrochloride (Atabrine) is the drug of choice; metronidazole (Flagyl) is proving to be an effective alternative drug.

C. Epidemic measures: Any cluster of cases from a single area or institution requires epidemiological investigation to determine source of infection and mode of transmission. If a common vehicle is indicated, such as water, take appropriate measures to correct the situation. If the epidemiological evidence points to person-to-person transmission, emphasis is on personal cleanliness and sanitary disposal of feces.

D. International measures: None.

GONOCOCCAL DISEASE

Urethritis, salpingitis, proctitis and cervicitis of adults, vulvovaginitis of children and ophthalmia of newborn and adults are inflammatory conditions caused by *Neisseria gonorrhoeae.* All are maintained in a population by the continued presence of gonorrhea; together they constitute an epidemiologic entity and similar principles of control apply to the group.

Clinically indistinguishable infections of the same anatomic structures are caused by a number of other infectious agents. This presentation relates specifically to gonococcal disease, but the final paragraph under identification of each of the 3 gonococcal conditions gives the general characteristics of these other infections. They occur frequently and methods of control are often ill-defined.

A. GONORRHEA (GONOCOCCAL URETHRITIS)

1. Identification—An infectious disease of venereal origin, initiated by the gonococcus, limited to columnar and transitional epithelium and accordingly differing between male and female in course, in seriousness and in ease of identification. In males, a thick yellow purulent discharge from the anterior urethra appears 3 to 9 days after infecting exposure, usually self-limited, but infection may extend to posterior urethra and result in epididymitis and prostatitis, and a chronic carrier state may occur. In females, the disorder is in 3 stages: (1) a few days after exposure, an initial urethritis or cervicitis, often so mild as to pass unnoticed; (2) a stage of pelvic invasion, at the first, second, or later menstrual period, with mild or severe symptoms of salpingitis or pelvic peritonitis; (3) a stage of residual and often chronic infection. Septicemia may occur, with arthritis and endocarditis. Death is rare, but early and late manifestations, especially complications, are common and seriously incapacitating. Synonym: Clap.

Bacteriologic culture on special media (e.g. Thayer-Martin media) confirms diagnosis; in females, repeated cultures or cervical smears stained with fluorescent antibody are often needed to detect residual infection.

Widespread and frequent nongonococcal urethritis, possibly also of sexual origin, seriously complicates the clinical diagnosis of gonorrhea in the male. In some countries the incidence exceeds that of gonorrhea and the condition is reportable. It is notoriously resistant to treatment; may be initiated by a number of infectious agents.

2. Occurrence—A common disease everywhere, particularly among persons of low economic status; affects both sexes and practically all ages, especially younger groups of greatest sexual activity; seriously underreported. In recent years, incidence has increased worldwide.

3. Infectious agent—*Neisseria gonorrhoeae*, the gonococcus.

4. Reservoir—Man is the only reservoir.

5. Mode of transmission—Almost wholly by sexual contact with exudates from mucous membranes of infected persons, even in children.

6. Incubation period—Usually 3 or 4 days, sometimes 9 days or longer.

7. Period of communicability—For months or years unless interrupted by specific therapy, which ends communicability within hours or days.

8. Susceptibility and resistance—Susceptibility is general. Acquired immunity after attack has not been demonstrated.

9. Methods of control—

   A. Preventive measures: Except for measures applying specifically to gonorrhea, primarily the use of chemoprophylactic agents in the eyes of the newborn (C9A1) and special attention (suppressive treatment) to contacts of infectious patients (9B6), the preventive measures are those of Syphilis (pp. 245–246).

B. Control of patient, contacts, and the immediate environment:

1) Report to local health authority: Case report is required in many states and countries, Class 2B (see Preface).

2) Isolation: None; antibiotics in adequate dosage promptly render discharges noninfectious. Refrain from sexual intercourse with untreated previous sexual partners to avoid reinfection.

3) Concurrent disinfection: Care in disposal of discharges from lesions and articles soiled therewith.

4) Quarantine: None.

5) Immunization of contacts: Not applicable (see 9B6).

6) Investigation of contacts: Interview of patients and tracing of contacts are fundamental features of a program for control. Trained interviewers obtain the best results. All sexual contacts within 10 days of onset should be treated at once. Examine serologically for syphilis, initially and 4 months after starting treatment for gonorrhea.

7) Specific treatment: Aqueous procaine penicillin G in 1 intramuscular injection on clinical, laboratory or epidemiological grounds. Females require much higher dosage than males. Repository preparations (benzathine penicillin G) contraindicated. For patients sensitive to penicillin and for infections resistant to penicillin, use tetracyclines. Rule out concurrent syphilis (see 9B6 above).

C. Epidemic measures: Intensification of routine procedures, especially therapy on epidemiologic grounds.

D. International measures: See Syphilis 9D, p. 247.

B. GONOCOCCAL VULVOVAGINITIS OF CHILDREN

1. Identification—An inflammatory reaction of the urogenital tract of prepubescent females, characterized by redness and swelling of mucous membrane and mucopurulent discharge of varying degree; in severe infections, excoriation of labia and thighs and extension to urethra and bladder. A self-limited disease; more than three-fourths of patients recover spontaneously within 3 to 6 months; a carrier state sometimes persists.

Diagnosis is established by bacteriologic culture of exudates; stained smears are unreliable.

Gonococcal vulvovaginitis is to be differentiated from acute vulvovaginitis due to a variety of other infectious agents. The several diseases are usually indistinguishable clinically; recognition is by bacteriological means. Outbreaks occur in institutions for children.

2. Occurrence—Extent not known but presumably widespread, particularly in families of lower social and economic levels where standards of personal, sexual and general hygiene are low. Epidemics are most frequent in institutions for children.

3. Infectious agent—*Neisseria gonorrhoeae,* the gonococcus.

4. Reservoir—The reservoir is man.

5. Mode of transmission—Intimate direct contact with exudates from infected adult patients in the home, direct sexual contact, infrequently contact with contaminated moist articles, insertion of contaminated instruments and foreign bodies in vagina and rectum, and indiscriminate use of rectal thermometers. The existence of transient inapparent gonococcal infection among children has been demonstrated.

6. Incubation period—Usually 3 to 9 days.

7. Period of communicability—While discharges persist, usually 3 to 6 months; may continue after clinical manifestations cease.

8. Susceptibility and resistance—Susceptibility is related to type of epithelium lining the vagina; until puberty, columnar or transitional epithelium; after puberty, stratified squamous type not attacked by gonococci. One attack does not protect against subsequent infection.

9. Methods of control—

A. Preventive measures:

1) Fundamentally dependent on control of gonorrhea (see above) ; general measures are those of Syphilis (see pp. 245–246).

2) Proper supervision of institutions for children, with rigid enforcement of hygienic principles and early sex education.

B. Control of patient, contacts, and the immediate environment:

1) *Report to local health authority:* Case report is required in most states and countries, Class 2B (see Preface).

2) *Isolation:* Until 24 hours after administration of antibiotics.

3) *Concurrent disinfection:* Care in disposal of discharges from lesions and articles soiled therewith.

4) *Quarantine:* None.

5) *Immunization of contacts:* None; chemotherapy on suspicion of infection.

6) *Investigation of contacts:* The proved importance of sexual transmission among children calls for trained interviewers to elicit history of sexual contact among playmates, family members and older males within the family group and outside. Histories are unreliable; actual search for gonorrhea among persons in the environment of the child is necessary.

7) *Specific treatment:* Aqueous procaine penicillin G in a single dose.

C. Epidemic measures:

1) Prompt search for source of infection within the institution or group affected and introduction of measures to protect preadolescent girls.

2) Education of those in charge of children as to causes of outbreaks and the sources and development of the disease,

with special emphasis upon personal hygiene of children. The importance of probable sexual transmission should be emphasized.

D. International measures: None.

C. GONOCOCCAL OPHTHALMIA NEONATORUM

1. Identification—Acute redness and swelling of the conjunctiva of one or both eyes, with mucopurulent or purulent discharge in which gonococci are identifiable by microscopic and cultural methods. Corneal ulcer, perforation and blindness are common if specific treatment is not given promptly.

Gonococcal ophthalmia neonatorum is only one of a number of acute inflammatory conditions of the eye or of the conjunctiva occurring within the first 3 weeks of life, and collectively known as ophthalmia neonatorum. Differentiation is bacteriological. Gonococcus is the most important but not always the most frequent infectious agent. Others are meningococci, hemophilic bacilli, a bedsonia (inclusion conjunctivitis, pp. 62–63), and others. All purulent inflammation of the conjunctiva is to be regarded as gonococcal until proved otherwise. Synonyms: Gonorrheal ophthalmia, Acute conjunctivitis of the newborn.

2. Occurrence—Varies widely according to measures for prevention of infection of eyes of the newborn by attendants at delivery. Infrequent where care is adequate; globally, the disease continues to be an important cause of blindness.

3. Infectious agent—*Neisseria gonorrhoeae,* the gonococcus.

4. Reservoir—Man is the only reservoir.

5. Mode of transmission—Contact with the maternal birth canal of an infected person during childbirth.

6. Incubation period—Usually 36 to 48 hours.

7. Period of communicability—For 24 hours following specific treatment or in its absence until discharges from infected membranes have ceased.

8. Susceptibility and resistance—Susceptibility is general. Immunity to subsequent gonococcal disease does not follow attack.

9. Methods of control—

A. Preventive measures:

1) Use of an established effective preparation for protection of the eyes of babies at birth; instillation of 1% silver nitrate solution stored in individual wax capsules remains the preferred prophylactic agent for general use.
2) Depends fundamentally on control of gonorrhea (see above), especially diagnosis and treatment of gonorrhea of the mother during prenatal period; general preventive measures are those of Syphilis (see pp. 245–246).

B. *Control of patient, contacts, and the immediate environment:*

1) *Report to local health authority:* Case report is required in most states and countries, Class 2B (see Preface).

2) *Isolation:* For the first 24 hours after administration of antibiotic.

3) *Concurrent disinfection:* Care in disposal of conjunctival discharges and articles soiled therewith.

4) *Quarantine:* None.

5) *Immunization of contacts:* Not applicable; prompt treatment on recognition or clinical suspicion of infection.

6) *Investigation of contacts:* Examination and treatment of mothers and their sexual partners.

7) *Specific treatment:* Parenteral penicillin; 1% tetracycline solution or oily suspension may be applied locally as an adjunct and as a safeguard against penicillin sensitization.

C. *Epidemic measures:* None; a sporadic disease.

D. *International measures:* None.

GRANULOMA INGUINALE

1. Identification—A mildly communicable, nonfatal, chronic, and progressive autoinoculable disease of skin and mucous membrane of external genitalia. A small nodule, vesicle or papule becomes a creeping, exuberant, ulcerative, or cicatricial process of the skin, frequently painless and extending peripherally with characteristic rolled edges and formation of fibrous tissue, in many cases actively granulomatous. Extragenital lesions have predilection for warm and moist surfaces such as folds between scrotum and thighs or labia and vagina. If neglected, may result in serious destruction of genital organs and spread to other parts of body. Synonyms: Donovaniasis, Granuloma venereum.

Laboratory confirmation by demonstrating infectious agent and pathognomonic cell in stained spreads of punch biopsy tissue taken from lesions, and by histologic examination of biopsy specimens.

2. Occurrence—An infrequent disease of tropical, subtropical and temperate areas; apparently more frequent among males than females, and among persons of lower social status; predominantly at ages 20 to 40 years.

3. Infectious agent—*Donovania granulomatis,* Donovan body.

4. Reservoir—Reservoir is man.

5. Mode of transmission—Unknown; sexual transmission unproved but presumably by direct contact with active lesions during intercourse.

6. Incubation period—Unknown; presumably between 8 and 80 days.

7. Period of communicability—Unknown; probably for the duration of open lesions of the skin or mucous membranes.

8. Susceptibility and resistance—Susceptibility variable; immunity apparently does not follow attack.

9. Methods of control—

A. *Preventive measures:* Except for measures specific for syphilis, preventive measures are those for syphilis. See Syphilis 9A (pp. 245–246).

B. *Control of patient, contacts, and the immediate environment:*

1) *Report to local health authority:* In selected endemic areas (U.S.A., some states); not a reportable disease in most states and countries, Class 3B (see Preface).

2) *Isolation:* None; avoid close personal contact until lesions are healed.

3) *Concurrent disinfection:* Care in disposal of discharges from lesions and articles soiled therewith.

4) *Quarantine:* None.

5) *Immunization of contacts:* Not applicable; prompt treatment on recognition or clinical suspicion of infection.

6) *Investigation of contacts:* Examination of sexual contacts.

7) *Specific treatment:* Streptomycin and tetracyclines are effective; recurrence expected in some instances, usually responding to a second course. Antimony compounds effective but healing slow and therapy must be continued for some months after apparent recovery.

C. *Epidemic measures:* Not applicable.

D. *International measures:* See Syphilis 9D, p. 247.

HEMORRHAGIC FEVERS OF ARGENTINIAN AND BOLIVIAN TYPES

1. Identification—Acute febrile illnesses, duration 7 to 15 days. Onset is gradual with malaise, headache, fever and sweats, followed by prostration. Exanthem appears on thorax and flanks 3 to 5 days after onset; may later show petechiae. Enanthem with petechiae on soft palate is frequent. Severe infections result in epistaxis, hematemesis, melena, hematuria, and gingival hemorrhage; encephalopathies are frequent. Bradycardia and hypotension are important findings, and leukopenia and thrombocytopenia are characteristic. Moderate albuminuria is present with many cellular and granular casts and vacuolated epithelial cells. Relapses occur.

Diagnosis is by isolation of virus from blood, or throat washings, and serologically by complement-fixation or neutralization test.

2. Occurrence—First described in Argentina in 1955, in rural areas among laborers in corn fields. Occurs from March to October (autumn and winter) with peak in May or June, and mainly at ages 15 to 44 years, males 5 times as frequently as females. Estimated case fatality from 5% to 30%, greatest among older patients. A similar disease was subsequently described in a series of epidemics in urban areas (small villages) of Bolivia.

3. Infectious agent—The Junin virus of the Tacaribe group for the Argentinian disease, and the closely related Machupo virus for the Bolivian.

4. Reservoir—In Argentina, wild rodents of corn fields are vertebrate hosts. Domestic rodents, particularly *Calomys callosus,* involved in Bolivia.

5. Mode of transmission—Saliva and excreta of infected rodents contain the virus. Possibly food-borne. Laboratory infections occur. There is no proof of arthropod transmission.

6. Incubation period—Commonly 10 to 14 days.

7. Period of communicability—Probably not often directly transmitted from man to man; evidence suggests this has occurred for the Bolivian disease.

8. Susceptibility and resistance—All ages appear susceptible but immunity of as yet unknown duration follows infection.

9. Methods of control—Specific rodent control where reservoir host has been identified.

HEMORRHAGIC FEVER WITH RENAL SYNDROME

1. Identification—An acute infectious disease characterized by fever of 3 to 6 days' duration, conjunctival injection, prostration, anorexia, vomiting, hemorrhagic manifestations which begin about the third day, proteinuria about the fourth day, and hypotension about the fifth; renal abnormalities, varying from mild to acute renal failure, continue for several weeks. About one-fourth of cases show an alarming hypotension and the majority of deaths (fatality about 6%) occur during shock; other deaths from renal shutdown. Convalescence is usually rapid during the third week. Synonym: Hemorrhagic nephrosonephritis, Epidemic hemorrhagic fever.

Specific laboratory tests are not available; clinical laboratory findings such as proteinuria, leukocytosis, thrombocytopenia, and elevated nonprotein nitrogen assist in establishing the diagnosis.

2. Occurrence—In Korea in the vicinity of the 38th parallel among United Nations troops and civilians since 1951. Earlier Japanese and Russian experience in Manchuria and Siberia along the Amur River indicates that women and children acquire the malady as well as men.

Recently recognized in European USSR in the Yaroslavl region north of Moscow and suspected elsewhere. A few cases occur throughout the year, but in Korea two seasonal outbreaks, in May–June and in October–November. The majority of cases are isolated events but outbreaks have involved 5 to 20 persons within a small area, all apparently acquired at the same time and place. This is a rural disease.

3. Infectious agent—Unknown; Berkefeld and Seitz filtrates of human materials induce hemorrhagic fever in experimentally inoculated volunteers. The agent has not been established in laboratory animals. Tissue culture fluorescent antibody reported positive in USSR.

4. Reservoir—Assumed to be maintained in nature by rodent, with man only an accidental host.

5. Mode of transmission—Unknown; epidemiologic observations in Korea suggested an analogy to scrub typhus and implicated a non-flying arthropod vector of limited motility; trombiculid mites were suggested. Presently, transmission from rodent excreta is suspected.

6. Incubation period—Usually 12 to 16 days but varying from 9 to 35.

7. Period of communicability—Apparently not directly transmitted from man to man.

8. Susceptibility and resistance—Newcomers to endemic areas are uniformly susceptible; indigenous populations probably have some acquired resistance. Mild or inapparent infections are suspected but unproved. Second attacks have not been observed.

9. Methods of control—

    A. Preventive measures: Without adequate information of etiologic agent and mode of transmission, preventive measures employed are those of disease with a field rodent host.

    B. Control of patient, contacts, and the immediate environment:

        1) Report to local health authority: In selected endemic areas; in most countries not a reportable disease, Class 3A (see Preface).

        2) Isolation: None.

        3) Concurrent disinfection: None.

        4) Quarantine: None.

        5) Immunization of contacts: None.

        6) Investigation of contacts: None.

        7) Specific treatment: None. Appropriate treatment for shock or for renal shutdown.

    C. Epidemic measures: Rodent control.

    D. International measures: None.

HEPATITIS, VIRAL

Introduction

Viral hepatitis is a generic term which embraces both *infectious hepatitis* and *serum hepatitis,* and avoids the often difficult problem of differential diagnosis. Indeed, individual cases of either disease are frequently indistinguishable on clinical grounds alone, because the dominant physical finding is jaundice and biochemical tests of liver function reveal similar abnormalities.

The two diseases can usually be distinguished on epidemiological grounds. For example, a history of contact with another case of jaundice within an incubation period of 15 to 50 days, or occurrence in a localized epidemic associated with person-to-person spread in a school, housing project or defined neighborhood, or with a common exposure to contaminated water, food or raw shellfish, strongly supports the diagnosis of infectious hepatitis. In contrast, a history of parenteral inoculation of blood or blood products, or exposure to contaminated syringes or needles, within a period of 50 to 160 days strongly supports the diagnosis of serum hepatitis. When groups of cases of either disease are studied in well-defined epidemics, subtle clinical differences between the two diseases may be recognized that are not apparent in the study of individual cases. These differences are outlined in the sections below.

It is generally accepted that these two diseases are caused by viruses. Extensive controlled human-transmission studies have established that the causative agents are submicroscopic. Many reports of the isolation of viruses in various tissue cultures and of transmission of the disease to various species of animals—particularly to primates—have been published but none has yet been confirmed.

Recently a particulate antigen termed the hepatitis-associated antigen (HAA) and also referred to as the Australia or SH antigen has been found in the circulating blood of many persons and convalescents of viral hepatitis and in serum and plasma known to transmit the disease. This antigen is less commonly found in association with chronic hepatitis and a few other diseases not directly related to hepatitis. The significance of HAA is not yet clarified, but several studies strongly suggest that HAA is associated with persons infected with serum hepatitis and not with infectious hepatitis. This discovery may lead to new and useful procedures for differential diagnosis and for the identification of contaminated blood.

Included within the broad classification, viral hepatitis, is *posttransfusion hepatitis,* an epidemiologic term in common use which also avoids the problem of differentiating between serum and infectious hepatitis. This form of jaundice develops anywhere from 10 days to 180 days following transfusion of blood, pooled plasma or other blood products. It has often been assumed that posttransfusion hepatitis was a composite of cases of the two subject infections. In several large series of cases, however, there was no evidence of a biphasic distribution of incubation periods, and therefore no way to determine the relative importance of the two infections in causing posttransfusion cases. The failure of large doses of immune serum globulin to protect against posttransfusion hepatitis and experimental evidence that the viremia in infectious hepatitis is of short duration (a few weeks) but in serum hepatitis may be prolonged (months or years) suggest that most cases of posttransfusion hepatitis are caused by the virus of serum hepatitis. Nevertheless, the wide range of incubation periods of posttransfusion hepatitis remains unexplained.

A. INFECTIOUS HEPATITIS

1. Identification—Onset is usually abrupt, with fever, malaise, anorexia, nausea and abdominal discomfort, followed within a few days by jaundice. Severity varies from a mild illness lasting 1 to 2 weeks, to a severely disabling disease lasting several months with prolonged convalescence. In general, severity increases with age, but complete recovery without sequelae or recurrences is the rule. Many cases are mild, without jaundice, especially in children, and recognizable only by liver function or serum enzyme tests. Case fatality is less than 1%. Synonyms: Epidemic hepatitis, Epidemic jaundice, Virus A hepatitis.

There are no specific diagnostic measures. Differential diagnosis depends on clinical and epidemiological evidence for the exclusion of other causes of febrile jaundice.

2. Occurrence—Worldwide, sporadic and, in epidemics, with a tendency to cyclic recurrences. Periods of high incidence in the U.S.A. were recognized in 1954 and 1961. Outbreaks are commonest in institutions, in low-cost housing projects, in rural areas, and in military forces, particularly during war. Epidemics often evolve slowly, involve wide geographic areas, and last many months. Incidence in rural areas is higher than in cities. Most common among school-age children and young adults. In temperate zones incidence is two to three times higher during autumn and winter than during spring and summer.

3. Infectious agent—A filterable agent commonly assumed to be a virus has been demonstrated in experimental infection of human subjects.

4. Reservoir—Man and, perhaps rarely, chimpanzees and certain other nonhuman primates.

5. Mode of transmission—Person-to-person contact presumably by the fecal-oral route. The infectious agent may be found in feces and urine. Presence of the infectious agent in nasal and pharyngeal discharges has not been established but is assumed on epidemiologic grounds. Some well-defined epidemics have suggested airborne spread. Common-vehicle outbreaks have been related to contaminated water and food, including milk, sliced meats, salads, raw or undercooked clams and oysters, and bakery products. The infectious agent is present in circulating blood prior to onset of jaundice and for a few days later. Therefore, spread by parenteral inoculation of infected blood or blood products, or by contaminated needles and syringes, may occur, particularly among illicit drug users.

6. Incubation period—10 to 50 days, commonly about 30 to 35.

7. Period of communicability—Human-transmission studies and epidemiological evidence indicate maximum infectivity during the latter half of the incubation period continuing through a few days after onset of jaundice (or during peak transaminase activity in anicteric cases).

8. Susceptibility and resistance—Susceptibility is general. Low incidence among exposed infants and preschool children suggests that mild and anicteric illnesses may prevail at this age. Degree and duration of immunity after attack are unknown but presumed to be long lasting.

9. Methods of control—

A. *Preventive measures:*

1) Health education directed toward good sanitation and personal hygiene, with special emphasis on sanitary disposal of feces.
2) Proper sterilization of syringes and needles and other equipment, or the use of disposable units, for parenteral injections (see Serum Hepatitis 9A, pp. 109–110).
3) Travelers to highly endemic areas, North Africa, the Middle East, and Asia may be given prophylactic doses of immune serum globulin (ISG). For expected exposures up to 2 months, a single dose of 0.02 ml per kg of body weight is recommended; for more prolonged exposures, 0.06 ml per kg should be repeated at intervals of 4 to 6 months.

    Staff and attendants in mental institutions, notably homes for retarded children, who experience intensive prolonged exposure may be given ISG in doses of 0.04 to 0.1 ml per kg of body weight repeated at a 4 to 6 month interval. It is difficult, however, to differentiate infectious hepatitis from serum hepatitis in these situations, and the degree of protection provided is problematic.

B. *Control of patient, contacts, and the immediate environment:*

1) *Report to local health authority:* Reporting obligatory in all states of the U.S.A., although not now required in many countries; Class 2A (see Preface).
2) *Isolation:* During first 2 weeks of illness and at least 1 week after onset of jaundice.
3) *Concurrent disinfection:* Sanitary disposal of feces and urine.
4) *Quarantine:* None.
5) *Immunization of contacts:* No vaccine for active immunization exists. Passive immunization with ISG, 0.02 ml per kg of body weight, should be given intramuscularly as soon

as possible after exposure. Recommended for all household contacts regardless of age. Larger doses give longer protection and should be limited to contacts suffering prolonged exposure such as in institutions.

6) *Investigation of contacts:* Search for missed cases and maintain surveillance of contacts.

7) *Specific treatment:* None.

C. *Epidemic measures:*

1) Epidemiologic investigation to determine mode of transmission, whether from person to person or by common vehicle, and to identify the population exposed to increased risk of infection. Search for suspicious illnesses among food handlers. Eliminate any common sources of infection. Provide ISG for exposed contacts.

2) Special efforts to improve sanitary and hygienic practices, to reduce fecal contamination of foods and water, and to prevent careless disposal of urine.

3) Focal concentration of disease in institutions may warrant mass prophylaxis with ISG of heavily exposed populations.

D. *International measures:* None.

B. SERUM HEPATITIS

1. Identification—Onset is usually insidious, with anorexia, vague abdominal discomfort, nausea and vomiting often progressing to jaundice. Fever may be absent or mild. Severity varies in the extreme—from inapparent cases detectable only by biochemical tests of liver function to fulminating fatal cases of acute hepatic necrosis. Case fatality also varies widely in different situations, from 1% or less (e.g., after use of yellow fever vaccine containing human plasma in World War II) to 40% or greater following common exposure to a particular lot of human serum. Case fatality following blood transfusion commonly ranges from 6 to 12%. Synonyms: Homologous serum jaundice, Virus B hepatitis.

Differential diagnosis depends on clinical and epidemiological evidence for the exclusion of other forms of jaundice. Demonstration of HAA is supportive evidence.

2. Occurrence—Worldwide distribution, endemic with little seasonal variation, most common in adults rather than children. Presently recognized among recipients of blood or blood products, and among individuals heavily exposed to these products such as employees of renal dialysis centers. Incidence is high among narcotic addicts and others who use drugs illicitly. Serious outbreaks have occurred in clinics and physicians' offices among patients who have received parenteral inoculations from contaminated and inadequately sterilized syringes and needles. Cases have been traced to tattoo parlors.

3. Infectious agent—A filterable agent commonly assumed to be a virus has been demonstrated in experimental infection of human subjects (see 4th par. under Introduction preceding, p. 105).

4. Reservoir—Man is the only known reservoir.

5. Mode of transmission—By parenteral (intravenous, intramuscular or subcutaneous) inoculation of human blood, plasma, serum, thrombin, fibrinogen, packed red cells and other blood products from an infected person. Immune serum globulin, heat-treated albumin, plasma protein fractions, and fibrinolysin do not transmit the disease. Contaminated needles, syringes and other intravenous equipment are also an important mode of spread. The infection may be spread through contamination of wounds or lacerations (track finder's hepatitis). Recent experimental studies indicate that serum hepatitis can be transmitted by ingestion of infective blood. This finding confirms published reports of the occurrence of hepatitis following exposure to patients with serum hepatitis.

6. Incubation period—From 50 to 180 days, usually 80 to 100 days. In posttransfusion hepatitis the incubation period may range from 10 days to over 180 days (see Introduction, 5th paragraph, p. 105).

7. Period of communicability—Blood from experimentally inoculated volunteers has been shown to be infective many weeks before onset of first symptoms. Blood remains infective through the acute clinical course of disease and in many instances the chronic carrier state persists for years. Some persons may be carriers without having experienced a clinically recognized attack.

8. Susceptibility and resistance—Poorly understood, but believed to be general; mechanism of recovery and immunology of the disease have not been defined.

9. Methods of Control—

A. *Preventive measures:*

1) Limit administration of whole blood or any blood products known to be potentially hazardous to those patients in clear need of such therapeutic measures.

2) Enforce strict discipline in blood banks, rejecting as donors all individuals who have a history of viral hepatitis, who show evidence of drug addiction, or who have received a blood transfusion within the preceding 6 months.

3) Maintain surveillance of all cases of posttransfusion hepatitis, including a register of all persons who donated blood for each case. Notify blood banks of these potential carriers, so that future donations may be promptly identified and scheduled for processing into useful blood products instead of being administered to patients.

4) Heat-sterilize thoroughly all syringes and needles and stylets for finger puncture. A fresh sterile syringe and needle is essential for each individual receiving skin tests, other parenteral inoculations, or venipuncture. Use dis-

posable equipment whenever possible. Discourage tattooing.

5) Immune serum globulin (ISG) is of no demonstrated value for the prevention of serum hepatitis, the most common cause of posttransfusion hepatitis.

B. Control of patient, contacts, and the immediate environment:

1) *Report to local health authority:* Official report is obligatory in the U.S.A., although not now required in many countries; Class 2A (see Preface).

2) *Isolation:* As required for infectious hepatitis Section A preceding (9B2).

3) *Concurrent disinfection:* Of equipment contaminated with blood.

4) *Quarantine:* None.

5) *Immunization of contacts:* None.

6) *Investigation of contacts:* See 9C below.

7) *Specific treatment:* None.

C. Epidemic measures: When two or more cases occur in association with some common exposure, conduct extensive search for additional cases among personal associates, such as drug addicts, or among patients who have attended in common a particular clinic or have been admitted to a particular hospital ward where parenteral inoculations have been given. Institute strict aseptic techniques. If a blood product such as pooled plasma, thrombin or fibrinogen is implicated, trace all recipients of the same lot in a search for additional cases. Recall all outstanding vials from any infective lots.

D. International measures: None.

HERPANGINA AND VESICULAR STOMATITIS WITH EXANTHEM

1. Identification—Herpangina is an acute infectious disease of childhood, with sudden onset, fever and small vesicular lesions on soft palate and anterior pillars of pharynx, which promptly ulcerate and cause moderate discomfort; lasts 3 to 5 days, with occasional recurrence of fever 1 week later; no deaths. In adults, illness may be severe and the meninges may be involved.

Vesicular Stomatitis with Exanthem is similar, but differs in that oral lesions are more diffuse and occur on the buccal surface of the cheeks and gums. Papulovesicular lesions also occur commonly on hands, feet, legs and buttocks and may persist for 7 to 10 days. Synonym: Hand, foot and mouth disease.

ACUTE LYMPHONODULAR PHARYNGITIS is also similar, but differs in that lesions are firm nodules occurring predominantly on uvula and posterior pharynx and occasionally on conjunctiva, with no exanthem.

Clinical diagnosis is facilitated by epidemic occurrence. Virus may be isolated in suckling mice from lesions and stool specimens. Serologic and virologic diagnostic procedures are not routinely available.

These diseases are not to be confused with vesicular stomatitis in man caused by the virus found in cattle and horses, which usually occurs in dairy workers, animal husbandrymen and veterinarians. Foot-and-mouth disease of cattle, sheep and swine rarely affects man except for laboratory workers handling the virus. Man can be a mechanical carrier of foot-and-mouth disease virus and can be the source of animal outbreaks.

Herpetic stomatitis requires differentiation; it has larger, deeper, more painful lesions commonly located in the front of the mouth.

2. Occurrence—Throughout the world, both sporadically and in epidemics, with greatest incidence in summer and early autumn. Mainly in children under 10 years, but adult cases are relatively frequent.

3. Infectious agents—Coxsackie virus, Group A, Types 2, 4, 5, 6, 8, 10 and perhaps Type 3 commonly cause herpangina; Type A-16 has been associated with vesicular stomatitis with exanthem, and Type A-10 with acute lymphonodular pharyngitis.

4. Reservoir—Man is the reservoir.

5. Mode of transmission—Direct contact with nose and throat discharges and feces of infected persons (who may be asymptomatic) and by droplet spread. Contaminated flies have been found. No reliable evidence of spread by insects, water, food or sewage.

6. Incubation period—Usually 3 to 5 days.

7. Period of communicability—During the acute stage of illness and perhaps longer, since the virus persists in stools for several weeks.

8. Susceptibility and resistance—Susceptibility to infection is general. Immunity is acquired by infection, either clinical or inapparent; duration unknown. Second attacks occur with Group A Coxsackie virus of a different immunological type.

9. Methods of control—

A. *Preventive measures:* Measures to reduce person-to-person contact.

B. *Control of patient, contacts, and the immediate environment:*

  1) *Report to local health authority:* Obligatory report of epidemics; no case report, Class 4 (see Preface).
  2) *Isolation:* None.
  3) *Concurrent disinfection:* Of nose and throat discharges, feces, and articles soiled therewith.
  4) *Quarantine:* None.

     5) Immunization of contacts: None.

     6) Investigation of contacts and source of infection: Of no practical value.

     7) Specific treatment: None.

C. *Epidemic measures:* General notice to physicians of increased incidence of the disease, together with a description of onset and clinical characteristics. Isolation of all children with fever, pending diagnosis.

D. *International measures:* WHO Reference Centres (see Preface).

HERPES SIMPLEX

    1. Identification—Herpes simplex is a viral infection marked by latency and repeated, recurrent localized lesions. The primary infection usually is asymptomatic and occurs in early childhood. In perhaps 10% of primary infections, overt disease may appear as a mild or severe illness marked by fever and malaise lasting a week or more, and associated with a gingivostomatitis accompanied by vesicular lesions in the oropharynx, or a severe keratoconjunctivitis, a vulvo-vaginitis, a generalized cutaneous eruption complicating chronic eczema (Kaposi's varicelliform eruption), a meningoencephalitis, or a fatal panvisceral infection as seen in newborn infants.

    Reactivation of the latent infection commonly results in *herpes labialis* (fever blisters or cold sores) manifested by superficial clear vesicles on an erythematous base, involving the face and lips, which crust and heal within a few days. Reactivation is precipitated by various forms of trauma, physiological changes, or intercurrent disease such as pneumococcal pneumonia, bacterial meningitis, and malaria. Reactivation may also involve other body tissues, particularly ectodermal tissues. It occurs in the presence of circulating antibodies and these are not elevated by reactivation.

    Central nervous system involvement occurs usually as a primary infection but may appear as a recrudescence. Serological studies indicate that 5 to 7% of cases of meningoencephalitis are due to this virus. Fever, headache, leucocytosis, signs of meningeal irritation, drowsiness, confusion, stupor, coma, and lateralizing signs usually referable to one or the other temporal region may occur. The condition can be confused with a variety of other intracranial lesions and requires differentiation from brain abscess and tuberculous meningitis.

    Diagnosis is confirmed by isolation of the virus from lesions or from the spinal fluid or surgical tissue in CNS cases; or by a rise in specific neutralizing antibodies. However, virus can frequently be isolated from healthy persons

2. Occurrence—Worldwide in distribution; 70 to 90% of adults possess circulating antibodies. Infection is most prevalent before the 5th year of life.

3. Infectious agent—*Herpesvirus hominis.*

4. Reservoir—Man.

5. Mode of transmission—Direct contact with virus in saliva of carriers is probably the most important mode of spread. Direct inoculation of the hands of attendants handling infants with the eczematoid disease occurs. Preexisting lesions in the recipient may play a significant role. Transmission to nonimmune adults is often by some form of sexual contact.

6. Incubation period—Up to 2 weeks.

7. Period of communicability—Secretion of virus in the saliva for as long as 7 weeks after recovery from stomatitis has been reported; virus can be isolated from the saliva of asymptomatic adults.

8. Susceptibility and resistance—Probably man is universally susceptible.

9. Methods of control—

A. *Preventive measures:*
1) Personal hygiene and health education directed toward minimizing the transfer of infectious material.
2) Particular care to avoid contaminating the skin of eczematous patients with infectious material.

B. *Control of patient, contacts, and the immediate environment:*
1) Report to local health authority: Official case report ordinarily not justifiable, Class 5 (see Preface).
2) Isolation, 3) Concurrent disinfection, 4) Quarantine, and *5) Immunization of contacts:* None.
6) Investigation of contacts: Seldom of practical value.
7) Specific treatment: None, except that topical 5-iodo-2'-deoxyuridine (Idoxuridine) may modify the acute manifestation of herpetic keratitis and early dendritic ulcers. Corticosteroids should never be used for this ocular involvement unless administered under the control of a skilled ophthalmologist. The value of Idoxuridine for treatment of encephalitis is under evaluation.

C. *Epidemic measures:* Not applicable.

D. *International measures:* None.

B-VIRUS INFECTION, or *Herpesvirus simiae* encephalomyelitis— caused by *Herpesvirus simiae,* a closely related virus—is an ascending encephalomyelitis occurring in veterinarians, laboratory workers and other individuals having close contact with monkeys or monkey cell cultures. After an incubation period of up to 3 weeks, there is an acute febrile onset, with headache, lymphocytic pleocytosis, and a variable neurological pattern, usually ending in death 1 day to 3 weeks after onset of symptoms. An occasional recovery has been associated with considerable residual disability. The virus causes a natural infection of monkeys analogous to *Herpesvirus hominis* infection in man. Human disease is acquired by the bite of apparently normal monkeys, or by exposure of naked skin to infected saliva or to monkey tissue cultures. There is no treatment. Prevention depends on use of proper gauntlets and care to minimize exposure to monkeys. If there has been exposure to monkey saliva, wash thoroughly with soap and water.

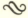

HISTOPLASMOSIS

Two clinically different mycoses have been designated as histoplasmosis because the two pathogens, when growing on culture media as a mold, cannot be distinguished morphologically. Detailed information will be given for the infection caused by *Histoplasma capsulatum*, followed by a brief resumé of histoplasmosis caused by *Histoplasma duboisii*.

1. **Identification**—A systemic mycosis of varying severity, with the primary lesion usually in the lungs. Infection is common, but clinical disease uncommon. Five clinical forms are recognized: (a) *Asymptomatic:* Detectable only by acquired hypersensitivity to histoplasmin. Calcification of primary lung lesion may occur. (b) *Acute benign respiratory:* Probably common in endemic areas but easily overlooked; varies from mild respiratory illness to temporary incapacity with general malaise, weakness, fever, chest pains, dry or productive cough. Erythema multiforme may occur. Recovery is slow and spontaneous, with or without multiple, small scattered calcifications in lung, hilar lymph nodes and spleen. (c) *Acute disseminated:* Varying degrees of hepatosplenomegaly, with septic-type fever, prostration, and rapid course. Often resembles miliary tuberculosis. Most frequent in infants and young children. Without therapy, usually fatal. (d) *Chronic disseminated:* Symptoms variable, depending on organs infected. May present as unexplained fever, anemia, patchy pneumonia, hepatitis, endocarditis, meningitis, or mucosal ulcers of mouth, larynx, stomach or bowel. Adrenal infection common but usually asymptomatic. More common in the adult male. Cytotoxic and corticosteroid therapies predispose. Course usually subacute; with variable progression over weeks up to a few years, usually having fatal outcome unless treated. (e) *Chronic pulmonary:* Clinically and radiologically resembles chronic pulmonary tuberculosis. More common in males over 40 years old. Disease progresses over months or years, with periods of quiescence and sometimes spontaneous cure. Death may result from respiratory insufficiency or cor pulmonale.

Clinical diagnosis is most rapid if the fungus can be seen in Giemsa's or Wright's stained smears of ulcer exudates, bone marrow, sputum or blood. Special stains are necessary to demonstrate the fungus in biopsies of ulcers, liver, lymph nodes or lung. Several serologic tests for serum anti-*Histoplasma* antibody are available and can be used to suggest but not prove the diagnosis. Both false-positive and false-negative serologic reactions occur. Prior positive skin tests with histoplasmin can cause false-positive serologic test results. Final diagnosis rests upon demonstration of the fungus in cultures of body fluids or biopsies on modified Sabouraud's agar or more enriched media.

2. Occurrence—Infection is common focally over wide areas of the Americas, Europe, Africa and the Far East; clinical disease is far less frequent, severe progressive disease rare. Histoplasmin hypersensitivity, sometimes to the extent of 80% of a population, indicating antecedent infection, is prevalent in parts of eastern and central U.S.A. Prevalence can vary widely within a few miles. The frequency of positive reactors increases from childhood to 30 years of age; differences by sex are not observed. Outbreaks have occurred in families or in groups of workmen with common exposure to bird or bat droppings; airborne epidemics in areas where contaminated soil has recently been disturbed. Histoplasmosis occurs also in dogs, cats, rats, skunks, opossums, foxes and other animals.

3. Infectious agents—*Histoplasma capsulatum*, a dimorphic fungus growing as a mold in soil, and as a yeast in animal and human hosts.

4. Reservoir—Soil around old chicken houses, in caves and starling roosts; around houses sheltering the common brown bat; and other soils with high organic content.

5. Mode of transmission—Inhalation of airborne spores in dust.

6. Incubation period—In reported epidemics, symptoms appear within 5 to 18 days after exposure, commonly 10 days.

7. Period of communicability—Not directly transmitted from man to man.

8. Susceptibility and resistance—Susceptibility is general. Inapparent infections are extremely common in endemic areas, with resulting resistance except to heavy exposure.

9. Methods of control—

A. *Preventive measures:* Minimize unavoidable exposure to a contaminated and circumscribed environment, such as chicken coops and surrounding soil, by spraying with water or disinfectant (3% formalin) to reduce dust; masks may be worn.

B. *Control of patient, contacts, and the immediate environment:*

1) *Report to local health authority:* Obligatory report of epidemics, Class 4 (see Preface).
2) *Isolation:* None.
3) *Concurrent disinfection:* Of discharges from skin lesions, sputum, and articles soiled therewith. Terminal cleaning.

4) *Quarantine:* None.

5) *Immunization of contacts:* None.

6) *Investigation of contacts:* Household contacts, for evidence of infection from a common environmental source.

7) *Specific treatment:* For disseminated or chronic pulmonary cases, amphotericin B (Fungizone) is the drug of choice; side effects require that it be used with caution. Sulfonamides in high doses may benefit an occasional case.

C. **Epidemic measures:** Occurrence of grouped cases of acute pulmonary disease in or outside an endemic area, particularly with history of exposure to dust within a closed space, should arouse suspicion of histoplasmosis. Suspected sites such as chicken houses, barns, silos, caves, starling roosts or basements should be investigated.

D. **International measures:** None.

AFRICAN HISTOPLASMOSIS—Usually presents as subacute granuloma of skin or bone. Infection may be localized in skin or bone, or disseminated in the skin, subcutaneous tissue, lymph nodes, bones and joints, lungs and abdominal viscera. Disease is more common in males and may occur at any age, though more common in the second decade of life. Thus far, the disease has been recognized only in Africa. Diagnosis is made by culture and by demonstrating in smear or biopsy the yeast cells of *H. duboisii.* These cells are much larger than the yeast cells of *H. capsulatum.* True prevalence of African histoplasmosis, its reservoir, mode of transmission and incubation period are unknown. Not communicable from man to man. Amphotericin B (Fungizone) is frequently an effective therapy.

HYDATIDOSIS

This disease is produced by the presence of space-occupying tapeworm cysts; symptoms are determined by the location and size of the cyst, which is the larval stage of *Echinococcus,* whose adult worms are found in *Canidae* hosts. There are 2 different but closely related species causing different clinical manifestations: (1) unilocular echinococcosis or hydatid disease, and (2) multilocular alveolar hydatid disease. Synonyms: Hydatid disease, Echinococcosis.

Microscopic examination for hooklets, protoscolices (scolices) and cyst membranes in sputum, vomitus, urine or feces after rupture of cysts, or in discharges from a sinus, aids in diagnosis. Complement fixation, indirect hemagglutination, latex flocculation and intradermal tests are helpful. Confirmation is by examination of tissues obtained surgically or at necropsy.

A. INFESTATION BY ECHINOCOCCUS GRANULOSUS (UNILOCULAR ECHINOCOCCOSIS)

1. Identification—The cysts of *Echinococcus granulosus* are found in the liver and lungs and less commonly in the kidney, heart, bone, central nervous system and thyroid. No tissue or organ of the body is exempt from infection. Symptoms are variable and depend upon the location of the slowly growing cyst, which may attain great size. In the liver and the lungs, as well as other tissues, cysts may give no symptoms throughout life and calcified cysts may be found incidentally during x-ray examination or at autopsy. In vital organs the cysts cause severe symptoms and death.

2. Occurrence—This parasite is common in grazing countries where human association with dogs is intimate. The Middle East, Greece, Italy, Australia, New Zealand, Argentina, Uruguay, southern Brazil and Chile are heavily infected. Infections acquired in continental U.S.A. are relatively rare.

3. Infectious agent—*Echinococcus granulosus,* the dog tapeworm.

4. Reservoir—Reservoirs are carnivores infected with adult worms, especially dog, wolf, dingo and other *Canidae;* these are the primary hosts.

5. Mode of transmission—By ingestion of infective eggs in foods and water contaminated with feces of infected animals, by hand-to-mouth transfer of dog feces and through objects soiled with feces. Eggs may survive for several years in pastures, gardens and around households. Ingested eggs hatch in intestine and larvae migrate to various organs to produce cysts. The dog-sheep-dog cycle is important in most areas where *E. granulosus* is endemic. In other regions it is the dog-pig-dog cycle. In northwest Canada, a moose-wolf-moose sylvan cycle maintains the disease.

6. Incubation period—Variable, from months to several years depending upon the number of cysts and how rapidly they grow.

7. Period of communicability—Not directly transmitted from man to man or from one intermediate host to another. Dogs begin to pass eggs of the parasite approximately 6 weeks after infection; in the absence of reinfection this ends in about 8 to 12 months.

8. Susceptibility and resistance—Man is universally susceptible to infection with the larval stage but does not harbor the adult worm.

9. Methods of control—

A. Preventive measures:

1) Rigid control of slaughtering of herbivorous animals so that dogs have no access to uncooked viscera. Dogs become infected by eating hydatid cysts, principally those present in food mammals, but also in wild animals.
2) Licensing and treatment of dogs, to reduce their numbers in areas of endemic prevalence so far as may be compatible with occupational requirements.
3) Education of school children and of the general public in

endemic areas to the dangers of close association with dogs, and of the need for controlled slaughtering of animals.
4) Incineration or deep burial of dead animals.

B. *Control of patient, contacts, and the immediate environment:*

   1) *Report to local health authority:* In selected endemic areas; not a reportable disease in most states and countries, Class 3B (see Preface).
   2) *Isolation:* None.
   3) *Concurrent disinfection:* None.
   4) *Quarantine:* None.
   5) *Immunization of contacts:* None.
   6) *Investigation of contacts and source of infection:* Examination of familial associates for suspicious tumors. Search for source of infection in dogs kept in and about the house.
   7) *Specific treatment:* None. Surgical removal of isolated cyst is sometimes curative.

C. *Epidemic measures:* In highly endemic areas, destruction of wild and stray dogs, wolves, coyotes and foxes. Mass antihelminthic treatment of dogs has varied effectiveness and must be repeated periodically.

D. *International measures:* Coordinated programs by neighboring countries where the disease is endemic, to control infection in animals and movement of dogs from known enzootic areas.

B. INFESTATION BY ECHINOCOCCUS MULTILOCULARIS (ALVEOLAR HYDATID DISEASE)

1. Identification—This disease, primarily of the liver, is due to the poorly circumscribed cysts of *Echinococcus multilocularis.* The cysts may also be found in the lungs and other organs. As the cyst's development is unhampered by a strong and intact laminated membrane, it may proliferate into the liver and even disseminate by metastasis. The clinical effects of this infection depend upon the size and location of the cyst.

2. Occurrence—In Central Europe, Siberia, North Pacific Islands and Alaska.

3. Infectious agent—*Echinococcus multilocularis.*

4. Reservoir—*E. multilocularis* is commonly maintained in nature in a fox-vole-fox cycle. The adult tapeworms are found in foxes, wolves and dogs.

5. Mode of transmission—By ingestion and hand-to-mouth transfer of infective eggs from dogs' feces contaminating their fur, harnesses and the living environment of man.

6. Incubation period, 7. Period of communicability, 8. Susceptibility and resistance and **9. Methods of control**—As in Section A, Echinococcosus Granulosis, preceding.

INFLUENZA

1. Identification—An acute infectious disease of the respiratory tract characterized by abrupt onset of fever, chills, headache, myalgia, and sometimes prostration. Coryza and sore throat are common, especially in later stages of the disease. Cough is almost universal, often severe and protracted. Usually a self-limited disease, with recovery in 2 to 7 days. Recognition is commonly by epidemiologic characteristics; sporadic cases can be identified only by laboratory procedures.

Influenza derives its importance from the rapidity with which epidemics evolve, the height of the attack rates, and the seriousness of complications—notably bacterial pneumonia. Deaths predominate among the elderly and persons debilitated by chronic cardiac, pulmonary, renal or metabolic disease. Case fatality is low, but epidemics are associated with a general mortality much in excess of nonepidemic expectancy; approximately 62,000 excess deaths occurred in the U.S.A. during the pandemic of influenza type A2 in 1957–1958, and 57,000 excess deaths were estimated during the epidemic of 1963.

Laboratory confirmation is by recovery of influenza viruses from pharyngeal or nasal secretions during the early febrile stage of disease in embryonated hen's eggs or tissue culture, and by demonstration of a specific serologic response using acute and convalescent sera.

2. Occurrence—In pandemics, epidemics, localized outbreaks, and as sporadic cases. During the past 75 years, pandemics began in 1889, 1918, 1957, and 1968. Attack rates during epidemics range from less than 15% to 40% or higher. Major epidemics show a periodic tendency: Influenza A appears in the U.S.A. at intervals of 2 to 3 years; influenza B at longer intervals, usually not less than 4 to 6 years. A major exception to this periodic pattern occurred in 1968, when the pandemic of influenza A2 (Hong Kong strain) followed one year after a major epidemic in the United States. In temperate zones, epidemics tend to occur in winter; in the tropics, often without reference to season.

Influenza viral infections also occur in swine, horses, and other animals in many parts of the world, but transmission from animals to man has not been demonstrated.

3. Infectious agent—Three types of influenza virus are recognized: A, B and C. Types A and B have long been associated with epidemics; type C virus has thus far appeared only in sporadic cases and in minor localized outbreaks. Three subtypes of influenza A virus have been isolated from man, the prototype strains being AO (PR8, 1934), A1 (FM1, 1947), and A2 (Japan 305, 1957). Within periods as short as 10 to 15 years, the prevailing influenza A subtype has been replaced by a new and antigenically distinct family of influenza A viruses. The Hong Kong strain of type A virus, which appeared with the pandemic of 1968, is presently classed as a major variant of type A2 virus, not as a new subtype. Strains of influenza B virus also show antigenic variation, but due to complex interrelationships, subtypes have not been designated.

Identification of the broad types of influenza virus, A, B, and C, is determined by complement-fixation test. The subtypes are identified by hemagglutination-inhibition and neutralization tests.

4. Reservoir—Man is the reservoir, although mammalian reservoirs, such as swine and horses, and even avian reservoirs are suspected.

5. Mode of transmission—By direct contact, through droplet infection, or by articles freshly soiled with discharges of the nose and throat of infected persons; probably airborne among crowded populations in enclosed spaces such as barracks, ships, or school buses.

6. Incubation period—Short, usually 24 to 72 hours.

7. Period of communicability—Probably limited to 3 days from clinical onset.

8. Susceptibility and resistance—Susceptibility is universal. Infection produces immunity to the specific infecting virus. Infection with related viruses broadens the base of immunity. Immunization produces serologic responses specific for the subtypes present in the vaccine, and booster responses to related strains with which the individual has had prior experience.

Age-specific attack rates during an epidemic reflect existing immunity from past experience with strains related to the epidemic subtype. Attack rates are also markedly influenced by the degree of exposure. In general, incidence is highest in school-age children. Rates decrease progressively among adults as age increases, though exceptions occur: In the 1962–1963 epidemic in the U.S.A., the third major recurrence of A2 influenza, incidence was rather uniform for all ages.

9. Methods of control—

A. Preventive measures:

1) Active immunization is moderately effective when vaccine is potent and contains antigens which closely match the prevailing strain of virus. Because of the uncertainty in any given year that epidemic influenza will occur and that vaccines will be effective, immunization should be limited to persons at greatest risk of serious complication or death (see par. 1 preceding). During years when widespread epidemics of influenza A are anticipated, immunization may also be considered for those engaged in essential community services. Vaccination should be accomplished before the influenza season is expected. Routine inoculation of healthy children and young adults or mass community-wide immunization programs should be discouraged.

2) Education of the public in basic personal hygiene (Definition 31), also stressing avoidance of crowds during epidemic periods.

B. Control of patient, contacts, and the immediate environment:

1) Report to local health authority: Obligatory reporting after January 1, 1971, as a *Disease under Surveillance by WHO,*

Class 1 (see Preface). Until then, report of epidemics resembling influenza; no individual case report; Class 4 (see Preface). Supplementary report of identity of epidemic agent as determined by laboratory examination.

2) *Isolation:* As practical during the acute illness, primarily for protection of the patient against secondary bacterial infections.

3) *Concurrent disinfection:* Of discharges from nose and throat of patients.

4) *Quarantine:* None.

5) *Protection of contacts:* Too late for immunization to be effective. A role for antiviral chemoprophylaxis in public health has not yet been defined.

6) *Investigation of contacts:* Of no practical value.

7) *Specific treatment:* None. Sulfonamides and antibiotics have no effect on the uncomplicated disease; they should be employed only after bacterial complications arise.

C. Epidemic measures:

1) The severe and often disrupting effects of epidemic influenza on community activities may be mitigated in part by effective health planning and education, particularly at the local level. Continued community surveillance by local health authorities of the extent and progress of outbreaks within areas of their jurisdiction is essential, followed by prompt report to state and national health agencies of the prevailing epidemic pattern. Current measurement of excess mortality from pneumonia, influenza, bronchitis and other respiratory diseases is an economical and effective index of the progress, extent and severity of epidemic influenza in large population groups. Such reports permit evaluation of the epidemic as a whole and are useful to health officers and all others responsible for the control of influenza.

2) The unnecessary aggregation of large numbers of people during epidemic periods should be discouraged. Closing of schools is not an effective control measure but may be unavoidable in the face of great pupil or teacher absenteeism.

3) Hospital administrators should anticipate the increased demand for space and staff during epidemic periods. Elective admissions as well as unnecessary hospitalization of mild uncomplicated influenza should be discouraged during these periods, and some curtailment of visiting privileges may be warranted.

D. International measures: In accordance with a Resolution of the 22nd World Health Assembly, influenza is now a *Disease*

under Surveillance by WHO. The following measures are recommended:

1) Prompt report to WHO of epidemics within a country and complete description of epidemiologic characteristics.

2) Prompt identification of the causative virus in individual epidemics, with immediate report and submission of prototype strains to WHO. Throat washings and blood samples may be sent to one of the 85 WHO national influenza centers located in 55 countries throughout the world. WHO maintains Reference Centres (see Preface).

3) Continuing epidemiologic studies and prompt identification of viruses by national health agencies; exchange of information with WHO in order to increase understanding of the basic epidemiology of influenza, to establish the broad movements of an epidemic, and to aid in early recognition of outbreaks in previously uninvaded territory.

4) Continuing effort to insure commercial or governmental facilities for the rapid production of sufficient quantities of vaccine should epidemic influenza due to a major antigenic variant of the virus appear anywhere in the world.

KERATOCONJUNCTIVITIS, INFECTIOUS

1. Identification—An acute infectious disease of the eye with unilateral or bilateral inflammation of conjunctivae, and edema of lids and periorbital tissues. Onset is sudden, with low-grade fever, headache, malaise and tender preauricular lymphadenopathy. Opacities of the cornea are evident within 4 to 14 days. Duration of illness is 2 to 4 weeks; complete recovery is usual although keratitis with impairment of vision may persist in some patients. Synonyms: Infectious punctate keratitis, Epidemic keratoconjunctivitis, Shipyard conjunctivitis.

Diagnosis is confirmed by recovery of virus from conjunctival scrapings in appropriate cell cultures or by serum neutralization tests.

2. Occurrence—Presumably worldwide. Both sporadic cases and large outbreaks occur in the Far East, Hawaii, North America and Europe. Outbreaks among industrial employees in temperate climates commonly involve only a small part of the population at risk.

3. Infectious agent—Type 8 adenovirus, occasionally other types.

4. Reservoir—Man is the only known reservoir.

5. Mode of transmission—Direct contact with discharges from eye of an infected person or with articles freshly soiled with conjunctival or nasal discharges. In industrial plants, from trauma to the conjunctivae from dust and dirt with subsequent introduction of the virus into the eye, in first aid stations and dispensaries where proper aseptic techniques are not employed. Outbreaks have originated in eye clinics and offices of physicians.

6. Incubation period—Probably 5 to 7 days.

7. Period of communicability—Indefinite, but certainly during acute stage of the disease.

8. Susceptibility and resistance—No natural immunity. Some degree of resistance follows attack but reinfections have been reported.

9. Methods of Control—

A. Preventive measures:

1) Education as to personal cleanliness and the danger in using common towels and toilet articles.
2) Use of safety measures such as goggles in industrial plants.
3) Rigid asepsis in ophthalmological procedures in industrial dispensaries and ophthalmic clinics to prevent spread of infection by hands of attendants or by instruments.

B. Control of patient, contacts, and the immediate environment:

1) *Report to local health authority:* Obligatory report of epidemics; no individual case report, Class 4 (see Preface).
2) *Isolation:* Advisable during the acute stage of the disease.
3) *Concurrent disinfection:* Of conjunctival and nasal discharges and articles soiled therewith. Terminal cleaning.
4) *Quarantine:* None.
5) *Immunization of contacts:* None.
6) *Investigation of contacts and source of infection:* Locate other cases and institute precautions at home or place of work.
7) *Specific treatment:* None.

C. Epidemic measures:

1) Intensify educational efforts with respect to hygiene of the eye.
2) Organize convenient facilities for prompt diagnosis and treatment.

D. International measures: WHO Reference Centres (see Preface).

LARVA MIGRANS

A. VISCERAL LARVA MIGRANS

1. Identification—A chronic and usually mild disease due to migration of certain nematode larvae in the organs and tissues. It is characterized by marked eosinophilia, anemia, hepatomegaly, hyperglobulinemia and fever. In severe cases the white cell count may reach 80,000 or more, with 80–90% eosinophils. Symptoms may persist for as long as a year. Endophthalmitis, caused by larvae entering the eye, occurs with some frequency in older children; pneumonitis or neurological disturbances may occur. Rarely a fatal disease.

Demonstration of larvae of *Toxocara* or typical eosinophilic granulomatous lesions by liver biopsy confirms the clinical diagnosis. Serodiagnostic tests are helpful but not generally available.

Aberrant larvae of *Ascaris lumbricoides, Strongyloides stercoralis, Necator americanus, Ancylostoma duodenale* and *Capillaria hepatica* are found occasionally in tissues, including some ectopic sites; they do not persist or migrate in the tissues for long periods as do the larvae of *Toxocara,* the usual causative agent.

2. Occurrence—Probably worldwide. Has had most attention in U.S.A. but prevalence is probably no greater than in most countries. Occurs sporadically as isolated cases in a family, mainly affecting children aged 14 to 40 months; occurs uncommonly at an older age among mentally retarded children. The next older or younger sibling often shows eosinophilia or other evidence of light or residual infection. Epidemics are unknown.

3. Infectious agents—Larvae of *Toxocara canis* and *Toxocara cati.*

4. Reservoir—Reservoirs are dog and cat.

5. Mode of transmission—By direct or indirect transmission of infective *Toxocara* eggs from contaminated soil to the mouth; directly related to eating of dirt by young children. Eggs reach the soil in feces from infected cats and dogs. They then require several weeks' incubation to become infective. After ingestion, embryonated eggs hatch in intestine, larvae penetrate the wall and migrate to liver and lungs by lymphatic and circulatory systems. From the lungs, larvae are spread by the systemic circulation to various organs, causing damage by their wanderings and through granulomatous tissue formation.

6. Incubation period—Probably weeks or months, depending upon intensity of infection, reinfection and sensitivity state of the patient.

7. Period of communicability—Not directly transmitted from man to man.

8. Susceptibility and resistance—Lower incidence in older children and adults probably relates to less exposure. Dogs may acquire infection as puppies; infection often ends on reaching sexual maturity. Sex and age differences are less marked for cats; older animals somewhat less susceptible than young.

9. Methods of control—

A. Preventive measures:

1) Prevent contamination of soil by feces of dogs and cats in areas immediately adjacent to houses and play areas of children, especially in multiple housing projects.

2) Bury deeply, or otherwise dispose of stools of dogs and cats passed in play areas. Children's sand boxes offer an attractive site for defecating cats; cover when not in use.

3) Deworm dogs and cats less than 6 months old and thereafter as indicated. Destroy worms and feces passed as a result of treatment.

4) Health education of the family as to source and origin of the infection, particularly the danger of eating dirt; and of children to wash hands after play in the soil and before eating.

B. Control of patient, contacts, and the immediate environment:

1) *Report to local health authority:* Official report not ordinarily justifiable, Class 5 (see Preface).

2) *Isolation:* None.

3) *Concurrent disinfection:* None.

4) *Quarantine:* None.

5) *Immunization of contacts:* None.

6) *Investigation of contacts and source of infection:* (See 9A3). Treat premises with raw salt or borax. Since these agents destroy lawns or any vegetation, this is applicable particularly to beaches, playgrounds and areas under houses.

7) *Specific treatment:* None. Thiabendazole and diethylcarbamazine under study.

C. Epidemic measures: Not applicable.

D. International measures: None.

B. CUTANEOUS LARVA MIGRANS

Infective larvae of cat and dog hookworm *(Ancylostoma brasiliense* and *Ancylostoma caninum)* cause a dermatitis in man, called "creeping eruption." This is a disease of utility men, gardeners, children, sea-bathers and others who come in contact with sandy soil contaminated with cat and dog feces; in the U.S.A., most prevalent in the Southeast. The larvae, which enter the skin, migrate intracutaneously but are unable to penetrate to deeper tissues. Each larva causes a serpiginous track, advancing several mm to a few cm a day. Self-limited, with spontaneous cure after several weeks or months. Individual larva can be killed by freezing the area with ethyl chloride spray; thiabendazole systemically or as a topical ointment is considered effective.

Differentiate from "swimmer's itch" caused by intracutaneous invasion by cercariae of bird or mammalian schistosomes, which reaches maximal intensity in 2–3 days and heals in a week or more.

LEISHMANIASIS, CUTANEOUS

1. Identification—A polymorphic disease of skin and mucous membranes characterized by ulcerating, indolent lesions; occasionally nodular lesions predominate (diffuse type). Clinical nature and distribution and course of lesions tend to be constant within a geographic area but may differ greatly from the characteristics that pertain in another area. Extensive involvement of nose, mouth and pharynx may be life threatening. Synonyms: In Old World: Aleppo, Baghdad, or Delhi boil, Oriental sore; in New World: Espundia, Uta, Chiclero or Bauru ulcer.

Diagnosis is by microscopic identification of *Leishmania* bodies in stained smears of scrapings from edges of lesions; also by culture on suitable media such as Novy, MacNeal & Nicolle's (NNN). An intradermal test using material derived from leptomonads generally becomes positive early in the disease and remains so thereafter; no serological test is of practical value.

2. Occurrence—Old World: Northwest India, West Pakistan, the Middle East, southern Russia, the Mediterranean littoral, North, West, and Central Africa. New World: endemic in Mexico (especially Yucatan), most of Central America, and every country of South America except Chile. In some areas the population at risk may be large, including young children while in other areas the disease is restricted to occupational groups such as those involved in work in forested areas. Generally more common in rural than urban areas.

3. Infectious agents—Old World, *Leishmania tropica;* New World, *Leishmania brasiliensis* and *Leishmania mexicana*—flagellate protozoa.

4. Reservoir—Unknown in some areas, but certain wild animals, especially rodents, or dogs are proven reservoirs in other areas.

5. Mode of transmission—Commonly through bite of infective female sandflies, *Phlebotomus;* possibly by direct contact of abraded skin with lesion of another person; or questionably through mechanical transmission by other flies.

6. Incubation period—From a few days to many months.

7. Period of communicability—As long as parasites remain in lesions; in untreated cases, a year or more. Spontaneous healing is the rule except for destructive lesions of mucous membrane. Duration of infectivity of vector unknown.

8. Susceptibility and resistance—Susceptibility is probably general. Immunity is usual after spontaneously healed infection.

9. Methods of control—

A. Preventive measures:

1) There is much variation from area to area, depending on the habits of the vector *Phlebotomus* and mammalian hosts. Where these habits are known, intelligent action may follow. Appropriate measures commonly include:

a) Periodic application of insecticides with residual action. *Phlebotomus* flies have a short flight range (under 200 yards) and are highly susceptible to control by systematic spraying with residual insecticides. Spraying should cover exterior and interior of doorways and other openings if infection occurs in dwellings, as well as possible breeding places, such as stone walls, animal houses, rubbish heaps, etc.

b) Elimination of rubbish heaps and other breeding places.

c) Destruction of animals implicated locally as reservoirs.

d) Avoidance of sandfly-infested areas after sundown.

e) Use of insect repellents and protective clothing if exposure to sandflies is unavoidable.

2) Health education concerning modes of transmission and methods of controlling *Phlebotomus*.

B. Control of patient, contacts, and the immediate environment:

1) *Report to local health authority:* Official report ordinarily not justifiable, Class 5 (see Preface).

2) *Isolation:* None. Where necessary reduce patient-*Phlebotomus* contact by using fine mesh (25–30 holes to the linear inch—aperture size not more than 0.035 inches) screening or application of residual insecticide to patient's surroundings.

3) *Concurrent disinfection:* None.

4) *Quarantine:* None.

5) *Immunization of contacts:* None.

6) *Investigation of contacts and source of infection:* Determine local transmission cycle and interrupt it in most practical fashion.

7) *Specific treatment:* A variety of agents including pentavalent antimonials, pyrimethamine (Daraprim), quinacrine (Atabrine hydrochloride), amphotericin B and cycloguanil pamoate (CL-501 or Camolar) are reported to be effective in certain geographic areas. Antimony sodium gluconate (Pentostam), the recommended drug, is available in the U.S.A. from the National Communicable Disease Center, Atlanta, Ga., on an investigational basis. In the Americas, a combination of pyrimethamine and cycloguanil pamoate has given good results.

C. Epidemic measures: In areas of high incidence, intensive efforts to control the disease by provision of diagnostic facilities, by mass treatment campaigns and by appropriate measures against *Phlebotomus* flies and the mammalian reservoir hosts.

D. International measures: WHO Reference Centres (see Preface).

LEISHMANIASIS, VISCERAL

1. Identification—A chronic systemic infectious disease characterized by fever, hepatosplenomegaly, lymphadenopathy, anemia with leucopenia, and progressive emaciation and weakness. Untreated, a highly fatal disease. Fever is of gradual or sudden onset, long continued and irregular, often with 2 daily peaks; alternating periods of apyrexia and low-grade fever follow. Chemotherapy may lead to cutaneous lesions containing *Leishmania*. Synonym: Kala azar.

Diagnosis is by demonstrating Leishman-Donovan bodies in stained smears from bone marrow, spleen, liver, lymph node or blood; by recovery of the parasite by culture of these materials on appropriate media such as NNN, or after injection into hamsters.

2. Occurrence—A rural disease of most tropical and subtropical areas of the world; Asia, the Middle East, Africa, South and Central America. In Europe: southern Russia, the Caspian littoral, Portugal and Mediterranean islands. In many affected areas, a relatively common disease, mainly as scattered cases among infants, children and adolescents, but occasionally in epidemic waves. Incidence modified by the use of antimalarial insecticides.

3. Infectious agent—*Leishmania donovani (Leishmania infantum)*; a flagellated protozoan.

4. Reservoir—Known or presumed reservoir hosts include man, dogs and other canines, cats and wild rodents. The relative importance of one or the other of these animals is strikingly different from one geographic area to another.

5. Mode of transmission—Through bite of infective sandflies of the genus *Phlebotomus*. The fly is infected by sucking the peripheral blood or by ingesting parasites present in skin of an infected reservoir host.

6. Incubation period—Generally 2 to 4 months; as short as 10 days or as long as 24 months.

7. Period of communicability—As long as parasites persist in the circulating blood or skin of the mammalian reservoir host. If man is the reservoir host, infectivity for *Phlebotomus* may extend beyond treatment and clinical recovery. Direct transmission from man to man, transmission by blood transfusion, through sexual contact, and by bite of infected laboratory animals has been reported.

8. Susceptibility and resistance—Susceptibility is general. Apparent lasting immunity, but recovery from cutaneous leishmaniasis does not confer immunity against kala azar or vice versa.

9. Methods of control—

    A. Preventive measures: Prevention of disease is accomplished by eliminating transmission of infection to man. Method will vary according to the local ecology and resources. Anti-*Phlebotomus* measures such as applications of residual insecticide to the area of sandfly-man contact are generally the most practical. (See Cutaneous Leishmaniasis 9A, pp. 126–127.)

B. Control of patient, contacts, and the immediate environment:

1) *Report to local health authority:* In selected endemic areas; in many countries not a reportable disease, Class 3B (see Preface).
2) *Isolation:* None. Protect patient from bites of *Phlebotomus* by fine-mesh screen and by spraying quarters with insecticide having residual action, and by use of repellents.
3) *Concurrent disinfection:* None.
4) *Quarantine:* None.
5) *Immunization:* None.
6) *Investigation of contacts and source of infection:* Ordinarily none.
7) *Specific treatment:* The pentavalent compounds of antimony (Neostibosan, Solustibosan, and urea stibamine) are effective. Antimony-resistant and antimony-sensitive cases may be treated by diamidine compounds such as stilbamidine, pentamidine isethionate. These are not used routinely because of their toxicity. In Mediterranean areas and the Sudan the parasite is more resistant than in India.

C. Epidemic measures: Epidemic measures must include a study of the local life cycle followed by selection of measures that will affect mammalian and *Phlebotomus* hosts so as to stop transmission. No method suitable for mass application will detect the infected individual in the absence of overt disease.

D. International measures: Coordinated programs of control among neighboring countries where the disease is endemic. WHO Reference Centres (see Preface).

LEPROSY

1. Identification—A chronic, mildly communicable disease characterized by lesions of the skin—infiltration, macules, plaques, papules and nodules—by involvement and often palpable enlargement of peripheral nerves, with consequent anesthesia, muscle weakness and paralysis, and trophic changes in skin, muscle and bone. Two distinct major types occur: lepromatous and tuberculoid. In lepromatous leprosy there are diffuse skin lesions and invasion of mucous membranes of the upper respiratory tract as well as of some viscera; skin lesions may ulcerate. The tuberculoid form is usually localized, with discretely demarcated skin lesions, relatively early nerve involvement, and frequently spontaneous healing in 1–3 years. Residual paralysis and anesthesia leading to trophic ulcers and other complications may result from either form of leprosy. Progress of the disease is slow; death is usually due to other causes. Synonym: Hansen's disease.

Diagnosis is supported by the demonstration of acid-fast bacilli in suspected lesions. Large numbers of bacilli are characteristically present in lepromatous lesions. Bacilli are sparse and occasionally not demonstrable in tuberculoid lesions, but these lesions are nearly always anesthetic. Diagnosis of leprosy is best confirmed by biopsy of suspected skin lesion with evaluation by a pathologist knowledgeable in the disease.

2. Occurrence—Mostly in the tropics and subtropics. Prevalence rates of 5 per 1000 or higher are found only in the tropics; however, socioeconomic conditions are probably more important than climate. A few countries with temperate climates have estimated rates of 1 per 1000, including China and Korea. India and China have about one-half of the estimated world total of 12 to 20 million cases. In Europe, low endemicity in Greece, Portugal and Spain; in several other countries, residual foci only. About 2600 known cases live in the U.S.A. Disease is endemic but decreasing in Hawaii; endemic foci exist in southeastern Texas and to a lesser extent in Louisiana and Florida. In the 1963–1968 period, an average of 100 newly diagnosed cases was reported annually, with an average of 26 annually from California, 21 from Texas, 15 from Hawaii, 9 from Florida, 9 from Puerto Rico, and 7 from New York City; the remainder were scattered. Approximately 70% were acquired outside the U.S.A.

3. Infectious agent—*Mycobacterium leprae,* the leprosy (Hansen's) bacillus, which has been cultured in the footpads of mice but not in artificial media.

4. Reservoir—Man is the only known reservoir.

5. Mode of transmission—Not established; bacilli from skin lesions or nasal discharges of infectious patients gain entrance presumably through the skin or respiratory tract. Close household contact important.

6. Incubation period—Shortest known is 7 months; probably average 3 to 5 years, although long periods often elapse before recognition.

7. Period of communicability—As long as bacilli are demonstrable, infectiousness should be considered possible unless treatment is known to be regular and effective. Clinical and laboratory evidence suggests that in previously untreated patients infectiousness is lost in most instances within 3 months of continuous therapy with DDS (dapsone, 4,4'-diaminodiphenylsulfone); although often present, bacilli which stain irregularly are probably noninfectious.

8. Susceptibility and resistance—No proven racial immunity. Reactivity to lepromin is absent in the lepromatous type, usually present in the tuberculoid type and in healthy adults. Lepromin test of no value in diagnosis, but is sometimes of value for purposes of classification.

9. Methods of control—

A. *Preventive measures:*

1) The effectiveness of DDS in terminating infectiousness and the ease of treatment of early cases have shifted the emphasis in leprosy control from isolation to early detection and treatment of infectious cases and surveillance of household and other close contacts for disease. Hospital facilities should be available for initiating treatment, and for surgical correction of deformities.

2) Health education stressing the availability of effective therapy and the absence of infectivity of patients under continuous treatment.

3) In a large controlled study in Uganda, prophylactic BCG apparently effected a considerable reduction in the incidence of tuberculoid leprosy among child contacts. Controlled studies in New Guinea showed less protection, and in Burma no measurable protection, but findings of these 3 important studies not yet final. Prophylactic DDS therapy also appeared to confer good protection to child contacts in a smaller study in Madras, India and to those under 25 in a study in Andhra Pradesh, India.

B. *Control of patient, contacts, and the immediate environment:*

1) *Report to local health authority:* Case reporting obligatory in most states and countries and desirable in all (Class 2B, see Preface).

2) *Isolation:* Formerly, patients were confined involuntarily in hospitals or colonies until consistently bacteriologically negative, but this practice results in concealment of cases. Hospitalization is encouraged only for initiation of treatment, if indicated; thereafter ambulatory treatment. No special isolation procedures are required when cases are hospitalized. No restrictions in employment and attendance at school are indicated from the public health standpoint for patients whose disease is regarded as noninfectious; medical indications (anesthesia, etc.) may require a change in type of employment.

3) *Concurrent disinfection:* Of nasal discharges and discharges from lesions. Terminal cleaning.

4) *Quarantine:* None.

5) *Immunization of contacts:* BCG vaccination and prophylactic DDS therapy may be used but are still under study (see 9A3 above).

6) *Control of contacts:* Periodic examination of household and other close contacts at 6 to 12 month intervals for at least 10 years after last contact with an infectious case; if feasible, separate newborn infants from infectious parents until therapy is well established.

7) *Specific treatment:* DDS orally, initial small doses being increased slowly to optimum therapeutic dosage and continued at maintenance levels for prolonged periods, preferably for life, for lepromatous leprosy. Tuberculoid leprosy is treated for shorter periods (up to several years). Patients whose bacilli have become sulfone resistant are best treated with B663, a riminophenazine compound. An injectable repository sulfone (DADDS) is being studied which would minimize the possible irregularities inherent in daily oral medication.

C. *Epidemic measures:* Not applicable.

D. *International measures:* International controls should be limited to infectious cases only.

WHO Reference Centres (see Preface).

LEPTOSPIROSIS

1. Identification—A group of acute infections with fever, headache, chills, severe malaise, vomiting, muscular aches and conjunctivitis; meningeal irritation occasionally; infrequently jaundice, renal insufficiency, hemolytic anemia and hemorrhage in skin and mucous membranes. Rash occurs occasionally. Clinical illness lasts from a few days to 3 weeks; relapses may occur. Infections may be asymptomatic. Fatality is low but increases with advancing age; may reach 20% or more in patients with jaundice and kidney damage. Synonyms: Weil's disease, Canicola fever, Hemorrhagic jaundice, Mud fever, Swineherd's disease.

Diagnosis by agglutination and complement-fixation tests and culture of leptospires in blood during the acute illness or in urine after the first week, in special media such as Fletcher's, or by inoculation of guinea pigs.

2. Occurrence—Outbreaks among swimmers exposed to water contaminated by urine of domestic or wild animals. An occupational hazard to rice field workers, sugarcane field workers, farmers, sewer workers, miners, veterinarians, animal husbandmen, abattoir workers, fish workers and military troops. Distribution of reservoirs of infection and of one or another serotype of *Leptospira* is worldwide, in urban and rural, developed and primitive areas.

3. Infectious agents—Many serotypes of *Leptospira*, such as *Leptospira icterohaemorrhagiae, Leptospira pomona, Leptospira canicola* and *Leptospira autumnalis,* have been recovered from human cases in U.S.A.; others are probable. At present 18 serogroups and more than 100 serotypes are recognized from various parts of the world.

4. Reservoir—Reservoirs among farm animals include cattle, dogs and swine. Rats and other rodents are frequently infected as are wild animals, including deer, foxes, skunks, racoons, opossums and even reptiles and amphibia (frogs).

5. Mode of transmission—Contact with water contaminated with urine of infected animals, as in swimming or accidental or occupational immersion; direct contact with infected animals. Infection presumably results from penetration of abraded skin or mucous membrane, or possibly through ingestion.

6. Incubation period—4 to 19 days, usually 10 days.

7. Period of communicability—Direct transmission from man to man is negligible.

8. Susceptibility and resistance—Susceptibility of man is general, varying with serotype.

9. Methods of control—

A. Preventive measures:

1) Protection of workers in hazardous occupations by provision of boots and gloves.
2) Identification of potentially contaminated waters.
3) Education of the public on modes of transmission, avoidance of swimming or wading in potentially contaminated waters, and need for proper protection when work requires such exposure.
4) Rodent control in human habitations, especially rural and recreational. Firing of cane fields before harvest.
5) Segregation of domestic animals, and the prevention of contamination of living, working and recreational areas of man by urine of infected animals.
6) Vaccination of farm and pet animals is valuable in prevention of disease. The vaccine must represent the dominant local strains.

B. Control of patient, contacts, and the immediate environment:

1) Report to local health authority: Obligatory case report in many states and countries, Class 2B (see Preface).
2) Isolation: None.
3) Concurrent disinfection: None.
4) Quarantine: None.
5) Immunization of contacts: None.
6) Investigation of contacts: Search for exposure to infected animals or history of swimming in contaminated waters.
7) Specific treatment: Penicillin, streptomycin, and tetracycline antibiotics are leptospirocidal, but they are not of demonstrated value in the treatment of human disease.

C. Epidemic measures: Search for source of infection, such as a pond used for swimming; eliminate contamination or prohibit use. Investigate industrial or occupational sources, including direct animal contact.

D. *International measures:* WHO Reference Centres (see Preface).

LISTERIOSIS

1. Identification—An acute meningitis with or without associated septicemia; less frequently, septicemia only. Onset of meningitis is usually sudden, with fever, intense headache, nausea, vomiting and signs of meningeal irritation; delirium and coma often appear early, occasionally collapse and shock. Abortion, endocarditis, granulomatous lesions in liver and other organs, localized internal or external abscesses, and pustular or papular cutaneous lesions occur irregularly. Septicemic listeriosis is an acute, mild, febrile illness, sometimes with influenza-like symptoms, which in pregnant women usually results in infection of the fetus and interrupted pregnancy. Infants may be stillborn, born with a massive septicemia, or develop meningitis in the neonatal period. Postpartum course of the mother is usually uneventful. Case fatality is 50% in newborn infants, approaching 100% when onset occurs in the first 4 days.

Diagnosis is confirmed by isolation of the infectious agent from spinal fluid, blood or lesions. Microscopic examination permits presumptive diagnosis. Fluorescent antibody tests are useful in the examination of tissues and spinal fluid. Serologic tests are unreliable.

2. Occurrence—Typically sporadic, rarely in small epidemics. Occurs in all seasons, slightly more often in males than females. About 40% of clinical cases occur within the first 3 weeks of life; in adults, mainly after age 40. Inapparent infections occur at all ages although of consequence only in gravidae. Abortion occurs as early as the 2nd month of pregnancy but mainly in the 5th or 6th month; perinatal infection, during last trimester. Incidence unknown, but in U.S.A. estimate is at least 100 cases annually.

3. Infectious agent—*Listeria monocytogenes,* a bacterium.

4. Reservoir—Reservoir is infected domestic and wild mammals, fowl and man. The organism is frequently found to be free living in water, mud and ensilage.

5. Mode of transmission—Unknown, except for infections transmitted from mother to unborn infant in utero, or during birth, and for papular lesions on hands and arms from direct contact with infectious material. Venereal transmission and infection from ingested contaminated food are possibilities.

6. Incubation period—Unknown; probably 4 days to 3 weeks. Fetus usually infected within several days after maternal disease.

7. Period of communicability—Rarely communicable from man to man except congenitally. Mothers of infected newborn infants may shed infectious agent in vaginal discharges or urine for 7 to 10 days after delivery, rarely longer.

8. Susceptibility and resistance—Unborn child and newborn highly susceptible. Children and young adults generally resistant, adults less so after age 40. Disease is frequently superimposed on other debilitating illnesses, especially in patients receiving steroids. Little evidence of acquired immunity, even after prolonged severe infection.

9. Methods of control—

A. Preventive measures:

1) Health education of pregnant women to avoid contact with infective materials on farms where the disease is endemic among livestock, and with known infected persons.
2) Proper precautions by veterinarians and farmers in handling aborted fetuses.

B. Control of patient, contacts, and the immediate environment:

1) Report to local health authority: Official report not ordinarily justifiable, Class 5 (see Preface).
2) Isolation: Of infected infants and their mothers until infectious agents are no longer present in body discharges.
3) Concurrent disinfection: Of discharges from the vagina of mothers, of discharges from eyes, nose and mouth of infants, of meconium, and of articles soiled therewith. Terminal cleaning.
4) Quarantine: None.
5) Immunization of contacts: None.
6) Investigation of contacts and source of infection: Of no practical value.
7) Specific treatment: Tetracycline antibiotics, ampicillin and chloramphenicol are effective.

C. Epidemic measures: Not applicable; usually a sporadic disease.

D. International measures: None.

LOIASIS

1. Identification—A chronic filarial disease characterized by migration of the adult worm through subcutaneous or deeper tissues of the body, causing transient "fugitive swelling" or calabar swelling of the trunk and extremities. Migration under the bulbar conjunctivae is attended by pain and edema.

Female worms produce larvae (microfilariae) which have a diurnal periodicity; best demonstrated in stained thick blood smears or stained sediment of laked blood. The intradermal test using *Dirofilaria* antigen is diagnostically useful although nonspecific.

Infection with other filariae such as *Wuchereria bancrofti, Brugia malayi, Onchocerca volvulus,* or *Acanthocheilonema perstans* requires differentiation in endemic areas.

2. Occurrence—Widely distributed in tropical West and Central Africa. In the Congo River basin up to 90% of indigenous inhabitants of some villages are infected.

3. Infectious agent—*Loa loa,* a nematode worm.

4. Reservoir—Reservoir is an infected person harboring microfilariae in the blood.

5. Mode of transmission—Transmitted by "mangrove fly" of the genus *Chrysops. Chrysops dimidiata, C. silacea* and other species ingest blood and microfilariae. The larvae develop within 10 to 20 days in the muscles and connective tissues of the fly. The developed filariform larva migrates to the proboscis and is transferred to a human host by bite of the infective fly.

6. Incubation period—Symptoms usually do not appear until several years after repeated infection but may occur as early as 4 months. Microfilariae do not appear in the peripheral blood until a year or more after infection.

7. Period of communicability—The adult worm may live in man as long as 17 years and microfilariae may be present in the blood during this time; in the fly, communicability is from 10 to 20 days after its infection and until all infective larvae have migrated or until the fly dies.

8. Susceptibility and resistance—Susceptibility is universal; repeated infections occur and immunity, if present, has not been demonstrated.

9. Methods of control—

A. Preventive measures:

1) Measures directed against the aquatic fly larvae have not proved practical or effective, as breeding areas are usually extensive.
2) Diethyltoluamide (DEET) or dimethylphthalate applied to exposed skin are effective repellants.

B. Control of patient, contacts, and the immediate environment:

1) *Report to local health department:* Official report ordinarily not justifiable, Class 5 (see Preface).
2) *Isolation:* Not practicable. So far as possible, patients with microfilariae in the blood should be protected from *Chrysops* bites as a means of reducing transmission.
3) *Concurrent disinfection:* None.

4) Quarantine: None.

5) Immunization of contacts: None.

6) Investigation of contacts: None; a community problem.

7) Specific treatment: Diethylcarbamazine (Hetrazan) causes disappearance of microfilariae, reduces frequency and intensity of calabar swellings, and may kill adult worm, with resulting cure. Surgical removal of adult worm for relief of acute bulbar conjunctivitis.

C. *Epidemic measures:* Not applicable.

D. *International measures:* WHO Reference Centres (see Preface).

LYMPHOCYTIC CHORIOMENINGITIS

1. Identification—A viral disease of animals, especially mice, transmissible to man, with a marked diversity of clinical manifestations. May begin with an influenza-like attack and terminate by recovery, or after a few days of more or less complete remission, meningeal symptoms suddenly appear. Attack sometimes begins with meningeal symptoms. Patients with severe meningoencephalitis have somnolence, disturbed deep reflexes, paralysis, and anesthesia of skin. Course is usually short, with recovery in a few weeks; occasionally fatal. Spinal fluid has from a few hundred to more than 3,500 cells per cu mm mostly lymphocytes.

Laboratory diagnostic methods include isolation of virus from blood, urine, nasopharynx or spinal fluid early in attack by inoculation of guinea pigs or LCM-free mice and rising titers of neutralizing or complement-fixing antibodies in paired sera.

Requires differentiation from other aseptic meningitides.

2. Occurrence—Uncommon. Foci of infection often persist within limits of a city block for months or years, resulting in sporadic clinical disease.

3. Infectious agent—The virus of lymphocytic choriomeningitis.

4. Reservoir—Reservoir is the infected house mouse, *Mus musculus;* naturally infected guinea pigs, monkeys, dogs, and swine have been observed.

5. Mode of transmission—Virus is excreted in urine and feces of infected animals, usually mice. Transmission to man is probably through contaminated food or dust, possibly by arthropods. Biological products of animal origin have been found contaminated.

6. Incubation period—Probably 8 to 13 days, 15 to 21 days to meningeal symptoms.

7. Period of communicability—Not known to be directly transmitted from man to man. Naturally infected mice may carry the virus through life; the infected female transmits virus to offspring.

8. Susceptibility and resistance—Unknown. Blood serum of persons recovered from the disease neutralizes virus, as occasionally does the serum of persons without history of recognized attack.

9. Methods of control—

A. *Preventive measures:* Cleanliness of home and place of work; elimination of mice and disposal of other diseased animals.

B. *Control of patient, contacts, and the immediate environment:*

1) *Report to local health authority:* Official report not ordinarily justifiable, Class 5 (see Preface).
2) *Isolation:* None.
3) *Concurrent disinfection:* Of discharges from the nose and throat, of urine and feces, and of articles soiled therewith.
4) *Quarantine:* None.
5) *Immunization of contacts:* None.
6) *Investigation of contacts and source of infection:* Home and place of employment for presence of house mice.
7) *Specific treatment:* None.

C. *Epidemic measures:* Not applicable.

D. *International measures:* None.

LYMPHOGRANULOMA VENEREUM

1. Identification—A venereally acquired infectious disease of lymph channels and lymph nodes manifest in bubo formation, ulceration, elephantiasis of genitalia, and rectal stricture. May begin with small painless evanescent erosion, papule, or herpetiform lesion, followed shortly by acute, subacute or chronic adenitis, usually with multiple foci of suppuration; bubo commonly first manifestation. Fever, chills, headache, vague abdominal aches, joint pains, and anorexia often occur during lymphatic progression. Spontaneous regression of buboes does not indicate recovery; course often long, disability great, but generally not fatal. Synonyms: Lymphogranuloma inguinale, Lymphopathia venereum, Climatic bubo.

Diagnosis by skin test with Frei antigen or by complement-fixation test; neither conclusive.

2. Occurrence—Commoner than ordinarily believed; widespread throughout world, especially in tropical and subtropical areas. Endemic in southern U.S.A., particularly among lower social classes; age incidence that of greatest sexual activity; most frequent among sexually promiscuous persons, including homosexuals; sex difference not pronounced; all races affected.

3. Infectious agent—A bedsonia (chlamydia) closely related to that of psittacosis.

4. Reservoir—Reservoir is man.

5. Mode of transmission—Direct contact during sexual intercourse with open lesions of infected persons; indirect contact with articles, including clothing, contaminated by discharges; children commonly infected from bedfellows.

6. Incubation period—Five to 21 days to primary lesion, usually 7 to 12; if bubo is first manifestation, 10 to 30 days, sometimes several months.

7. Period of communicability—Variable, from weeks to years, during presence of active lesions.

8. Susceptibility and resistance—Susceptibility general; no evidence of natural or acquired resistance.

9. Methods of control—

A. *Preventive measures:* Except for measures which are specific for syphilis, preventive measures are those for venereal diseases. See Syphilis 9A (pp. 245–246).

B. *Control of patient, contacts, and the immediate environment:*

1) *Report to local health authority:* In selected endemic areas (U.S.A., some states); in most states and countries not a reportable disease, Class 3C (see Preface).
2) *Isolation:* None. Refrain from sexual contact until lesions are healed.
3) *Concurrent disinfection:* None; care in disposal of discharges from lesions and of articles soiled therewith.
4) *Quarantine:* None.
5) *Immunization of contacts:* Not applicable; prompt treatment on recognition or clinical suspicion of infection.
6) *Investigation of contacts:* Search for sexual contacts of patient before and after appearance of disease.
7) *Specific treatment:* Tetracycline antibiotics are effective for all stages—for buboes and ulcerative lesions. Administer orally for 10 days or longer as indicated by clinical response. Do not incise bubo; drain by aspiration.

C. *Epidemic measures:* Not applicable.

D. *International measures:* See Syphilis 9D, p. 247.

MALARIA

1. Identification—The 4 diseases that constitute the human malarias can be sufficiently similar in symptomatology that they are difficult to differentiate without laboratory studies. The most serious, malignant tertian or aestivo-autumnal, may present a very varied clinical picture including fever not characterized by classical recurrence, chills and sweating, headache, icterus, coagulation defects, shock, renal failure, acute encephalitis and coma. It should be considered as a possible cause of coma in any person recently returned from a tropical area. Prompt treatment is essential (since irreversible complications may appear suddenly) even in apparently mild forms of the infection; case fatality among untreated children and nonimmune adults exceeds 10%.

The other human malarias, benign tertian, quartan and ovale, generally not life threatening except in the very young or in patients with concurrent disease, may begin with indefinite malaise followed by a shaking chill and rapidly rising temperature, usually accompanied by headache and nausea and ending with profuse sweating. After an interval free of fever, the cycle of chills, fever, and sweating is repeated, either daily, every other day or every 3rd day. Duration of untreated primary attack varies from a week to a month or longer. Relapses are common and may occur at irregular intervals for several years.

Individuals who have been taking prophylactic drugs may show a wide variation in the incubation period and in the initial clinical picture.

Laboratory confirmation should always be sought through demonstration of malaria parasites in blood films by microscopic examination. Repeated examinations may be necessary; the thick film method is most likely to reveal the parasite; parasites are often not demonstrable in films from patients recently or actively under treatment. Antibodies, demonstrable by fluorescent antibody test, persist many years after infection.

2. Occurrence—Epidemic malaria essentially has disappeared from many countries. Numerous countries in the tropics, with a tradition of hyperendemic malaria, have now greatly reduced the incidence by modern control measures. In certain tropical countries where malaria programs have been interrupted or suspended, malaria rates have risen in some instances to epidemic proportions. Still a major cause of ill health in many parts of tropical and subtropical Africa, Asia, Central and South America, and the Southwest Pacific.

3. Infectious agents—*Plasmodium vivax* for vivax (benign tertian) malaria, *Plasmodium malariae* for malariae (quartan) malaria, *Plasmodium falciparum* for falciparum malaria (malignant tertian) (aestivo-autumnal) and *Plasmodium ovale* for the less common ovale malaria. Mixed infections occur not infrequently in endemic areas.

4. Reservoir—Man is the only important reservoir of human malaria, although higher apes may harbor *P. malariae*. Monkeys are naturally infected by *Plasmodium knowlesi* and *Plasmodium cynomolgi,* which can infect man.

5. Mode of transmission—Transmitted by an infective female anopheline mosquito. Certain species of *Anopheles* ingest human blood containing plasmodia in the gametocyte stage and act as definitive hosts. The parasite develops into sporozoites in from 8 to 35 days, depending on species of parasite and temperature to which the vector is exposed. Sporozoites concentrate in the salivary glands and are injected into man as the insect thereafter takes blood meals. In the susceptible host, gametocytes usually appear in the blood within 3 to 14 days after onset of symptoms, according to species of parasite. Malaria may also be transmitted by injection or transfusion of blood of infected persons or by use of contaminated hypodermic syringes, as by drug addicts. Congenital transmission may occur.

6. Incubation period—Average 12 days for *P. falciparum,* 14 days for *P. vivax* and *P. ovale,* and 30 days for *P. malariae.* With some strains of *P. vivax,* there may be a protracted incubation period of 8 to 10 months, the period of latency. With infection by blood transfusion, incubation is usually short, but varies with the dose of parasites.

7. Period of communicability—For mosquito infection, as long as infective gametocytes are present in the blood of patients; varies with species and strain of parasite and with response to therapy. In untreated or insufficiently treated cases, infective gametocytes may persist indefinitely in quartan malaria, from 1 to 3 years in vivax, and generally not more than 1 year in falciparum malaria. The mosquito remains infective for the rest of its life, a few days to a month or more; only the female takes blood meals.

8. Susceptibility and resistance—Susceptibility is universal, the degree sometimes lessened by previous infection. Tolerance to infection develops in highly endemic communities where exposure to infective anophelines is continuous over many years. There is racial resistance to *P. vivax* in African Negroes.

9. Methods of control—

A. Preventive measures:

1) Application of residual insecticide (chlorinated hydrocarbons such as DDT, benzene hexachloride or dieldrin) in suitable formula and dosage on the inside walls of dwellings and on other surfaces upon which vector anophelines habitually rest will generally result in effective malaria control, except where resistance to these insecticides has appeared. When this occurs, the chlorinated hydrocarbons can be replaced by organophosphates (such as Malathion) or carbamate compounds. These are effective in residual application, but may be more toxic to man in certain formulations (such as Arpocarb). Entire communities should be treated in a spraying project, to be

carried forward year after year until malaria ceases to be endemic, after which surveillance activities may be used to eliminate the residual parasites in man. Countrywide effort over at least 4 consecutive years followed by adequate surveillance has in some instances eradicated malaria in local regions.

2) Where residual insecticide is not available, nightly spraying of living and sleeping quarters with a liquid or an aerosol preparation of pyrethrum or other space sprays is useful.

3) In endemic areas, install screens in living and sleeping quarters and use bed nets.

4) Insect repellents (such as diethyltoluamide 50% solution or dimethylphthalate; or 2-ethylhexane-diol, 1, 3, commonly called "612") applied to uncovered skin and impregnated in the clothing of persons exposed to bites of vector anophelines, are useful.

5) Sanitary improvements, such as filling and draining to eliminate breeding places of vector anophelines, should not be neglected. Larvicides (such as oil and Paris green) are now not commonly used where residual spraying is effective but may be useful under special conditions. The chlorinated hydrocarbons are not recommended as larvicides, but organophosphorus compounds such as Abate or Fenthion may be of value. Effectiveness of antilarval methods varies with the particular vector species involved.

6) Regular use of suppressive drugs in malarious areas (see 9B7 below).

7) Effective treatment of acute and chronic cases is an important adjunct to malaria control and essential in attempted eradication, with case detection methods to locate those still infected.

8) Blood donors should be questioned for a history of malaria or possible exposure to the disease, and should be rejected if they have a history of malaria at any time, or of drug prophylaxis within the preceding 2 years.

B. Control of patient, contacts, and the immediate environment:

1) Report to local health authority: Obligatory case report as a *Disease under Surveillance by WHO,* after January 1, 1971, Class 1. Until then, Class 2B (see Preface), in nonendemic areas, desirably limited to authenticated cases (U.S.A.) ; Class 3C (see Preface) is the more practical procedure in endemic areas.

2) Isolation: None; patients should be protected at night by mosquito proofing.

3) Concurrent disinfection: A single concurrent residual spraying of the neighborhood may be useful if a primary or relapsing case occurs in an area not under control, previously free from the disease, and where potential vectors are active.

4) Quarantine: None.

5) Immunization of contacts: Not applicable.

6) Investigation of contacts: Determine history of previous infection among household members or of exposure to anophelines. In advanced stages of eradication, attempt to determine source of infection in every detected case by mass blood survey in the neighborhood; treat persons with pyrexia by "presumptive" single-dose therapy even before result of blood examination is known.

7) Specific treatment for all forms of malaria in adults:

  a) For acute cases in nonimmune subjects, except *P. falciparum* infections acquired in South America or Southeast Asia: chloroquine base, 1500 to 2400 mg, orally over 3 to 5 days (600 mg base initially, 300 mg base 6 hours later, and 300 mg on each of the next 2 to 4 days); or amodiaquine base, 1400 mg, orally over 3 days (600 mg base initially, and 400 mg base on each of the next 2 days); or quinine sulfate or dihydrochloride, 15,000 mg (230 grains) orally over 10 days (650 mg every 8 hours for 3 days, then every 12 hours for the next 7 days).

  b) For acute cases, emergency treatment of grave infections, or persons unable to retain orally administered medication: chloroquine hydrochloride,* 300 mg base, intramuscularly, repeated if needed in 6 hours but not more than 900 mg base per 24 hours; or quinine dihydrochloride,* 650 mg (10 grains) diluted in a liter of normal saline, glucose or plasma, administered intravenously and slowly, repeated if needed in 6 hours but not more than 3 injections per 24 hours; or chloroquine hydrochloride, 300 mg base in 500 ml of normal saline administered intravenously and slowly, once in 24 hours. Intravenous chloroquine administration is seldom required, as intramuscular chloroquine produces a rapid response. If there is evidence of renal failure, quinine dosages should be reduced. All parenteral drugs should be discontinued as soon as oral drug administration can be initiated.

  c) For *P. falciparum* infections acquired in South America or Southeast Asia: These infections respond poorly or not at all to the synthetic drugs described above. For such persons or any patient developing clinical malaria while on chloroquine prophylaxis: quinine,

---

* Available in U.S.A. from National Communicable Disease Center if not available locally.

orally (or parenterally if required), should be used in the dosage and on the schedules noted in the previous paragraphs. Concurrently, for the first 3 days of treatment, administer pyrimethamine, 25 mg twice daily by mouth (for a total of 150 mg). In instances of repeated reappearance of clinical illness despite therapy as indicated above, or when quinine is not tolerated, some good results have been obtained with a combination of sulfonamides and pyrimethamine given over a 3–5 day period.

d) For acute attacks in semi-immune subjects: Chloroquine or amodiaquine in a single oral dose of 600 mg base will often terminate the acute attack, but further treatment as under 9B7 is desirable.

e) For prevention of relapses in vivax, malariae and ovale infections acquired by mosquito bites, treated as in 9B7a or 9B7b: the oral administration of primaquine, 15 mg base, daily for 14 days, usually is adequate to eradicate the secondary tissue forms of the parasite, but in some areas, i.e., New Guinea, it has to be increased to 22.5 mg daily. Primaquine may be administered concurrently with the other drug or following completion of the primary therapy. Certain individuals, particularly those originating from the eastern Mediterranean and African areas, may develop hemolysis from this dosage of primaquine.

f) For suppression or prophylaxis of nonimmune persons temporarily residing in or traveling through endemic areas, chloroquine (Aralen) or amodiaquine (Camoquin), 300 mg base, once weekly; or pyrimethamine (Daraprim), 25 mg once weekly, always on the same day each week; or proguanil monohydrochloride (chlorguanide) (Paludrine), 100 mg daily. To prevent breakthrough of resistant strains in South and Middle America and Southeast Asia, a tablet containing 300 mg chloroquine base and 45 mg primaquine may be given once a week. Suppressive treatment should be continued for 2 months after patient leaves endemic area. For persons who have been on suppressive drugs and are leaving an endemic area, primaquine base, 45 mg, may be administered once a week for 8 weeks concurrently with the suppressive chloroquine. Alternately, 15 mg primaquine may be given daily for 14 days, the suppressive drug being continued on the original schedule.

All doses in the above paragraph are for adults of average weight. Doses of antimalarial drugs for children should be adjusted according to age and especially weight.

C. *Epidemic measures:* A field survey to determine nature and extent of the epidemic situation is the point of departure. Intensify residual spraying, find and treat acute cases, and use suppressive drugs. Sometimes the breeding places of anophelines responsible for an epidemic can be eliminated. Mass chemoprophylaxis must be considered.

D. *International measures:*

1) Disinsection of aircraft, ships or other vehicles on arrival in an area free from malaria or any of its vectors, if the health authority at place of arrival has reason to suspect importation of malaria vectors.

2) Disinsection of aircraft before departure or in transit from an area where vectors have become resistant to a particular insecticide or insecticides, using an insecticide of a type to which the vectors are still susceptible.

3) Strong effort to maintain rigid antimosquito sanitation within the mosquito flight range of all ports and airports.

4) In special circumstances, administration of antimalarial drugs to migrants, seasonal workers or persons taking part in periodic mass movement into an area or country where malaria has been eliminated. Primaquine, 45 mg base, given as a single dose on a weekly basis, renders the gametocytes of the human malarias (including some of the drug-refractory strains from South America and Southeast Asia) noninfectious for mosquitoes.

5) WHO is supporting a worldwide eradication program; WHO Reference Centres (see Preface).

6) In accordance with a Resolution of the 22nd World Health Assembly, malaria is now a *Disease under Surveillance by WHO,* and a scheme for the collection and distribution of information on an international basis has been developed.

MEASLES

1. Identification—An acute, highly communicable viral disease with prodromal fever, conjunctivitis, coryza, bronchitis, and Koplik spots on the buccal mucosa. A characteristic dusky-red blotchy rash appears on the 3rd or 4th day, beginning on the face, becoming generalized, lasting 4 to 6 days and sometimes ending in branny desquamation. Leucopenia is usual. More severe in adults. In U.S.A., death from uncomplicated measles is rare; such deaths as occur are from secondary pneumonia mainly in children less than 2 years old; occasionally from postinfection encephalitis. Measles is a severe disease among malnourished children of developing countries, with fatality of 5 to 10% or more. Synonyms: Morbilli, Rubeola, Red measles.

Virus isolation from blood, conjunctivae and nasopharynx by tissue culture, or demonstration of a rise in specific hemagglutination-inhibiting, complement-fixing, or neutralizing antibodies is possible, but the necessary laboratory facilities are often not available.

2. Occurrence—Common in childhood; probably 80 to 90% of persons surviving to age 20 years have had measles; few persons go through life without an attack. Endemic and relatively mild in large metropolitan communities, attaining epidemic proportions about every other year. In smaller communities and areas, outbreaks tend to be more widely spaced and somewhat more severe. With long intervals between outbreaks, as in the Arctic and some island areas, measles often affects large portions of the population and case fatality may be high. In temperate climates, it is prevalent in all seasons except summer, but primarily in spring.

3. Infectious agent—The virus of measles.

4. Reservoir—Reservoir is man.

5. Mode of transmission—By droplet spread or direct contact with secretions of nose, throat and urine of infected persons; indirectly and less commonly airborne, and by articles freshly soiled with secretions of nose and throat. One of the most readily transmitted communicable diseases.

6. Incubation period—About 10 days, varying from 8 to 13 days, from exposure to initial fever; about 14 days until rash appears; uncommonly longer or shorter. Late inoculation with measles immune serum globulin in attempted passive protection may extend incubation to 21 days.

7. Period of communicability—From the beginning of the prodromal period to 4 days after appearance of the rash.

8. Susceptibility and resistance—Practically all persons are susceptible; permanent acquired immunity is usual after attack. Babies born of mothers who have had the disease are ordinarily immune for roughly the first 6 months of life.

9. Methods of control—

A. Preventive measures:

1) Live attenuated and inactivated measles virus vaccines have been used.

a) Live attenuated vaccine: Several types are in use. A single injection induces active immunity in 95% of susceptible children for over 7 years. Majority have mild or inapparent noncommunicable infection with minimal symptoms: 10–40% develop fever, 103 F rectal, on 4th to 10th day, lasting 2–5 days but little disability; of these, 10–40% have modified measles rash as fever subsides; a few have coryza, mild cough and Koplik spots. Symptoms sharply reduced by measles immune globulin (human) (see 9B5) administered at the same time but at different site with separate syringe; fever exceeding 103 F in 15%, of shorter duration, rash less frequent. Serological conversion the same, but antibody level slightly lower, persisting an observed 4 years and protecting against natural disease for known 3 years. Rare reports of encephalitis or serious reactions in normal children; convulsions uncommon, without known sequelae, probably febrile.

Indications for use: Primarily children with no history of measles, at 12 months of age or as soon thereafter as possible. Adult vaccination rarely indicated, nearly all immune; reactions approximate those of children. Recommended especially for institutionalized children and for those with cystic fibrosis, tuberculosis, heart disease, asthma and other chronic pulmonary diseases.

Contraindications to the use of live attenuated vaccine are: pregnancy, leukemia, lymphomas, other generalized neoplasms; resistance-depressing therapy (steroids, irradiation, alkylating agents, antimetabolites); severe illness; active tuberculosis not under treatment; egg sensitivity; and following transfusion of whole blood or injection of immune serum globulin (human), in which event administration should be delayed 12 weeks.

b) Inactivated vaccine: Use not recommended in the U.S.A. because of short-lived protection and because of unusual and severe reactions observed when individuals inoculated with inactivated vaccine developed natural measles infection later. Live vaccine should be given to prevent this aggravated infection; occasionally followed in 1 to 6 days by localized reaction and possible fever, malaise and regional lymphadenopathy.

2) Education as to special danger of exposing young children to those exhibiting any fever or acute catarrhal symptoms, particularly during years and seasons of epidemic measles.

3) Encouragement by health departments and by private physicians of administration of measles vaccine to all susceptible infants and children. Those under 3 years of age in families or institutions where measles occurs for whom vaccine is contraindicated should be protected by measles immune globulin (human).

B. Control of patient, contacts, and the immediate environment:

1) Report to local health authority: Obligatory case report in most states and in many countries, Class 2B (see Preface). Early report permits better isolation and adequate care for the underprivileged child and provides opportunity for passive protection of contacts.

2) *Isolation:* From diagnosis until 7 days after appearance of rash, to reduce the patient's risk against secondary invaders and to minimize transfer of measles to susceptible contacts, especially children less than 3 years old.

3) *Concurrent disinfection:* All articles soiled with secretions of nose and throat.

4) *Quarantine:* Impractical and of no value in large communities. Exclusion of exposed susceptible school children and teachers from school and from all public gathering until 14 days from the last exposure may be justifiable in sparsely settled, nonendemic rural areas. If date of single exposure is reasonably certain, an exposed susceptible child may be allowed to attend school for the first 7 days of incubation. Quarantine of institutions, wards or dormitories for young children is of value; strict segregation of infants if measles occurs in an institution.

5) *Protection of contacts:* Live attenuated vaccine given before or on the day of exposure usually prevents natural measles; no known adverse effect if given later in incubation period but, in case of delay, administration of measles immune serum globulin (human) especially indicated for children less than 2 years old. Given within 3 days after first exposure to known measles, globulin will avert the attack in most instances and almost certainly modify it; maximum duration of immunity about 3 weeks. Given between 4 and 6 days after 1st exposure, modification may be expected and probably the usual lasting immunity; given after the 6th day, little effect. For protection, the dosage of measles immune globulin (human) is 0.25 ml per kg of body weight; for modification, 0.05 ml per kg.

6) *Investigation of contacts:* Search for exposed susceptible children under 3 years of age is profitable. Carriers are unknown.

7) *Specific treatment:* None. Treat complications with an appropriate antibiotic after bacteriologic confirmation.

C. Epidemic measures:

1) Prompt community vaccination program to cover all potential susceptibles. If vaccination not feasible, daily examination of exposed children and known susceptible adult contacts, with recording of body temperature. Promptly isolate susceptible persons exhibiting a rise of temperature of 0.5 C (1.0 F) or more, pending diagnosis.

2) Schools should not be closed nor classes discontinued; provide daily observation of children by physician or nurse and remove sick children promptly.

3) In institutional outbreaks, protective doses of measles immune serum globulin (human), to all susceptibles whose

vaccination is contraindicated. New admissions should be vaccinated or protected passively.

4) In many less developed countries measles is a highly fatal disease. If vaccine is available, prompt use at the beginning of an epidemic will limit spread, especially among young children to whom risk is greatest.

D. International measures: None.

MELIOIDOSIS

1. Identification—An uncommon disease, with a range of clinical manifestations from inapparent infection to a rapidly fatal septicemia. The picture may simulate typhoid fever or, more commonly, tuberculosis, including pulmonary cavitation, empyema, chronic abscesses, and osteomyelitis.

Diagnosis will depend upon isolation of the causative agent, although acute and convalescent agglutination titers may be of confirmatory value. The possibility of melioidosis should be kept in mind in any unexplained suppurative disease, especially cavitating pulmonary disease, in a patient living in, or recently returned from, Southeast Asia.

2. Occurrence—Clinical disease is uncommon, generally occurring in individuals who have had intimate contact with soil and water. It may appear as a complication of an overt wound or may follow aspiration of water. Cases have been recorded in Southeast Asia, Iran, northeast Australia, Ecuador, Panama, Guam and Aruba. In certain of these areas, 5–10% of agricultural workers have demonstrable antibodies but no history of overt disease.

3. Infectious agent—*Pseudomonas pseudomallei (Loefflerella whitmori),* Whitmore's bacillus.

4. Reservoir—Various animals, including sheep, goats, horses, swine, monkeys and rodents (and a variety of animals in zoological gardens) can become infected. There is no evidence that they are important reservoirs except in transfer of the agent to new foci. The organism is saprophytic in certain soils and waters.

5. Mode of transmission—By contact with contaminated soil or water through overt or inapparent skin wounds, or by aspiration or ingestion of contaminated water.

6. Incubation period—Can be as short as 2 days. However, several months or years may elapse between the presumed exposure and the appearance of clinical disease.

7. Period of communicability—Man-to-man transmission, except by direct inoculation, is not known. Laboratory infections are uncommon.

8. Susceptibility and resistance—Despite close contact with known contaminated soils and waters, disease in man is rare. Many cases have severe associated injuries or burns, or a history of diabetes or other systemic disease.

9. Methods of control—

A. *Preventive measures:* Unknown.

B. *Control of patient, contacts, and the immediate environment:*

1) *Report to local health authority:* Optional report, Class 3B (see Preface).
2) *Isolation:* Wound isolation precautions.
3) *Concurrent disinfection:* None.
4) *Quarantine:* None.
5) *Immunization of contacts:* None.
6) *Investigation of contacts and source of infection:* Human carriers are not known.
7) *Specific treatment: In vitro* tests show susceptibility to sulfonamides, chloramphenicol and tetracyclines, and a favorable outcome may be expected in many subacute and chronic cases. The method of treatment for septicemic cases has not been established, although recovery has been recorded following administration of drug combinations in heroic amounts.

C. *Epidemic measures:* Not applicable to man; a sporadic disease.

D. *International measures:* None, although livestock should be examined for evidence of disease when being moved to non-endemic areas.

GLANDERS

Glanders is a highly communicable disease of horses, mules and donkeys which has disappeared from most areas of the world, although enzootic foci are known to exist in Mexico and Mongolia. Human infection has occurred rarely and sporadically, almost exclusively in those whose occupations involve contact with animals, and laboratory workers. The etiological organism, *Malleomyces mallei (Actinobacillus mallei),* the glanders bacillus, cannot be differentiated serologically from *Pseudomonas pseudomallei;* differentiation from melioidosis can only be accomplished by study of the isolated organism. Prevention depends on control of glanders in the equine species and care in handling organisms. Susceptibility of man is low; cases in man have been rare even among those having close association with infected animals.

MENINGITIS, ASEPTIC

1. Identification—A common nonfatal clinical syndrome with multiple viral etiology characterized by sudden onset of febrile illness with signs and symptoms of meningeal involvement, spinal fluid findings of pleocytosis, usually mononuclear (may be polymorphonuclear in early stages), increased protein, normal or low sugar and absence of bacteria. Active illness seldom exceeds 10 days. Transient paresis and encephalitic manifestations may occur. Paralysis is unusual. Residual signs lasting a year or more may include weakness, muscle spasm, insomnia and personality changes. Recovery is usually complete. Various viral agents cause the syndrome. A morbilliform rash resembling rubella typifies certain types caused by ECHO and Coxsackie viruses. Vesicular and petechial rashes occur. Gastrointestinal symptoms may be associated with the enterovirus group and respiratory manifestations may occur. Synonyms: Nonbacterial or abacterial meningitis, Viral meningitis, Serous meningitis.

Under optimal conditions, specific identification, using serologic and isolation techniques, can be made in more than half of patients. Viral agents may be readily isolated in early stages from specimens of blood, throat washings, stool or spinal fluid by tissue culture techniques or animal inoculation.

Differential diagnosis: Various diseases caused by nonviral agents may mimic aseptic meningitis, such as inadequately treated pyogenic meningitis, tuberculous and cryptococcal meningitis, meningitis caused by other fungal forms, cerebrovascular syphilis and lymphogranuloma venereum. Free-living amebae such as *Naegleria gruberi* have caused a group of fatal meningoencephalitis cases reported from Richmond, Va., Northern Bohemia, and Australia; all had swum in freshwater lakes or swimming pools. Postinfectious and postvaccinal reactions require differentiation, including sequelae to measles, mumps, varicella and variola, and postrabies and post-smallpox vaccination; these syndromes are usually encephalitic in type. Leptospirosis, listeriosis, lymphocytic choriomeningitis, viral hepatitis, infectious mononucleosis, influenza and others require differentiation (see Index).

2. Occurrence—Worldwide distribution, usually as sporadic cases, occasionally in epidemics as with Coxsackie, ECHO and other virus diseases. Actual incidence unknown. Commonly observed when other forms of meningitis are not present in the community.

3. Infectious agents—Caused by a wide variety of infectious agents, many of which are associated with other specific diseases. Many viruses are capable of producing the syndrome. A third or more of cases have no demonstrable agent. Mumps may be responsible for about 25% or more of cases in epidemic periods. In U.S.A., enteroviruses cause most cases; Coxsackie B, types 2, 3, 4, 5 cause about one-third and ECHO types 2, 5, 6, 7, 9 (most), 10, 11, 14, 18 and 30, about 10%. Poliovirus, Coxsackie A, types 2, 3, 7 and 9, arboviruses, measles, herpes simplex and varicella viruses, lymphocytic choriomeningitis, adenovirus and others are responsible for sporadic cases. Incidence of specific types varies with geographic locality and time.

4. Reservoir, 5. Mode of transmission, 6. Incubation period, 7. Period of communicability, 8. Susceptibility and resistance— These features vary with the specific infectious agent. (Refer to specific sections.)

9. Methods of control—

    A. *Preventive measures:* Dependent upon etiology. (See specific diseases.)

    B. *Control of patient, contacts, and the immediate environment:*

        1) *Report to local health authority:* In selected endemic areas (U.S.A.); in many countries not a reportable disease. Class 3B (see Preface). If confirmed by laboratory means, specify the infectious agent; otherwise report as cause undetermined.

        2) *Isolation:* Specific diagnosis depends upon laboratory data not usually available until recovery. Therefore isolate all patients during febrile period.

        3) *Concurrent disinfection:* Includes eating and drinking utensils and articles soiled by secretions and excretions of patient.

        4) *Quarantine:* None.

        5) *Immunization of contacts:* See specific diseases.

        6) *Investigation of contacts:* Not usually indicated.

        7) *Specific treatment:* None for the usual viral agents.

    C. *Epidemic measures:* See specific diseases.

    D. *International measures:* WHO Reference Centres (see Preface).

MENINGITIS, MENINGOCOCCAL

1. Identification—An acute bacterial disease characterized by sudden onset, with fever, intense headache, nausea and often vomiting, stiff neck, and frequently a petechial rash. Pink macules or, very rarely, vesicles may develop. Delirium and coma often appear; occasional fulminating cases exhibit sudden prostration, ecchymoses, collapse and shock at onset. Meningococcemia may occur without extension to the meninges and should be suspected in cases of otherwise unexplained acute febrile illness associated with petechial rash and leucocytosis. Septic monarthritis is not uncommon. Formerly fatality rates exceeded 50% but, with modern therapy and supportive measures, fatality should be less than 5%. In fulminating meningococcemia the death rate is high despite antibacterial treatment; promptness in instituting therapy is essential. There is variation in morbidity and mortality during endemic and epidemic cycles. Synonyms: Cerebrospinal fever, Meningococcal infection, Meningococcemia.

Diagnosis is confirmed by recovery of meningococci on special media from the blood, spinal fluid, and/or posterior nasopharynx. Microscopic examination of stained smears from petechiae may reveal the organism.

Purulent meningitides often are secondary to parameningeal or systemic involvement of the nose, middle ear, mastoid, accessory nasal sinuses, or the lung, endocardium, skin or other site may be involved. Clinical signs and symptoms may be indistinguishable from those caused by meningococci except for the latter's characteristic rash.

Differentiation is based on the results of smears and bacteriologic studies. The commoner infectious agents, which vary in frequency with age, are pneumococci, hemolytic and other streptococci, *Haemophilus influenzae, Staphylococcus aureus, Escherichia coli;* less commonly, but of increasing frequency in recent years, members of the colon-aerogenes-proteus group, *Salmonella, Pseudomonas aeruginosa,* and others.

Several mycoses cause subacute and chronic meningitis. *H. influenzae* meningitis occurs in infants and young children as a primary suppurative meningitis, i.e., without evidence of local or general disease other than of the meninges. Epidemiologic behavior and control are described herein under the individual diseases, e.g., the pneumonias, streptococcal diseases, staphylococcal diseases, and mycoses (see Index). Aseptic meningitis as well as meningismus must be considered.

2. Occurrence—Endemic and epidemic; no limits in geographic distribution. Common in both temperate and tropical climates, with sporadic cases throughout the year in both urban and rural areas and greatest prevalence during winter and spring. At irregular intervals epidemic waves occur, usually lasting 2 to 3 years. Meningococcal infection occurs in children and young adults, in males more than in females, and more commonly in adults under crowded living conditions, such as in barracks and institutions. Large epidemics have occurred in hot dry regions. A broad area of high incidence has existed for many years in the sub-Sahara region of mid-Africa.

3. Infectious agent—*Neisseria meningitidis (N. intracellularis),* the meningococcus. Group A organisms have caused the major epidemics in the U.S.A. and elsewhere; Group B and Group C generally produce sporadic cases and small outbreaks in interepidemic periods. Presently Group B and Group C are responsible for most cases in U.S.A.; Group A in Africa. Additional serogroups have been recognized in recent years but little is known of their importance.

4. Reservoir—Reservoir is man.

5. Mode of transmission—By direct contact, including droplet spread, with discharges from nose and throat of infected persons, more often with carriers rather than cases, causing an acute nasopharyngitis or a subclinical mucosal infection, with comparatively rare invasion sufficient to cause systemic disease. Carrier prevalence of 25% or more may exist without clinical cases. During epidemics more than half of a military unit may be healthy carriers of pathogenic meningococci. Indirect contact is of questionable significance because the meningococcus is highly susceptible to temperature changes and desiccation.

6. Incubation period—Varies from 2 to 10 days, commonly 3 to 4 days.

7. Period of communicability—Until meningococci are no longer present in discharges from nose and mouth. Susceptible meningococci usually disappear from the nasopharynx within 24 hours after institution of appropriate specific treatment.

8. Susceptibility and resistance—Susceptibility to the clinical disease is low, with a high ratio of carriers to cases. Type-specific immunity of unknown duration probably follows even subclinical infection; experimental vaccines are under investigation.

9. Methods of control—

A. Preventive measures:

1) Health education regarding personal hygiene and the necessity of avoiding direct contact or droplet infection.
2) Prevention of overcrowding in living quarters, public transportation, working places and especially in barracks, camps, ships and schools.

B. Control of patient, contacts, and the immediate environment:

1) Report to local health authority: Obligatory case report in most states and countries, Class 2A (see Preface).
2) Isolation: Until 24 hours after start of chemotherapy.
3) Concurrent disinfection: Of discharges from the nose and throat and of articles soiled therewith. Terminal cleaning.
4) Quarantine: No complete quarantine; surveillance is profitable.
5) Immunization of contacts: None available.
6) Investigation of contacts: Impractical.
7) Specific treatment: Penicillin given parenterally in adequate doses is the drug of choice. Parenteral ampicillin is effective; chloramphenicol is effective but should be reserved for penicillin-sensitive patients. If the outbreak is shown to be caused by sulfonamide-sensitive strains, sulfadiazine may be given intravenously; however, sulfonamide-resistant Groups B and C, and recently Group A, strains are commonplace in many parts of the world.

C. Epidemic measures:

1) When an outbreak occurs, major emphasis must be placed on careful surveillance, early diagnosis, and immediate treatment of suspected cases. A high index of suspicion is valuable.
2) Assure the separation of individuals and the ventilation of living and sleeping quarters of all persons who are espe-

cially exposed to infection because of their occupation or congested living conditions.

3) At present no single antimicrobial agent or combination of agents is satisfactory for mass or limited prophylaxis in outbreaks due to sulfonamide-resistant organisms. Because of the current widespread prevalence of sulfonamide-resistant meningococcal strains throughout the world, sulfonamide prophylaxis should not be instituted unless fewer than 5% of the strains obtained from a statistically valid sample of the carrier population show sulfonamide resistance (resistant strains are those resistant to more than 0.1 mg of sulfadiazine per 100 ml).

When the epidemic strain is sulfonamide-sensitive, mass chemoprophylaxis with sulfadiazine (0.5 g for children, 1.0 g for adults, every 12 hours, for 4 doses) reduces the carrier rate and limits spread of the disease in institutional and military outbreaks when entire community is treated. Piecemeal use through limitation to direct contacts or selected segment of a population serves no useful purpose and encourages the emergence of resistant strains. No satisfactory prophylactic agent exists for populations harboring a large proportion of resistant strains.

D. International measures: WHO Reference Centres (see Preface).

MONONUCLEOSIS, INFECTIOUS

1. Identification—An acute infectious disease characterized by irregular fever; sore throat (often with exudative pharyngotonsillitis) ; lymphadenopathy, especially posterior cervical; splenomegaly; and lymphocytosis exceeding 50%, including abnormal forms, and occasionally rash. In children, it is generally mild and difficult to recognize. Jaundice occurs in about 4% of young adult patients. Duration is from 1 to several weeks, rarely fatal. Synonyms: Glandular fever, Monocytic angina.

Laboratory diagnosis includes examination of blood smears for abnormal lymphocytes, tests for elevated sheep cell heterophile antibodies or tests for ox cell hemolysins. Liver function tests are also helpful.

2. Occurrence—Worldwide, usually as sporadic cases and localized epidemics; most commonly recognized in college students and hospital personnel. Probably common and widespread in childhood. In temperate climates, greatest incidence from October through May.

3. Infectious agent—A virus closely related to that of herpes morphologically, but distinct serologically. This virus is identical with or very closely related to virus isolated from Burkitt's tumor.

4. Reservoir—Reservoir apparently limited to man.

5. Mode of transmission—Unknown; probably person-to-person, spread by an oral-pharyngeal route. Kissing may facilitate spread among young adults.

6. Incubation period—Seemingly varies from 2 to 6 weeks.

7. Period of communicability—Unknown but presumably from before symptoms appear to end of fever and clearing of the oral-pharyngeal lesions.

8. Susceptibility and resistance—Susceptibility apparently general but incidence greatest among children and young adults. Infection appears to confer high degree of resistance; persistence of resistance from unrecognized childhood infection may account for low communicability among adults.

9. Methods of control—

A. *Preventive measures:* None.

B. *Control of patient, contacts, and the immediate environment:*
  1) *Report to local health authority:* Obligatory report of epidemics; no individual case report, Class 4 (see Preface).
  2) *Isolation:* None.
  3) *Concurrent disinfection:* Of articles soiled with nose and throat discharges.
  4) *Quarantine:* None.
  5) *Immunization of contacts:* None.
  6) *Investigation of contacts:* For the individual case, of little value.
  7) *Specific treatment:* None.

C. *Epidemic measures:* Field investigation of epidemics should be undertaken with the hope of adding to knowledge of the disease.

D. *International measures:* None.

MUCORMYCOSIS

1. Identification—A mycosis caused by members of the family *Mucoraceae* of the class *Phycomycetes*. These fungi have an affinity for blood vessels, causing thrombosis and infarction. Craniofacial form of disease usually presents as nasal or paranasal sinus infection, most often during diabetic acidosis. Gangrene of the turbinates, perforation of the hard palate, gangrene of the cheek, or orbital cellulitis, proptosis, and ophthalmoplegia may occur. Infection may penetrate to frontal lobe of brain, causing infarction. In the pulmonary form of disease.

the fungus causes thrombosis of pulmonary blood vessels and infarcts of the lung. In the gastrointestinal form, mucosal ulcers or thromboses and gangrene of stomach or bowel may occur.

Diagnosis confirmed by microscopic demonstration of distinctive broad, nonseptate hyphae in biopsies and by culture of biopsy tissue. Wet preparations and smears may be examined. Cultures alone are not diagnostic because these *Phycomycetes* are frequent in the environment as bread or fruit molds. Synonym: Phycomycosis. (See below.)

2. Occurrence—Infection is worldwide. Incidence is increasing because of longer survival of patients with diabetes mellitus and certain blood dyscrasias, especially leukemia.

3. Infectious agent—Species of *Rhizopus,* especially *Rhizopus oryzae* and *Rhizopus arrhizus,* have caused most of the craniofacial cases of mucormycosis from which the fungus has been cultured. Probably *Rhizopus* is the chief cause of the pulmonary and gastrointestinal forms of mucormycosis. *Mucor, Mortierella,* and *Absidia* have been reported from a few human cases of mucormycosis.

4. Reservoir—*Mucoraceae* are common saprophytes in the environment.

5. Mode of transmission—By inspiration or ingestion of fungus by susceptible individuals. Direct inoculation by minor trauma; intravenous catheter or cutaneous burns occasionally implicated.

6. Incubation period—One or 2 days. Fungus spreads rapidly in susceptible tissues.

7. Period of communicability—Not directly transmitted from man or animal to man.

8. Susceptibility and resistance—Scarcity of infection in healthy individuals despite abundance of *Mucoraceae* in environment indicates natural resistance. Corticosteroid therapy and bone marrow depressants predispose. Malnutrition predisposes to gastrointestinal form.

9. Methods of control—

> A. *Preventive measures:* Optimal control of diabetes mellitus. Avoid overtreatment of blood dyscrasias.
>
> B. *Control of patient, contacts, and the immediate environment:*
>
> > 1) *Report to local health authority:* Official report ordinarily not justifiable, Class 5 (see Preface).
> > 2) *Isolation:* None.
> > 3) *Concurrent disinfection:* Ordinary cleanliness. Terminal cleaning.
> > 4) *Quarantine:* None
> > 5) *Immunization of contacts:* None.
> > 6) *Investigation of contacts:* Ordinarily not profitable.
> > 7) *Specific treatment:* In cranial form, control of diabetic

acidosis, amphotericin B (Fungizone) and resection of necrotic tissue have been helpful.

C. Epidemic measures: Not applicable, a sporadic disease.

D. International measures: None.

PHYCOMYCOSIS designates all infections caused by fungi of the class *Phycomycetes.* This includes mucormycosis, subcutaneous phycomycosis and rhinoentomophthoromycosis. The latter two have been recognized principally in tropical and subtropical Asia and Africa, are not characterized by thromboses or infarction, do not usually occur in association with serious preexisting disease, do not usually cause disseminated disease, and seldom cause death.

SUBCUTANEOUS PHYCOMYCOSIS is a granulomatous inflammation caused by *Basidiobolus meristosporus,* a ubiquitous fungus occurring in decaying vegetation, soil and the gastrointestinal tract of reptiles. Disease presents as a firm subcutaneous mass, fixed to the skin, principally in children and adolescents, more commonly in males. Infection may heal spontaneously. Recommended therapy is oral iodide.

RHINOENTOMOPHTHOROMYCOSIS usually originates in the nasal mucosa and presents as nasal obstruction or swelling of the nose or adjacent structures. Lesions of the mucosa of the palate and pharynx also occur. Disease is uncommon, occurs principally in adult males. Recommended therapy is oral iodide or intravenous amphotericin B (Fungizone). The infectious agent, *Entomophthora coronata,* occurring in soil and decaying vegetation, also causes disease in insects. For both subcutaneous phycomycosis and rhinoentomophthoromycosis, incubation period and mode of transmission are unknown. Man-to-man transmission does not occur.

MUMPS

1. Identification—An acute viral disease characterized by fever, and by swelling and tenderness of one or more salivary glands, usually the parotid, sometimes the sublingual or submaxillary glands. Orchitis occurs in 20–35% of males and oophoritis in about 5% of females past puberty; sterility may follow orchitis. Pancreatitis, neuritis, arthritis, mastitis, and pericarditis may occur. The central nervous system is frequently involved either early or late in the disease. Orchitis and meningoencephalitis due to mumps virus may occur without involvement of a salivary gland. Death from mumps is exceedingly rare. Synonym: Infectious parotitis.

Serological tests are of value in confirming diagnosis. Virus may be isolated in chick embryo or cell cultures from saliva, blood, urine and cerebrospinal fluid during the acute phase of the disease.

2. **Occurrence**—Classical mumps is of less regular occurrence than other common communicable diseases of childhood, such as measles and chickenpox. About one-third of exposed susceptible persons have inapparent infections. Winter and spring are seasons of greatest prevalence; sporadic and epidemic except in large cities where the disease is endemic. Outbreaks are frequent and serious in aggregations of young adults.

3. **Infectious agent**—The virus of mumps, a myxovirus antigenically related to the parainfluenza group.

4. **Reservoir**—Man is the reservoir.

5. **Mode of transmission**—By droplet spread and by direct contact with saliva of an infected person, or indirectly through articles freshly soiled with saliva of such persons.

6. **Incubation period**—12 to 26 days, commonly 18 days.

7. **Period of communicability**—The virus has been isolated from saliva from 6 days before salivary gland involvement to as long as 9 days thereafter, but the height of infectiousness occurs about 48 hours before swelling commences. Urine positive as long as 14 days after onset of illness. Persons with inapparent infection can be infectious.

8. **Susceptibility and resistance**—Susceptibility is general. Immunity generally held to be lifelong and develops after inapparent as well as clinical attacks. The currently available skin test is not a reliable index of immunity.

9. **Methods of control**—

    A. *Preventive measures:* Live attenuated vaccine prepared in chick embryo cell culture is available. Protection against natural infection has continued for 4 years, and, in limited observations, antibody levels have persisted without decline. This vaccine is useful for children more than 12 months of age (to avoid interference by maternal antibody) and is of particular value in children approaching puberty, for adolescents and adults (especially males) who have not had mumps, and selected groups of susceptibles in the military or labor force likely to be exposed to the disease for a limited time. Withhold from egg- and neomycin-sensitive individuals, from patients with severe underlying disease such as lymphomas or generalized malignancies, from those on steroids, antimetabolites, alkylating drugs, and from those receiving radiation therapy.

    B. *Control of patient, contacts, and the immediate environment:*

        1) Report to local health authority: Selectively reportable. Class 3C (see Preface).

        2) Isolation: For 9 days from onset of swelling; less if swelling has subsided.

3) *Concurrent disinfection:* Of articles soiled with secretions of nose and throat.

4) *Quarantine:* None.

5) *Immunization of contacts:* Whether protection results from vaccination after exposure to natural mumps is not known; however, vaccination is not contraindicated under such conditions. Mumps hyperimmune globulin is of questionable effectiveness when administered following exposure.

6) *Investigation of contacts:* Not profitable.

7) *Specific treatment:* None.

C. Epidemic measures: Vaccination of susceptibles, especially those at risk of exposure.

D. International measures: None.

MYCETOMA

1. Identification—A clinical syndrome of diverse etiology characterized by swelling and suppuration of subcutaneous tissues, formation of sinus tracts and presence of small colonies of fungus (granules) in pus from sinus tracts. Lesions usually are on the foot or lower leg, sometimes on the hand, over the shoulders and back in burden bearers, and rarely in other sites. Synonym: Madura foot.

Isolation of the fungus in culture and study of the granules in fresh preparations or histopathologic slides are necessary for conclusive identification.

2. Occurrence—Rare in continental U.S.A.; common in Mexico, northern Africa, southern Asia and other tropical and subtropical areas, especially where people go barefoot.

3. Infectious agents—Actinomycetic mycetoma is caused by *Nocardia brasiliensis, Nocardia asteroides, Streptomyces madurae, Streptomyces pelletieri* or *Streptomyces somaliensis.* Mycotic mycetoma is caused by *Madurella mycetomi, Madurella grisea, Allescheria boydii (Monosporium apiospermum), Phialophora jeanselmei, Cephalosporium recifei, Cephalosporium falciforme, Leptosphaeria senegalensis, Neotestudina rosatii,* and *Pyrenochaeta romeroi.*

4. Reservoir—Presumably soil and decaying vegetation.

5. Mode of transmission—Subcutaneous implantation by penetrating wounds (thorns, splinters) of spores or hyphal elements from a saprophytic source.

6. Incubation period—Usually months.

7. Period of communicability—Not directly transmitted from man to man.

8. Susceptibility and resistance—Unknown.

9. **Methods of control—**

A. *Preventive measures:* Protection against small puncture wounds, as by wearing shoes or protective clothing.

B. *Control of patient, contacts, and the immediate environment:*

1) *Report to local health authority:* Official report ordinarily not justifiable, Class 5 (see Preface).

2) *Isolation:* None.

3) *Concurrent disinfection:* Ordinary cleanliness.

4) *Quarantine:* None.

5) *Immunization of contacts:* None.

6) *Investigation of contacts and source of infection:* Not profitable.

7) *Specific treatment:* None. Sulfones, long-acting sulfonamides, benefit some cases of actinomycetic mycetoma. Penicillin and other antibiotics are not useful. Intravenous or locally injected amphotericin B (Fungizone) may benefit an occasional case of mycotic mycetoma. Amputation of an extremity with advanced lesions may be required.

C. *Epidemic measures:* Not applicable, a sporadic disease.

D. *International measures:* WHO Reference Centres (see Preface).

NOCARDIOSIS

1. **Identification**—A chronic mycotic disease often initiated in the lungs, with hematogenous spread to produce abscesses of brain, subcutaneous tissue and other organs; high case fatality. The frequent occurrence of *Nocardia asteroides* in chronic pulmonary disease of other origin may represent a mild form of nocardiosis. Other species of *Nocardia* cause mycetoma (see p. 160), including a species indistinguishable from *N. asteroides*.

Microscopic examination of stained smears of sputum, pus or spinal fluid reveals partially acid-fast, branching hyphae; confirmation is by culture and pathogenicity for animals.

2. **Occurrence**—Occasional sporadic disease in man and animals in all parts of the world. No evidence of age, sex, or racial differences.

3. **Infectious agent**—*Nocardia asteroides,* an actinomycete.

4. **Reservoir**—Reservoir is soil.

5. **Mode of transmission**—Direct contact with contaminated soil through sometimes minor wounds and abrasions; pulmonary infections presumably occur through inhalation of organisms suspended in dust.

6. Incubation period—Unknown; probably weeks.

7. Period of communicability—Not directly transmitted from man or animals to man.

8. Susceptibility and resistance—Unknown.

9. Methods of control—

A. *Preventive measures:* None.

B. *Control of patient, contacts, and the immediate environment:*

1) Report to local health authority: Official report not ordinarily justifiable, Class 5 (see Preface).

2) Isolation: None.

3) Concurrent disinfection: Of discharges and contaminated dressings.

4) Quarantine: None.

5) Immunization of contacts: None.

6) Investigation of contacts: Not profitable.

7) Specific treatment: Sulfonamides in high doses are effective in systemic infections if given early and for prolonged periods.

C. *Epidemic measures:* Not applicable, a sporadic disease.

D. *International measures:* None.

ONCHOCERCIASIS

1. Identification—A chronic, nonfatal filarial disease with fibrous nodules in skin and subcutaneous tissues, particularly of head and shoulders (America) or pelvic girdle and lower extremities (Africa). The female worm discharges microfilariae which migrate through the skin, causing loss of skin elasticity. Microfilariae frequently reach the eye, causing ocular disturbances and blindness. Indurated, pigmented and inflamed lesions of the skin often occur.

Laboratory diagnosis is by superficial biopsy of skin with demonstration of microfilariae in fresh preparations by microscopic examination; by excision of nodule and finding adult worms; in ocular manifestations, by observation with ophthalmic microscope of microfilariae in cornea, anterior chamber or vitreous body.

Differentiation from other filarial diseases is required in endemic areas; filariasis (see p. 87), loiasis (see p. 135), dracontiasis (see p. 82), and others.

2. Occurrence—Geographical distribution in Western Hemisphere limited to Guatemala (principally western slope of continental divide), southern Mexico (states of Chiapas and Oaxaca), northern Venezuela and a very small area in Colombia; in Africa from Sierra Leone, south to Angola, and eastward in the area south of the Sahara through the

Republic of the Congo to Zambia, Malawi, Kenya, Uganda, Ethiopia and Sudan. In some localities, almost all of the population is infected.

3. Infectious agent—*Onchocerca volvulus,* a nematode worm.

4. Reservoir—Reservoir is infected persons.

5. Mode of transmission—By bite of infected black flies of the genus *Simulium* in Guatemala and Mexico; *Simulium ochraceum, Simulium callidum, Simulium metallicum,* and possibly other species; in Africa *Simulium damnosum* and *Simulium neavei.* Microfilariae penetrate thoracic muscles of the vector, develop into infective larvae, migrate to proboscis, and are liberated in the skin of man as the insect feeds.

6. Incubation period—Nodules commonly become visible after 3 to 4 months. Worms begin to discharge larvae 1 year or more after infection.

7. Period of communicability—Man infects flies as long as living microfilariae persist in the skin; probably for years. In Africa, vector is infective after 6 days; in Guatemala, measurably longer, up to 14 days, because of lower temperatures. Not directly transmitted from man to man.

8. Susceptibility and resistance—Susceptibility is universal.

9. Methods of control—

A. Preventive measures:

1) Avoid bites of *Simulium* flies by covering body and head as much as possible; or by use of an insect repellent, such as diethyltoluamide.
2) Control of vector larvae in rapidly running streams and in artificial waterways by DDT or other insecticide, and sometimes of adult *Simulium,* by aerial spray; feasibility depends on vector and terrain.
3) Provision of facilities for diagnosis and treatment.

B. Control of patient, contacts, and the immediate environment:

1) *Report to local health authority:* Official report not ordinarily justifiable, Class 5 (see Preface).
2) *Isolation:* None.
3) *Concurrent disinfection:* None
4) *Quarantine:* None.
5) *Immunization of contacts:* None.
6) *Investigation of contacts:* A community problem (see 9A).
7) *Specific treatment:* Diethylcarbamazine (Hetrazan) is useful, but causes severe reactions due to destruction of larvae; does not kill adult worms. Suramin sodium (Naphuride, Antrypol), which is available in the U.S.A. from the National Communicable Disease Center, Atlanta, Ga., kills the adult worms and leads to gradual disappearance of microfilariae; undesirable reactions may occur and

require close medical supervision. Neither drug is suited to mass treatment. Excision of nodules to eliminate adult worms reduces symptoms.

C. *Epidemic measures:* In areas of high prevalence make concerted effort to reduce incidence, taking measures listed under 9A.

D. *International measures:* Coordinated programs entered into by neighboring countries where the disease is endemic, designed to prevent migration of infected persons across international boundaries and to institute treatment and other control measures near such boundaries. WHO Reference Centres (see Preface).

PARAGONIMIASIS

1. Identification—Clinical manifestations of this trematode disease depend on path of migration and organs parasitized. Lungs are most frequently involved; symptoms are cough and hemoptysis. Worms become surrounded by an inflammatory reaction which eventually organizes into a fibrous, cystic lesion. Roentgenographic findings often closely simulate pulmonary tuberculosis. Development in other organs not infrequent, with worms maturing in such sites as intestinal wall, lymph nodes, genitourinary tract, subcutaneous tissue and brain. Infection usually lasts for many years, although patients often appear surprisingly well. Synonyms: Pulmonary distomiasis, Endemic hemoptysis, Lung fluke disease.

The sputum generally contains flecks of orange-brown pigment, sometimes diffusely distributed, in which masses of worm eggs are seen microscopically. Eggs are also found in feces, rarely in urine.

2. Occurrence—Extensive in the Far East, particularly Korea, Japan, Taiwan, scattered foci in Philippines, parts of mainland China, Southeast Asia, Africa and South America.

3. Infectious agent—*Paragonimus westermani,* a trematode, in the Orient; other species in Africa and South America.

4. Reservoir—Man, dog, cat, pig, and wild carnivores are definitive hosts and act as reservoirs.

5. Mode of transmission—Infection occurs when the flesh of fresh water crabs such as *Eriocheir* and *Potamon* and of crayfish such as *Cambaroides* containing infective larvae (metacercariae) is ingested raw, or partially cooked, by a susceptible mammal. The larvae emerge in the duodenum, penetrate the intestinal wall, migrate through the tissues, encyst in pairs, and develop into egg-producing adults. Eggs leave the definitive host via sputum and feces, gain entrance to fresh water, and embryonate in 2 to 4 weeks. A larva (miracidium) hatches and penetrates a suitable fresh water snail (*Semisulcospira, Thiara* or other species) and undergoes a cycle of development of approximately 3 months. Larvae (cercariae) emerge from the snail and penetrate and encyst in fresh water crustacea.

6. Incubation period—Flukes mature and begin to lay eggs approximately 6 weeks after man ingests infective larvae. The interval until symptoms appear is long, variable, poorly defined and depends on the organ involved.

7. Period of communicability—Eggs may be discharged by the human host for 20 years or more; duration of infection in mollusk and crustacean hosts unknown. Not directly transmitted from man to man.

8. Susceptibility and resistance—Susceptibility is general. Increased resistance possibly develops as a result of infection.

9. Methods of control—

A. Preventive measures:
1) Health education of people in endemic areas concerning the life cycle of the parasite; stress thorough cooking of crustacea.
2) Sanitary disposal of sputum and feces.
3) Control of snails by molluscicides is feasible in some areas, as well as destruction of crabs. Dinitro-o-cyclohexylphenol is effective against both amphibian and aquatic snails.

B. Control of patient, contacts, and the immediate environment:
1) *Report to local health authority:* Official report not ordinarily justifiable, Class 5 (see Preface).
2) *Isolation:* None.
3) *Concurrent disinfection:* Of sputum and feces.
4) *Quarantine:* None.
5) *Immunization of contacts:* None.
6) *Investigation of contacts:* None.
7) *Specific treatment:* Bithionol, available in U.S.A. from the Parasitic Disease Drug Service, National Communicable Disease Center, Atlanta, Ga., gives good results and is the drug of choice. Both emetine hydrochloride and chloroquine (Aralen) produce clinical improvement and an occasional cure.

C. Epidemic measures: In an endemic area, occurrence of small clusters of cases or even sporadic infections is an important signal for examination of local waters for infected snails, crabs and crayfish, and determination of reservoir mammalian hosts.

D. International measures: None.

PARATYPHOID FEVER

1. Identification—A generalized bacterial disease, often with abrupt onset, continued fever, involvement of lymphoid tissues of mesentery and of intestines, enlargement of spleen, sometimes rose spots on trunk, and usually diarrhea. While clinically similar, fatality is much lower than for typhoid fever. Many mild attacks are no more than a transient diarrhea (see p. 214 for Salmonella gastroenteritis).

Laboratory confirmation and individual type distinction is by bacteriologic examination of blood, feces and urine.

2. Occurrence—Occurs sporadically or in limited outbreaks. Probably more frequent than reports suggest because of the large number of unrecognized cases. In U.S.A., paratyphoid fever is not frequently identified; of the 3 varieties, paratyphoid B is commonest, A less frequent and C extremely rare. In Europe, incidence of paratyphoid A and B is somewhat greater, with C common in Eastern Europe and Asia.

3. Infectious agents—*Salmonella paratyphi, Salmonella schottmuelleri, Salmonella hirschfeldii* (paratyphoid bacilli A, B, and C), all of human origin; a number of phage types can be distinguished. A bacteremic infection with similar clinical reaction may be induced by any *Salmonella* of the group pathogenic for both man and animals.

4. Reservoir—Reservoir is man, both patients and carriers, with temporary carriers often frequent in epidemics.

5. Mode of transmission—Direct or indirect contact with feces or urine of patient or carrier. Vehicles of indirect spread are food, especially milk, milk products and shellfish, usually contaminated by hands of a carrier or missed case. Under some conditions, flies are vectors. A few outbreaks are related to water supplies.

6. Incubation period—One to 3 weeks for enteric fever, 1–10 days for gastroenteritis; somewhat longer for paratyphoid A than for B and C.

7. Period of communicability—As long as the infectious agent persists in excreta; usually from appearance of prodromal symptoms, throughout illness, and for varying periods after recovery.

8. Susceptibility and resistance—Susceptibility is general. Some species-specific immunity usually follows recovery.

9. Methods of control—

    A. Preventive measures: The preventive measures applicable to paratyphoid fever are those listed under Typhoid fever, 9A, 1–9 (see pp. 272–273).

    B. Control of patient, contacts, and the immediate environment:

        1) Report to local health authority: Case report in most states and countries, both suspect and confirmed infections, Class 2A (see Preface).

        2) Isolation: Exclusion of infected persons from food handling and from patient care and occupations involving nursing care of young children and the elderly until cultures of feces are free from *Salmonella* for at least 3 successive days.

3) *Concurrent disinfection:* Of feces and urine and of articles soiled therewith. In communities with a modern and adequate sewage disposal system, feces can be discharged directly into sewer without preliminary disinfection. Terminal cleaning.

4) *Quarantine:* Family contacts should not be employed as food handlers during period of contact with patient or carrier.

5) *Immunization of contacts:* None.

6) *Investigation of contacts:* Bacteriological investigation, especially of family contacts, for unrecognized mild cases and carriers. See (2) above.

7) *Specific treatment:* For overt enteric fever or septicemia, chloramphenicol is the drug of choice; ampicillin is the preferred alternative, but if it is necessary to use other antibiotics, sensitivity tests should be performed.

C. Epidemic measures: Those for Typhoid Fever, 9C (p. 274).

D. International measures: WHO Reference Centres (see Preface).

PEDICULOSIS

1. Identification—Infestation of the scalp, of the hairy parts of the body, or of clothing, especially along the seams of inner surfaces, with adult lice, larvae, or nits (eggs). Crab lice usually infest the pubic area. They may infest eyelashes. Synonym: Lousiness.

Identification is by direct microscopic examination of the louse.

2. Occurrence—Worldwide. The head louse is common in outbreaks among school children.

3. Infesting agents—*Pediculus humanus capitis,* the head louse, and *P. humanus humanus,* the body louse. Animal lice do not infest man.

4. Reservoir—Reservoir is infested persons.

5. Mode of transmission—Direct contact with an infested person and indirectly by contact with their personal belongings, especially their clothing and headgear.

6. Incubation period—Under optimum conditions the eggs of lice hatch in a week, and sexual maturity is reached in approximately 2 weeks.

7. Period of communicability—While lice remain alive on the infested person or in his clothing, and until eggs in hair and clothing have been destroyed.

8. Susceptibility and resistance—Any person may become lousy under suitable conditions of exposure. Repeated infestations often result in dermal hypersensitivity.

9. Methods of control—

A. Preventive measures:

1) Health education of the public in the value of using hot water and soap to maintain cleanliness, and laundering of clothing to destroy nits and lice.

2) Direct inspection of heads and, when necessary, of body and clothing, particularly of children in schools, institutions and summer camps.

B. Control of infested persons, contacts, and the immediate environment:

1) Report to local health authority: Official report not ordinarily justifiable; school authorities should be informed, Class 5 (see Preface).

2) Isolation: Not necessary after application of effective insecticide.

3) Concurrent disinfection: Of members of family or group.

4) Quarantine: None.

5) Immunization of contacts: Does not apply.

6) Investigation of contacts: Examination of household and other close personal contacts, with concurrent treatment as indicated.

7) Specific treatment: 10% DDT dusting powder for body and head lice; dust clothing, particularly along seams, and the hair; cover head with towel or cap for several hours; comb hair with fine tooth comb; repeat dusting in a week without washing hair or clothing in the interim. For crab lice, dust hairy parts of body and bathe after 12 to 24 hours; repeat treatment in one week; continue treatment at weekly intervals until lice or nits are no longer present.

For DDT-resistant lice, gamma benzene hexachloride (Lindane), 1% dusting powder or 1% ointment (Kwell), may be substituted; also effective and acceptable for head lice. No more than 60g as a 1% preparation should be used per person within a 7-day period, and should not be used in conjunction with insect repellents or other oily liquids applied to the skin. The insecticide Abate, which is nontoxic to man, is under evaluation.

C. Epidemic measures: Mass treatment as recommended in 9B7.

D. International measures: None.

PINTA

1. Identification—An acute and chronic nonvenereal treponematosis. Within 7 to 20 days after skin infection a scaling papule appears, usually on hands, legs or dorsum of feet, with a satellite bubo. In 5 to 12 months a maculopapular, erythematous secondary rash appears and may evolve into tertiary lesions, the dyschromic stage, with achromic or pigmented (blue, pink, yellow, violet) spots of variable size, mainly on distal portions of extremities but often including trunk and face. In rare instances the untreated disease may end fatally. Synonyms: Carate, Tina, Lota, Azul, and others.

Organisms demonstrable in lesions by dark-field examination. Serologic tests for syphilis usually become reactive during secondary rash and thereafter behave as in venereal syphilis.

2. Occurrence—Frequent among dark-skinned people of tropics and subtropics; in Western Hemisphere among Negroes, native Indians and those of mixed blood. Especially prevalent in Mexico, Colombia, Venezuela, and Ecuador. Pinta-like conditions are reported from east and west coasts of Africa, North Africa, the Middle East, and in India and the Philippines. Predominantly a disease of childhood.

3. Infectious agent—*Treponema carateum*, a spirochete.

4. Reservoir—Reservoir is man.

5. Mode of transmission—Unknown; evidence suggests transmission by direct and indirect contact with initial skin lesions and those of early dyschromic stage; location of primary lesions suggests an influence of trauma. Various biting and sucking arthropods have been implicated; rare reports of venereal and congenital transmission.

6. Incubation period—Seven to 20 days.

7. Period of communicability—Unknown; potentially communicable while skin lesions are active, sometimes for many years.

8. Susceptibility and resistance—Undefined; presumably as in other treponematoses. Rare in white persons, suggesting some natural resistance, but not distinguished clearly from factors of personal hygiene and social and economic status.

9. Methods of control—

    A. Preventive measures: Those applicable to other nonvenereal treponematoses apply to pinta, see Yaws 9A (pp. 285–286).

    B. Control of patient, contacts, and the immediate environment:

        1) Report to local health authority: In selected endemic areas; in most countries not a reportable disease, Class 3B (see Preface).

        2) Items 2 to 7: See Yaws 9B (p. 286).

    C. Epidemic measures: See Yaws 9C (p. 286).

    D. International measures: See Yaws 9D (p. 286).

PLAGUE

1. Identification—A highly infectious disease characterized classically by lymphadenitis, septicemia and petechial hemorrhages, often with toxemia, high fever, shock, fall in blood pressure, rapid and irregular pulse, restlessness, staggering gait, mental confusion, prostration, delirium and coma. Plague occurs mainly in three clinical forms: (a) *Bubonic plague,* the most common, with acutely inflamed and painful swellings of lymph nodes draining the site of original infection. Secondary invasion of the blood often leads to localized infection in diverse parts of the body including the meninges. A secondary, often terminal pneumonia has special significance as the means by which primary pneumonic plague is engendered. (b) *Primary septicemic plague,* proved by blood smear or blood culture, is rare; it is a form of bubonic plague in which the bubo is obscure and includes pharyngeal and tonsillar infections. (c) *Primary pneumonic plague* is the most serious form. It occurs in localized and sometimes devastating epidemics among persons living under crowded conditions. Untreated bubonic plague has a case fatality rate commonly reported to be 25 to 50%; occasionally it is no more than a localized infection of short duration (pestis minor). Untreated primary septicemic plague and pneumonic plague are usually fatal. Modern therapy materially reduces the case fatality rate of bubonic plague; pneumonic and septicemic plague also respond if recognized and treated early.

Diagnosis is confirmed by demonstrating the agent in fluid from buboes, in blood, spinal fluid or sputum. Fully virulent plague organisms have been recovered from throat cultures of apparently healthy contacts of plague patients. This temporary carrier state is not necessarily followed by overt disease, even in the absence of drug prophylaxis.

2. Occurrence—Sylvatic (wild rodent) plague is known to exist in the western third of U.S.A., in large areas of South America, in central and southern Africa, in the Near East, in Iranian Kurdistan and the frontier area between Yemen and Saudi Arabia, in Central and in parts of Southeast Asia. Plague in man in U.S.A. is limited to rare instances of exposure to wild rodents or their fleas. Urban plague has been controlled in most of the world. Rural bubonic plague of rat origin, until recently a serious health problem in India and Burma, presently shows a marked decline. However, epidemics have recently occurred in Indonesia and Nepal; since 1962 South Vietnam has experienced a marked increase in plague, with several thousands of cases of bubonic plague, both urban and rural, and scattered cases of pneumonic plague. In many areas of the world, plague continues to be potentially dangerous because of vast areas of persisting wild rodent infection and commingling of wild rodents with domestic rats.

3. Infectious agent—*Pasteurella pestis,* the plague bacillus.

4. Reservoir—Wild rodents and less often rabbits (lagomorpha) are natural reservoirs of plague; numerous species of rodents in many parts of the world are subject to periodic epizootics. The infection may transfer to domestic rats in urban or rural areas where rats and wild rodents commingle.

5. Mode of transmission—Bubonic plague is transmitted by the bite of an infective (blocked) flea, *Xenopsylla cheopis* (the oriental rat flea) and other species, or by handling the tissues, or from contact with the pus, of an infected animal. Pneumonic plague (and pharyngeal plague) are spread by the airborne route or by contact with exhaled droplets or sputum from patients with primary pneumonic plague or from patients with bubonic plague or from patients with bubonic plague who develop terminal plague pneumonia. Accidental infections may occur among laboratory workers.

6. Incubation period—From 2 to 6 days in bubonic plague; 3 to 4 days in pneumonic plague; may be shorter, rarely longer.

7. Period of communicability—Bubonic plague is not directly transmitted from person to person except through terminal plague pneumonia. Fleas may remain infected for days or weeks or months under suitable conditions of temperature and humidity, or may clear themselves of infection; infective (blocked) fleas are short-lived (3 to 4 days). Pneumonic plague is usually highly communicable under climatic or social conditions which lead to overcrowding, especially in unsanitary dwellings.

8. Susceptibility and resistance—Susceptibility is general. Immunity after recovery is temporary and relative.

9. Methods of control—

A. Preventive measures:

1) Active immunization with a vaccine of killed bacteria may confer some protection for several months when administered in 2 or 3 doses at weekly intervals; repeated booster injections are necessary for continued protection. Vaccination of persons traveling or living in areas of high incidence and of laboratory workers handling plague bacilli is justifiable but not to be relied upon as the principal preventive measure.

2) Periodic surveys in endemic and potentially epidemic areas to determine prevalence of rats and rat fleas; decrease attractiveness for rats by good housekeeping, e.g., control of food, garbage and refuse; suppress rats by poisoning or trapping in urban areas (see 9B6 below) ; continue inspection and survey of wild rodents and their ectoparasites in areas of known sylvatic plague. Where plague is present or threatening, a systematic search for infected fleas and serologic surveys of rodents can further delineate the extent of the problem.

3) Ratproofing of buildings and reduction of breeding places and harborages, particularly on docks and in warehouses.

4) Rat control on ships by ratproofing or periodic fumiga-

tion, combined when necessary with destruction of rats and their fleas in vessels, and in cargoes before shipment, especially containerized cargoes, and on arrival from plague localities.

5) Health education of the public in endemic areas on mode of transmission and protective measures against fleas and rats.

B. Control of patient, contacts, and the immediate environment:

1) *Report to local health authority:* Case report of suspect and confirmed cases universally required by International Sanitary and Health Regulations, Class 1 (see Preface).

2) *Isolation:* Rid patient, and especially his clothing and baggage, of fleas with an insecticide of tested effectiveness against local fleas, and hospitalize if practical; ordinary hospital isolation precautions suffice for patients with bubonic plague; strict isolation with precautions against airborne spread is required for patients with primary pneumonic plague or patients developing plague pneumonia until effective antibiotic therapy has been established.

3) *Concurrent disinfection:* Of sputum and purulent discharges, and articles soiled therewith, and with urine and feces of patients. Terminal cleaning. Bodies of persons dying of plague should be handled with strict aseptic precautions.

4) *Quarantine:* For contacts of bubonic plague, disinfestation with insecticide powder and surveillance for 6 days. For close contacts of pneumonic plague, dust with insecticide powder, institute chemoprophylaxis (9B5) and maintain surveillance for 6 days, observing closely for developing illness; hospitalize and start additional specific therapy as soon as fever or other clinical symptoms appear. (Contacts who have been taking antimalarial prophylaxis should continue this.)

5) *Protection of contacts:* The management of contacts should concentrate on surveillance and close observation, with prompt institution of specific treatment at first appearance of fever or other signs of disease. Close contacts of pneumonic cases should be given chemoprophylaxis and be observed closely. Chemoprophylaxis may be effected with broad-spectrum antibiotics such as tetracycline, 1.0 g per day for adults; or sulfonamides, 2.0 to 3.0 g per day, for 6 days. Postexposure immunization is not useful.

6) *Investigation of contacts and source of infection:* Search for infected rodents and fleas or persons exposed to plague pneumonia. Elimination of fleas should precede anti-rat measures, using an appropriate insecticide powder with residual effect. Dust rat runs and harborages in and about known or suspected plague premises or areas. Disinfect by dusting, or insecticide-spray the houses, outhouses and

household furnishings in the same areas. Dust the persons and clothing of immediate contacts and all other residents in the immediate vicinity. Suppress rat populations by energetic campaigns of poisoning or trapping.

7) *Specific treatment:* Streptomycin, tetracyclines, and chloramphenicol used early are highly effective. Results are good even in pneumonic plague if therapy is begun within 24 hours of onset, but poor thereafter. Streptomycin-resistant organisms have been described. After a satisfactory response to drug therapy some patients will show a self-limited brief febrile episode on the 5th or 6th day unaccompanied by any other evidence of illness. However, reappearance of fever at any time in association with other clinical or laboratory evidence of disease may show that the infectious agent is resistant, or that a complication has developed, such as secondary pneumonia due to other bacteria; sputum should be examined by stained smear and cultured immediately. Penicillin or other appropriate antibiotics may then be indicated. (Penicillin is not effective against plague itself.) When other antibiotics are not available, use sulfonamides.

C. Epidemic measures:

1) Investigate all deaths, with autopsy and laboratory examinations when indicated. Develop case-finding facilities. Establish the best possible provision for diagnosis and treatment. Alert all existing medical facilities toward immediate reporting and toward utilization of diagnostic and therapy services. Provide adequate laboratory services, kits containing appropriate bacteriologic transport media, and adequate supplies of antibiotics.

2) Institute intensive flea control in expanding circles from known foci.

3) Supplemental rodent destruction within affected areas.

4) Prophylactic administration of broad-spectrum antibiotics or sulfadiazine to all medical, nursing and public health personnel exposed to definite and repeated risk of infection may be considered if they cannot be kept under close and frequent observation. Restriction of hospital personnel and family contacts to the premises is desirable when patients with pneumonic plague are under treatment.

5) Personal protection of field workers against fleas by weekly dusting of clothing with insecticide powder to which fleas are sensitive. Daily application of insect repellents is a valuable adjunct.

6) A single dose of avirulent living plague bacillus vaccine has proved valuable among residents of endemic areas. There are no generally accepted standards for safety and potency testing of such a vaccine. Killed vaccine (see 9A1)

affords temporary protection; the need for repeated doses presents practical problems.

D. International measures:

1) Telegraphic notification by governments to WHO and to adjacent countries of the first imported, first transferred or first nonimported case of plague in any area previously free of the disease. Report newly discovered or reactivated foci of plague among rodents.

2) Measures applicable to ships, aircraft, and land transport arriving from plague areas are specified in International Health Regulations,* WHO, Geneva.

3) All ships should be free of rodents, or periodically deratted.

4) Ratproofing of buildings of seaports and airports; application of appropriate insecticide with residual effect every 6 months; deratting with effective rodenticide.

5) International travelers: Plague-infected persons or suspects are not permitted to depart from a country. International regulations require that prior to their departure on an international voyage from an area where there is an epidemic of pulmonary plague, those exposed to infection shall be placed in isolation for 6 days after last exposure. On arrival, travelers may be disinsected and kept under surveillance for a period of not more than 6 days reckoned from the date of arrival. No country currently requires immunization against plague for entry. Because protection by vaccines is brief, immunization should be completed just preceding anticipated exposure. (See 9A1 above.)

6) WHO Reference Centres (see Preface).

PLEURODYNIA

1. Identification—An acute viral disease with sudden onset of severe paroxysmal pain commonly localized at the costodiaphragmatic border, and accompanied by headache, anorexia, malaise and intermittent fever often recurring with exacerbations of pain. Duration 1 to 3 days; remissions frequent. A nonfatal illness usually recognized in localized epidemics. Important to differentiate from more serious medical or surgical conditions. Synonyms: Bornholm disease, Epidemic myalgia, Devil's grippe.

Diagnosis is aided by isolation of virus from feces in tissue culture and by rise in titer of type-specific neutralizing antibodies in blood sera of early and late illness.

---

* These will come into force on January 1, 1971. Until that date, *International Sanitary Regulations,* 3rd edition (Geneva: WHO, 1966) are applicable.

2. Occurrence—An uncommon disease occurring in summer and early autumn and at all ages but mainly in children and young adults. Multiple cases in a household are frequent. Usually observed in epidemics, with outbreaks reported in Europe, Australia, New Zealand and North America.

3. Infectious agents—Various Coxsackie Group B viruses, Types 1, 2, 3, 4 and 5, have been associated with the illness.

4. Reservoir—Reservoir is man.

5. Mode of transmission—Probably contact with an infected person or with articles freshly soiled with feces or throat discharges of infected persons, who may or may not have symptoms. Coxsackie Group B viruses have been found in sewage, on flies and mosquitoes; the relation to transmission of human disease is not clear.

6. Incubation period—Three to 5 days is usual.

7. Period of communicability—Apparently during the acute stage of disease.

8. Susceptibility and resistance—Susceptibility is probably general, and presumably a type-specific immunity results from infection.

9. Methods of control—

A. *Preventive measures:* None.

B. *Control of patient, contacts, and the immediate environment:*
1) *Report to local health authority:* Obligatory report of epidemics; no individual case report, Class 4 (see Preface).
2) *Isolation:* None.
3) *Concurrent disinfection:* Prompt and safe disposal of nose and throat discharges and of feces. Articles soiled therewith should be disinfected.
4) *Quarantine:* None.
5) *Immunization of contacts:* None.
6) *Investigation of contacts:* Of no practical value.
7) *Specific treatment:* None.

C. *Epidemic measures:* General notice to physicians of the presence of an epidemic and the necessity for differential diagnosis from more serious medical or surgical emergencies.

D. *International measures:* WHO Reference Centres (see Preface).

THE PNEUMONIAS

A. PNEUMOCOCCAL PNEUMONIA

1. Identification—An acute bacterial disease characterized by sudden onset with chills followed by fever, often pain in chest, and usually a productive cough, dyspnea, and leucocytosis. X-rays may provide the first evidence of consolidation. Pneumonia often is bronchial rather than lobar, especially in children, with vomiting and convulsions the first manifestations. Pneumococcal pneumonia is an important cause of death, with much variation in fatality according to serologic type of pneumococcus and age of patient, being highest for infants and the aged. Fatality, formerly 20 to 40% for hospital patients, has been greatly reduced by antibiotics and chemotherapy.

Early etiologic diagnosis is important to therapy. Presumptive diagnosis is by microscopic search for gram-positive diplococci in smears of lower respiratory tract secretions. Confirmation is by isolation of agent from blood or lower respiratory specimens.

2. Occurrence—A common disease, particularly in infancy and old age. Most frequent in industrial cities and lower economic groups. Occurs in all climates and seasons, but is most frequent in winter and spring in temperate zones. Usually sporadic in U.S.A., but epidemics occur in institutions and in barracks; consistently recurring epidemics have been described in South African mines. A rising incidence commonly accompanies epidemics of viral respiratory disease, especially influenza.

3. Infectious agent—*Diplococcus pneumoniae.* Pneumococci of Types I to XXXII account for about 95% of cases; the remainder are due to rarely recognized types.

4. Reservoir—Reservoir is man; patients and carriers. Pneumococci may be found in the upper respiratory tract of healthy members of most communities throughout the world.

5. Mode of transmission—By droplet spread, by direct oral contact with patients or carriers, or indirectly through articles freshly soiled with discharges of nose and throat of such persons. Airborne transmission may be possible but has not been established as important. Person-to-person transmission is common, but illness among contacts and attendants is infrequent.

6. Incubation period—Not well determined; believed to be 1 to 3 days.

7. Period of communicability—Unknown; presumably until discharges of mouth and nose no longer contain the infectious agent in appreciable numbers or in virulent form. Penicillin will eliminate the pneumococcus from most patients within 3 days.

8. Susceptibility and resistance—Resistance is generally high but may be lowered by wet, cold and exposure, physical and mental fatigue, and by alcoholism. Inapparent infection is extremely common, particularly with Type III pneumococcus and strains of higher types. Immunity to the homologous type usually follows an attack, may last for months or years and is highly specific; antibody response may be diminished by early antibiotic treatment.

9. Methods of control—

    A. *Preventive measures:* Whenever practicable and particularly in institutions and barracks and on shipboard, avoid crowding in living and sleeping quarters.

B. *Control of patient, contacts, and the immediate environment:*

1) *Report to local health authority:* Obligatory report of epidemics; no individual case report, Class 4 (see Preface).
2) *Isolation:* Of dubious value; unnecessary after 24 hours of antibiotic therapy.
3) *Concurrent disinfection:* Of discharges from nose and throat. Terminal cleaning.
4) *Quarantine:* None.
5) *Immunization of contacts:* None.
6) *Investigation of contacts:* Of no practical value.
7) *Specific treatment:* Penicillin intramuscularly; oral penicillin G is effective; tetracyclines are nearly comparable. In event of penicillin sensitivity or ineffective response to penicillin, substitute tetracycline, sulfonamide drug or erythromycin.

C. *Epidemic measures:* In outbreaks in institutions or in other limited or closed population groups, general hygienic measures may be supplemented by chemoprophylaxis with sulfonamides or antibiotics. Immunization with bacterial polysaccharides of prevailing types may be effective in high-risk populations such as mine workers or military units; effectiveness is under evaluation.

D. *International measures:* None.

B. BACTERIAL PNEUMONIA, OTHER THAN PNEUMOCOCCAL

1. Identification—An acute febrile disease with pulmonary involvement evidenced by symptoms, physical signs or roentgen-ray examination. Often occurs in association with other infections of the respiratory tract, particularly influenza. With adequate treatment, fatality is generally low but varies according to infectious agent and age of patient.

Bacteriologic examination of sputum, nasopharyngeal swabs and blood helps in diagnosis. Differentiate from Plague and Anthrax (see pp. 170 and 8, respectively).

2. Occurrence—Worldwide in distribution; a frequent disease in infancy and old age, and in winter months in temperate climates. Usually sporadic, but epidemics occur in association with influenza, measles and acute undifferentiated viral respiratory diseases.

3. Infectious agents—Various pathogenic bacteria commonly found in the mouth, nose and throat, as *Streptococcus pyogenes* (Group A hemolytic streptococci), *Staphylococcus aureus, Klebsiella pneumoniae* (Friedländer bacillus) and *Haemophilus influenzae*.

4. Reservoir—Man.

5. Mode of transmission—By direct droplet spread, by oral contact, or indirectly through articles freshly soiled with discharges of nose or throat of infected persons.

6. Incubation period—Variable, usually short, 1 to 3 days.

7. Period of communicability—Unknown; probably while the infectious agent is present in discharges of nose and throat of patients. For many agents, antibiotic therapy greatly decreases period of communicability.

8. Susceptibility and resistance—Resistance is generally high, except in debilitated persons and infection is often secondary to viral infections. Specific immunity varies with the infectious agent and is probably minimal except for type-specific immunity to Group A streptococci. Immunization procedures are not feasible.

9. Methods of control—

A. Preventive measures:

1) Good personal hygiene; avoid crowding in institutions and hospitals.
2) Immunization against influenza (p. 120) and chemoprophylaxis of streptococcal infections (p. 241) may be useful in closed or limited general populations when indicated.

B. Control of patient, contacts, and the immediate environment:

1) *Report to local health authority:* Obligatory report of epidemics; no individual case report, Class 4 (see Preface). Identification of an accompanying or preceding epidemic of acute respiratory disease is of public health significance.
2) *Isolation:* None.
3) *Concurrent disinfection:* Of discharges from mouth and nose and of articles soiled therewith. Terminal cleaning.
4) *Quarantine:* None.
5) *Immunization of contacts:* None.
6) *Investigation of contacts:* Of no practical value except for streptococcal pneumonias; contacts should be searched for and treated.
7) *Specific treatment:* For streptococcal, same as pneumococcal pneumonia. For staphylococcal, penicillinase-resistant penicillins. If organism proves resistant, use tetracycline antibiotics as in pneumococcal pneumonia. Sensitivity tests with the isolated organism are important in selecting the most suitable antibiotic. For *H. influenzae:* tetracyclines, ampicillin and chloramphenicol are effective; combined sulfadiazine-streptomycin is also used. For *K. pneumoniae* (Friedländer bacillus): streptomycin in combination with tetracyclines or chloramphenicol.

C. Epidemic measures: Applicable only in outbreaks in institutions or in other limited or closed population groups when associated with influenza, measles or other respiratory infection.

Immunization against influenza and of infants and children against measles may be useful. Individual chemoprophylaxis has no proven value.

D. International measures: None.

C. MYCOPLASMAL (PPLO) PNEUMONIA

1. Identification—A febrile upper respiratory infection which sometimes progresses to bronchitis or pneumonia. Onset is gradual, with headache, malaise, cough and usually substernal but no pleuritic pain. Sputum, scant at first, may increase later. Early patchy infiltration of the lungs revealed by roentgenographic examination is often more extensive than clinical findings suggest. In severe cases pneumonia may progress from one lobe to another. Leucocytosis may occur after the 1st week. Duration of illness varies from a few days to several weeks. Secondary bacterial infection and other complications are infrequent; fatality is about 0.1%. Synonyms: Primary atypical pneumonia, Eaton agent pneumonia.

Development of cold hemagglutinins during early convalescence or of agglutinins for *Streptococcus* MG, or both, supports diagnosis in one-half to two-thirds of cases. The infectious agent may be cultured on special agar; serological confirmation by immunofluorescence, complement fixation or growth inhibition test.

Differentiation required from pneumonitis due to adenovirus, respiratory syncytial virus or certain enteroviruses, influenza, parainfluenza, measles, psittacosis, Q fever, certain mycoses and early tuberculosis.

2. Occurrence—Worldwide distribution; sporadic, endemic, and occasionally epidemic, especially in institutions and military populations. Attack rates of 5 to over 50 per 1000 per annum in military and 1 to 3 per 1000 per annum in civilian populations. Incidence greatest during fall and winter months in temperate climates, with much variation from year to year and in different geographic areas. No selectivity for race or sex. Occurs at all ages, but recognized disease is most frequent among adolescents and young adults.

3. Infectious agent—*Mycoplasma pneumoniae,* Eaton agent, a member of the pleuropneumonia-like group of organisms (PPLO).

4. Reservoir—Man; patients and persons with mild, unrecognized infections.

5. Mode of transmission—Probably by droplet inhalation or by oral contact with an infected person or with articles freshly soiled with discharges of nose and throat. Secondary cases of pneumonia among contacts and attendants are infrequent; contacts may contract a mild respiratory disease. Rise in antibody titer among persons with no history of illness suggests inapparent infections, especially during periods of high prevalence.

6. Incubation period—7 to 21 days, commonly 12.

7. Period of communicability—Probably less than 10 days; occasionally longer with persisting febrile illness.

8. Susceptibility and resistance—Clinical pneumonia occurs in about 3 to 30% of infections with *M. pneumoniae*, depending on age. Attack varies from mild afebrile upper respiratory illness involving the upper or lower respiratory tract. Duration of immunity indefinite, but resistance has been correlated with presence of humoral antibodies and these remain for 1 or more years.

9. Methods of control—

A. *Preventive measures:* Avoid crowding in living and sleeping quarters whenever possible, especially in institutions, in barracks and on shipboard. Maintain general resistance by adequate food, sufficient sleep, fresh air and good personal hygiene.

B. *Control of patient, contacts, and the immediate environment:*

1) *Report to local health authority:* Obligatory report of epidemics; no individual case report, Class 4 (see Preface).
2) *Isolation:* None.
3) *Concurrent disinfection:* Of discharges from nose and throat. Terminal cleaning.
4) *Quarantine:* None.
5) *Immunization of contacts:* None.
6) *Investigation of contacts:* Of no practical value.
7) *Specific treatment:* Tetracycline antibiotics and erythromycin give good results, especially in severe mycoplasmal pneumonia. The infectious agent is highly resistant to penicillin, and variably, although in lesser degree, to streptomycin.

C. *Epidemic measures:* No reliably effective measures for control are available.

D. *International measures:* WHO Reference Centres (see Preface).

D. PNEUMOCYSTIS PNEUMONIA

1. Identification—An often fatal, subacute, pulmonary disease occurring early in life, especially in ill or premature infants. Also occurs in older children and adults as an opportunistic infection associated with debilitating conditions, diseases of immune mechanisms and the use of immunosuppressants. Clinically there is progressive dyspnea, tachypnea, cyanosis, and pallor with or without fever or auscultatory signs. X-ray reveals diffuse increased density and areas of emphysema. Postmortem examination reveals heavy airless lungs, thickened alveolar septa, and foamy material containing clumps of parasites in the alveolar spaces. Synonym: Interstitial plasma-cell pneumonia.

Diagnosis is established by demonstration of causative agent in material from lung biopsy, in smears of tracheobronchial mucus, or in histological sections or impression smears from affected lungs stained with Gomori's methenamine silver nitrate method. There are no satisfactory laboratory, cultural or serological methods.

2. Occurrence—The disease has been recognized in England, Europe, North America and Australia. The organism was first seen in animals in South America. Endemic and epidemic in infants in some European hospitals and institutions.

3. Infectious agent—*Pneumocystis carinii,* an organism of uncertain classification but generally regarded as a protozoan.

4. Reservoir—Organisms have been demonstrated in lungs of many animals, including man. The epidemiological significance of the various potential sources is unknown.

5. Mode of transmission—Unknown.

6. Incubation period—Analysis of institutional outbreaks among infants indicates 1 to 2 months.

7. Period of communicability—Unknown.

8. Susceptibility and resistance—Susceptibility enhanced by prematurity, by chronic debilitating illness, or by disease or therapy in which immune mechanisms are impaired.

9. Methods of control—

A. *Preventive measures:* None known.

B. *Control of patient, contacts, and the immediate environment:*

1) *Report to local health authority:* Official report ordinarily not justifiable, Class 5 (see Preface).
2) *Isolation:* Isolation wards have been used in European institutional outbreaks in infants. Prudence would suggest removal of patients from the environment of high-risk individuals.
3) *Concurrent disinfection:* Insufficient knowledge.
4) *Quarantine:* None.
5) *Immunization of contacts:* None.
6) *Investigation of contacts and source of infection:* None.
7) *Specific treatment:* Pentamidine isethionate (Lomidine) is useful. It is available in the U.S.A. from the National Communicable Disease Center, Atlanta, Ga., on an investigational basis.

C. *Epidemic measures:* Knowledge of source of organism and mode of transmission is so inadequate that there are no generally accepted measures.

D. *International measures:* None.

E. OTHER PNEUMONIAS

Among the known viruses, adenovirus, respiratory syncytial, and parainfluenza viruses, and probably others as yet unidentified, have the capacity to induce a pneumonitis. Because these infectious agents cause upper respiratory disease more often than pneumonia, they are presented under Acute febrile respiratory disease (pp. 199–203). See also Viral pneumonia of measles, Chickenpox and Influenza (pp. 145, 51, and 119). Pneumonia is also caused by infection with chlamydia (psittacosis) and rickettsiae (Q fever) and can be associated with the invasive phase of certain nematode infections (ascariasis).

POLIOMYELITIS

1. **Identification**—An acute viral illness with a wide range of severity, from inapparent infection to nonparalytic and paralytic disease. Symptoms include fever, headache, gastrointestinal disturbance, malaise and stiffness of neck and back, with or without paralysis. The virus invades the alimentary tract; viremia may then follow with invasion of central nervous system and selective involvement of motor cells resulting in flaccid paralysis, most commonly of lower extremities. Site of paralysis depends upon location of nerve cell destruction in spinal cord or brain stem; but characteristically asymmetrical. Nonparalytic poliomyelitis is one of the causes of aseptic meningitis (see p. 151). Incidence of inapparent infection usually exceeds clinical cases by more than a hundred fold. Case fatality for paralytic cases varies from 2 to 10% in epidemics and increases markedly with age. Synonym: Infantile paralysis.

Poliovirus can be isolated by tissue culture from feces or possibly throat secretions early in the course of infection; a rising titer of complement-fixing or neutralizing antibodies denotes recent infection.

The differential diagnosis of nonparalytic poliomyelitis includes other forms of aseptic meningitis, purulent meningitis, tuberculous meningitis, brain abscess, leptospirosis, lymphocytic choriomeningitis, the encephalitides and toxic encephalopathies.

Paralytic poliomyelitis can usually be recognized on clinical grounds, but can be confused with other paralytic conditions. Other enteroviruses (ECHO and Coxsackie, especially type A7) can cause an illness simulating paralytic poliomyelitis, though usually less severe and with negligible residual paralysis. Tick-bite paralysis occurs uncommonly, but worldwide, affecting man and animals, to give a flaccid ascending motor paralysis. In northwestern U.S.A., *Dermacentor andersoni* is most frequently involved; also other ticks in the east and south, mainly in spring and early summer. Patient usually recovers promptly when tick is removed.

2. **Occurrence**—Worldwide. Before the large-scale immunization programs were carried out, the highest incidence of clinically recognizable disease has been in temperate zones and the more developed countries. Occurs as sporadic cases and in epidemics; more common during summer and early autumn in temperate climates, but with wide variations from year to year and from region to region

Fairly large areas may experience low incidence for several years, with ultimate reappearance in large numbers. Characteristically a disease of children and adolescents; all ages are affected where artificial or natural immunity has not been acquired, with paralytic illness proportionately more frequent among older persons. In recent years, preschool children and their parents, fathers more than mothers, have been mainly involved in U.S.A. Improved living standards may be associated with emergence of paralytic poliomyelitis, as illustrated by increasing incidence in regions with decreasing infant mortality rates. Severe epidemics, formerly uncommon, now occur in lesser developed areas with increasing frequency, mainly involving young children. In lesser developed areas, antibodies to all 3 types of poliovirus are generally present by school age. In countries where artificial immunization has been widely practiced, paralytic cases are chiefly among the least vaccinated groups, mainly preschool children of lower social classes. The use of vaccines has resulted in a marked decrease in over-all incidence of paralytic disease.

3. Infectious agent—Poliovirus types 1, 2 and 3: type 1 is most commonly associated with paralytic illness, type 3 less frequently and type 2 uncommonly.

4. Reservoir—Reservoir is man, most frequently persons with inapparent infections, especially children.

5. Mode of transmission—Direct contact with pharyngeal secretions of infected persons through close association. In rare instances milk has been a vehicle. No reliable evidence of spread by other foods, insects or virus-contaminated sewage; water is rarely if ever involved. Whether feces or pharyngeal secretions have the greater importance in transmission has not been determined and may vary according to environmental circumstances. Virus is more readily detectable and for a longer period in feces than throat, but epidemiologic evidence suggests that oral-oral spread may be more important than fecal-oral spread where sanitation is good.

6. Incubation period—Commonly 7 to 12 days, with a range from 3 to 21 days.

7. Period of communicability—Poliovirus is demonstrable in throat secretions as early as 36 hours and in the feces 72 hours after infection in both clinical and inapparent cases. Virus persists in the throat for approximately one week and in the feces for 3 to 6 weeks or longer. Cases are most infectious from 7 to 10 days before and after the onset of symptoms.

8. Susceptibility and resistance—Susceptibility to infection is general but few infected persons develop paralysis. Type-specific resistance of long duration follows both clinically recognizable and inapparent infection. Second attacks are rare and usually result from infection with poliovirus of a different type. Infants born of immune mothers have transient passive immunity. Earlier removal of tonsils predisposes to bulbar involvement. Trauma and injection of precipitated antigens or certain other insoluble substances may provoke paralysis in an already infected but symptomless person, the paralysis tending to be localized in the affected limb or appearing there first. Excessive muscular fatigue in the prodromal period may likewise predispose to paralytic involvement. An increased susceptibility to paralytic poliomyelitis is associated with pregnancy.

9. Methods of control—

A. Preventive measures:

1) Active immunization of all susceptible persons against the 3 types of poliovirus. Give priority to ages with highest incidence and to selected groups at unusual risk. Follow by maintenance program to cover all infants. Two methods are available; immunization by either method may begin as early as 6 weeks of age although delay to 4 to 6 months avoids the depressive effect of maternal antibody on immune response.

   a) Oral poliovirus vaccines provide a high level of immunity by causing an alimentary infection with attenuated polioviruses. They are administered by mouth, generally in the form of trivalent combinations of the 3 types. The generally accepted pattern in the U.S.A. is of 2 doses of trivalent vaccine fed at an interval of 4 to 6 weeks with a third dose 6 to 12 months later. (Some recommend 3 initial doses at 4 to 6 week intervals and a fourth 6 to 12 months later.) In the United Kingdom and Canada, 3 doses of trivalent vaccine are recommended at intervals of 6 to 8 weeks between the 1st and 2nd doses and 6 months between the 2nd and 3rd doses.

   b) Formalin-inactivated poliovirus vaccine also provides protection but is less effective in preventing subsequent alimentary infection. In U.S.A., a basic series of 4 injections, preferably initiated in early infancy, is recommended, the first 3 about 6 weeks apart, the fourth 6 months or more after the third. In Sweden, 2 doses are given 2–4 weeks apart for primary vaccination and booster doses are given 1 and 4–5 years later. In order to maintain optimal antibody levels, regular booster doses every few years appear to be needed.

   c) Additional booster doses of either oral or inactivated vaccine are indicated with the threat of an epidemic, or travel to a hyperendemic area and at the time of entering school. If not previously immunized at school age, give a full series.

2) Health education of the public on the advantages of immunization in early childhood, on modes of spread, and on the desirability of avoiding excessive physical exertion during epidemic periods.

B. Control of patient, contacts, and the immediate environment:

1) *Report to local health authority:* Obligatory case report after January 1, 1971, as a *Disease under Surveillance by WHO,* Class 1; until then, Class 2A (see Preface). Each case is to be designated as paralytic or nonparalytic. Supplemental reports giving vaccine history, virus type, severity and persistence of residual paralysis 60 days or longer after onset are necessary measures for effective control.

2) *Isolation:* Isolation precautions for not more than 7 days in hospital management of the patient. Of little value under home conditions because spread of infection is greatest in the prodromal period.

3) *Concurrent disinfection:* Of throat discharges and feces and of articles soiled therewith. In communities with modern and adequate sewage disposal systems, feces and urine can be discharged directly into sewers without preliminary disinfection. Terminal cleaning.

4) *Quarantine:* Of no community value because of large numbers of unrecognized infections in the population.

5) *Protection of contacts:* Vaccination of familial and other close contacts contributes little to immediate control; ordinarily the virus is widely spread among them by the time the first case is recognized. Passive protection with immune serum globulin (human), giving 0.3 ml per kg of body weight, may have considerable value if given within a few days of known single exposure at a susceptible age. In the U.S.A., occurrence of a single paralytic case in a community may be regarded as sufficient cause for initiating a mass oral immunization program for individuals in the neighborhood.

6) *Investigation of contacts:* Thorough search for sick persons, especially children, to assure treatment of unrecognized and unreported cases. Footdrop, scoliosis and other deformities resulting in functional impairment may be late manifestations of initially mild or inapparent illness.

7) *Specific treatment:* None; attention during the acute illness to the complications of paralysis; may require expert knowledge, especially for patients in need of respiratory assistance.

C. Epidemic measures:

1) Institute mass vaccination with oral vaccine at the earliest indication of an outbreak. Use monovalent vaccine of the same virus type causing the outbreak. If typing facilities are not available, use trivalent vaccine.

2) Organize mass vaccination campaigns to achieve the most rapid and complete immunization of epidemiologically relevant groups, especially younger children. Locate vac-

cination centers in relation to population densities, taking advantage of normal social patterns; schools often meet these criteria.

3) With the use of mass immunization, it is no longer necessary to disrupt community activities by closing schools and other places of population aggregation.

4) Postpone elective nose and throat operations and other elective immunizations until after the epidemic has ended.

5) Provide facilities in strategically located centers for specialized medical care of acutely ill patients and rehabilitation of those with significant paralysis.

D. International measures:

1) In accordance with a Resolution of the 22nd World Health Assembly, poliomyelitis becomes a *Disease under Surveillance by WHO*. National health administrations are expected to inform WHO of outbreaks promptly by telegram or telex, and to supplement these reports as soon as possible with details of the source, nature and extent of the epidemic and of the identity of the type of epidemic virus involved.

2) Susceptible international travelers visiting areas of hyperendemic prevalence should be adequately immunized.

3) WHO Reference Centres (see Preface).

PSITTACOSIS

1. Identification—An acute generalized infectious disease with fever, headache and early pneumonic involvement; cough is initially absent or nonproductive; sputum mucopurulent, not copious; anorexia extreme; commonly constipation; pulse usually slow in relation to temperature; lethargy; occasional relapses. Human infections may be severe but are most often mild in character. Death is rare. Synonyms: Ornithosis, Parrot fever.

Laboratory diagnosis is by demonstrating significant increase in complement-fixing antibodies during convalescence; or, under suitably safe laboratory conditions only, by isolation of the infectious agent from sputum, blood or postmortem tissues in mice or eggs. Recovery of the agent may be difficult, especially if the patient has received broad-spectrum antibiotics.

2. Occurrence—Worldwide, as sporadic cases or household outbreaks among persons exposed to sick or seemingly healthy birds. In U.S.A. an occupational disease of persons associated with pet shops, aviaries, pigeon lofts, poultry farms, poultry processing and rendering plants.

3. Infectious agent—The filterable agent of psittacosis, a bedsonia (chlamydia) of the Psittacosis-LGV-Trachoma group.

4. Reservoir—Reservoirs are parakeets, parrots, pigeons, turkeys, domestic fowl, and other birds; occasionally man. Apparently healthy birds can be carriers and occasionally shed the infectious agent.

5. Mode of transmission—Infection is acquired usually by inhalation of the agent from desiccated droppings of infected birds in an enclosed space. This at times has been in the home, in pigeon lofts, or in poultry processing and rendering plants. Exposure has also apparently occurred through direct contact with infected birds on squab, turkey and duck farms. Household birds have been most frequent sources. Many laboratory infections have occurred. Transmission from man to man is rare, but occasional cases have occurred in nurses attending psittacosis patients.

6. Incubation period—From 4 to 15 days, commonly 10 days.

7. Period of communicability—Primarily during the acute illness, especially with paroxysmal coughing. Diseased birds may shed the agent intermittently throughout infection and sometimes continuously for weeks or months.

8. Susceptibility and resistance—Susceptibility is general; but older adults have a more severe illness; one attack does not always confer immunity.

9. Methods of control—

A. Preventive measures:

1) Regulation of importation and traffic of birds of parrot family to prevent or eliminate infections by quarantine or appropriate antibiotic treatment. Prevent exposure of previously noninfected birds to potentially infected birds or birds of unknown history.
2) Surveillance of pet shops and aviaries where psittacosis has occurred or where birds epidemiologically linked to cases were obtained. Infected birds should be treated or destroyed and the premises thoroughly cleaned. In instances where birds were treated, they should remain in quarantine until shown to be healthy.
3) Psittacine birds offered in commerce should be raised under psittacosis-free conditions and handled in such manner as to prevent infection. Tetracycline-impregnated birdseed has proved effective in controlling disease in parakeets.
4) Education of the public in the danger of household or occupational exposure to infected birds of the parrot family.

B. Control of patient, contacts, and the immediate environment:

1) *Report to local health authority:* Obligatory case report in most states and countries, Class 2A (see Preface).
2) *Isolation:* Important during acute febrile stage. Nurses

caring for patients with a cough should wear adequate masks.

3) Concurrent disinfection: Of all discharges. Terminal cleaning.

4) Quarantine: None.

5) Immunization of contacts: None.

6) Investigation of contacts and source of infection: Trace origin of suspected birds. Kill suspect birds and immerse bodies in 2% cresol or equivalent disinfectant. Place in plastic bag, close securely, and ship frozen (on dry ice) to nearest competent laboratory. Buildings housing infected birds should not be used by man until thoroughly cleaned and aired.

7) Specific treatment: Tetracycline antibiotics or chloramphenicol, continued for at least one week after temperature returns to normal.

C. Epidemic measures: Ordinarily not applicable to man because cases are usually sporadic or confined to family outbreaks. The epidemic problem concerns birds. Report outbreaks of ornithosis in flocks of turkeys to state agriculture and health authority. Large doses of tetracyclines will suppress but may not eliminate infection in poultry flocks. Identify susceptibles among employees on farms and in processing plants by serologic tests; workers preferably should be restricted to those with demonstrated antibodies.

D. International measures: Reciprocal respect for national regulations designed to control importation of psittacine birds.

Q FEVER

1. Identification—An acute febrile rickettsial disease; onset may be sudden, with chilly sensations, retrobulbar headache, weakness, malaise, and severe sweats; much variation in severity and duration. A pneumonitis occurs in most cases, with mild cough, scanty expectoration, chest pain, minimal physical findings, and little or no upper respiratory involvement. Chronic endocarditis and general infections have been reported; inapparent infections occur. Fatality of untreated patients is less than 1%; with treatment, negligible except in aged persons and individuals who develop endocarditis.

Laboratory diagnosis is by complement-fixation or agglutination tests, with demonstration of rise in antibody between acute and convalescent stages; or by recovery of the infectious agent from blood of patient, a procedure hazardous to laboratory workers.

2. Occurrence—Reported from all continents; endemic in many areas. In the U.S.A. endemic in California and several other states, affecting especially veterinarians, dairy workers, and farmers; rare in many areas where infection exists enzootically in animals; explosive epidemics among workers in diagnostic laboratories, stockyards, meat packing and rendering plants, and wool processing factories.

3. Infectious agent—*Coxiella burneti (Rickettsia burneti).*

4. Reservoir—Ticks, wild animals (bandicoots), cattle, sheep, and goats are natural reservoirs, with infection inapparent.

5. Mode of transmission—Commonly by airborne dissemination of rickettsiae in dust, in or near premises contaminated by placental tissues and birth fluids of infected animals, in establishments processing infected animals or their by-products, and in necropsy rooms. Also contracted by direct contact with infected animals or other contaminated materials such as wool, straw, fertilizer, and the laundry of exposed persons. Raw milk from infected cows may be responsible for some cases.

6. Incubation period—Dependent on size of infecting dose; usually 2 to 3 weeks.

7. Period of communicability—Direct transmission from man to man is very rare.

8. Susceptibility and resistance—Susceptibility is general. Immunity following recovery from clinical illness probably is permanent.

9. Methods of control—

A. *Preventive measures:*

1) Public education on sources of infection and the necessary hygienic practices of pasteurization of milk, and adequate disposal of animal placentas; also strict hygienic measures in cow sheds and barns (dust, urine, feces, rodents) during epizootics.

2) Pasteurization of milk from cows, goats and sheep at 62.9 C (145 F) for 30 minutes, or at 71.6 C (161 F) for 15 seconds by the high-temperature short-time method, or boiling of milk, inactivates rickettsiae.

3) Immunization with inactivated vaccine prepared from *C. burneti* infected yolk sac is useful in protecting laboratory workers and might be considered for others in hazardous occupations. However, since severe local reactions can occur, immunization should be preceded by a sensitivity test with a small dose of vaccine.

B. *Control of patient, contacts, and the immediate environment:*

1) *Report to local health authority:* In selected endemic areas (U.S.A.); in many countries not a reportable disease, Class 3B (see Preface).

2) *Isolation:* None.

3) *Concurrent disinfection:* Of sputum and blood, and articles freshly soiled therewith. Precautions at postmortem examination.

4) *Quarantine:* None.

5) *Immunization of contacts:* Unnecessary.

6) *Investigation of contacts and source of infection:* Search for history of contact with cattle, sheep, and goats, consumption of raw milk, or direct or indirect association with a laboratory handling *C. burneti.*

7) *Specific treatment:* Tetracyclines administered orally and continued for several days after patient is afebrile; reinstitute if relapse occurs.

C. Epidemic measures: Outbreaks are generally of short duration; control measures are essentially limited to observation of exposed persons and antibiotic therapy for those becoming ill.

D. International measures: Control of importation of goats, sheep, and cattle.

RABIES

1. Identification—An almost invariably fatal acute encephalitis. Onset begins with a sense of apprehension, headache, fever, malaise, and indefinite sensory changes often referred to site of a preceding local wound resulting from bite of a rabid animal. The disease progresses to paresis or paralysis; spasm of muscles of deglutition on attempts to swallow leads to fear of water (hydrophobia). Delirium and convulsions follow; death is due to respiratory paralysis—usual duration is 2 to 6 days, sometimes longer. Synonym: Hydrophobia.

Other diseases resulting from bites of animals include pasteurellosis *(Pasteurella multocida* and *P. haemolytica)* from cat and dog bites; B-virus from monkey bites; tularemia, rat-bite fever, tetanus, and cat-scratch fever.

2. Occurrence—Uncommon in man; primarily a disease of animals. Occurs throughout the world except Australia, New Zealand, Japan, Hawaii and other Pacific Islands, some of the West Indies, Great Britain and Ireland, and Norway and Sweden, which are presently rabies-free. Urban rabies is a problem of dogs and occasionally other pets; sylvatic or rural rabies is a disease of wild biting animals, with sporadic disease among dogs and domestic livestock. In the U.S.A., wildlife rabies is steadily increasing.

3. Infectious agent—The virus of rabies.

4. Reservoirs—Many wild and domestic *Canidae,* including dog, fox, coyote, wolf, jackal and also cat, skunk, racoon, mongoose, and other biting mammals. Vampire and fruit-eating bats are infected in South and Central America and Mexico; insectivorous bats in U.S.A., Canada, Europe, and Southeast Asia.

5. Mode of transmission—Virus-laden saliva of a rabid animal is introduced by a bite or rarely by entering a scratch or other fresh break in the skin. Transmission from man to man is not confirmed, though saliva may contain virus. Airborne spread from bats to man in caves where bats are roosting has been demonstrated but rarely occurs.

6. Incubation period—Usually 3 to 6 weeks, occasionally shorter or much longer; depends on extent of laceration, site of wound in relation to richness of nerve supply, amount of virus introduced, clothing, and other factors.

7. Period of communicability—In dogs and most biting animals, for 3 to 5 days before onset of clinical signs, and during the course of the disease. Bats may shed virus for many months without evidence of illness.

8. Susceptibility and resistance—Most warm-blooded animals are susceptible. Natural immunity in man is unknown.

9. Methods of control—

A. Preventive measures:

1) After animal bites, prevention of rabies is based on physical removal of the virus and specific immunological prevention.

   a. Perhaps the most effective rabies prevention is immediate and thorough cleansing—with water, soap and water, or detergent and water—of all types of wounds caused by bite or scratch of an animal with rabies or suspected rabies. If hyperimmune serum is used (see 9A4 below) part of the dose should be infiltrated beneath the bite wound. The wound should not be sutured for at least several days.

   b. Specific prevention of rabies in man is by administration of antirabies vaccine soon after injury, for at least 14 consecutive days; in severe or multiple bites, sometimes for 21 days. Booster doses should be given 10 days and at 20 or more days following the last daily dose of vaccine, in all cases. Non-nervous tissue vaccine, such as duck embryo killed vaccine, is preferred to the killed vaccines prepared from nervous tissue. Vaccination often is supplemented by passive immunization with hyperimmune serum. The following is a guide in different circumstances:

      (1) If the animal is apprehended, confine and observe for 7 to 10 days. Start administering vaccine to the

exposed person at the first physical sign or laboratory evidence of rabies in the observed animal.

(2) If the animal is not apprehended and rabies is known to be present in that species in the area, start vaccination immediately if attack by the animal was unprovoked.

(3) Rabies vaccination carries a small risk of post-vaccinal encephalitis. This must be weighed against the risk of contracting rabies. Vaccine should not be given unless the skin is broken or a mucosal surface has been contaminated by the animal's saliva. The schedule of inoculations may be reduced if the patient has had a previous full course of antirabic inoculations. If severe sensitivity appears in the course of vaccination, either with suspensions of nervous tissue or with duck embryo vaccine, complete the series with the other type.

(4) With severe exposure (multiple or deep puncture wounds or any bites on the head, face, neck, hands or fingers), if there is any likelihood that the animal is rabid, give a dose of rabies hyperimmune serum immediately, infiltrating the bite wound with serum if possible (see 9A-1a(3) below); follow promptly with a full 21-day course of vaccine (discontinue when the biting animal proves to be nonrabid), with booster doses of non-nervous tissue vaccine at 10, and again at 20 days, after initial series is completed. To avoid anaphylaxis, an intradermal or subcutaneous test dose should precede administration of serum. With mild exposure (scratches, lacerations or single bites on areas of the body other than the head, face, neck, hands or fingers, or open wounds such as abrasions, that are suspected of being contaminated with saliva), see the Guide for Post-Exposure Antirabies Prophylaxis in this section.

c. Management of an animal bite, adapted from Fifth Report of the WHO Expert Committee on Rabies by the USPHS Advisory Committee on Immunization Practices, is summarized thus:

CHECKLIST OF TREATMENTS FOR ANIMAL BITES

1. Flush Wound Immediately (First Aid).
2. Thorough Wound Cleansing Under Medical Supervision.
3. Antirabies Serum and/or Vaccine as Indicated.
4. Tetanus Prophylaxis and Antibacterial Treatment when Required.
5. No Sutures or Wound Closure Advised.

GUIDE FOR POSTEXPOSURE ANTIRABIES PROPHYLAXIS

(These recommendations are intended only as a guide. They may be modified according to knowledge of the species of biting animal and circumstances surrounding the biting incident.)

Biting Animal		Treatment		
		Exposure		
Species	Status at Time of Attack	No Lesion	Mild *	Severe *
Dog or Cat	Healthy	None	None[1]	S[1]
	Signs suggestive of rabies	None	V[2]	S+V[2]
	Escaped or unknown	None	V	S+V
	Rabid	None	S+V	S+V
Skunk, Fox, Racoon, Coyote, Bat	Regard as rabid in unprovoked attack	None	S+V	S+V
Other	Consider individually—see rationale of treatment in text.			

CODE: *=See definitions in text.
V=Rabies vaccine.
S=Antirabies serum.
1=Begin vaccine at first sign of rabies in biting dog or cat during holding period (preferably 7–10 days).
2=Discontinue vaccine if biting dog or cat is healthy 5 days after exposure, or if acceptable laboratory negativity has been demonstrated in animal killed at time of attack. If observed animal dies after 5 days and brain is positive, resume treatment.

SOURCE: Adapted from the Fifth Report of the WHO Expert Committee on Rabies (Technical Report Series No. 321, 1966), and from the USPHS Advisory Committee on Immunization Practices, DHEW.

2) Education of the public in the necessity of complying with restrictions on dogs; of vaccinating dogs; of seeking immediate medical attention if bitten by a dog; of confining and observing animals that have inflicted bites; of prompt reporting to the police of dogs manifesting strange behavior; and of reporting rabies in dogs and bites of persons by animals to the local health authority. Warn against picking up or handling sick or strangely acting bats or other animals.

3) Detention and clinical observation for 7 to 10 days of dogs or other animals known to have bitten a person or showing suspicious signs of rabies. Domestic animals need not be killed until existence of rabies is reasonably established by clinical signs, but wild animals should be sacrificed and the brain examined for evidence of rabies. Rabid dogs and cats usually show a change in behavior, with excitability or paralysis, followed by death; if animal was infective at the time of bite, signs of rabies in the animal will follow usually within 5 days.

4) Immediate submission to a laboratory of intact heads, packed in ice, of animals that died of suspected rabies. Confirmation of rabies is by demonstration of Negri bodies in the brain, by animal inoculation, or by demonstration of viral antigen by fluorescent antibody testing.

5) Immediate destruction or 6 months' detention in approved pound or kennel of unvaccinated dogs or cats bitten by known rabid animals. If previously vaccinated, revaccinate and restrain for 30 days.

6) Registration and licensing of all dogs. Dogs in congested areas should be kept on leash when not within the owner's premises. Collect and destroy stray dogs by public authority. Emphasize preventive vaccination of dogs; attenuated live vaccines administered intramuscularly confer longer lasting immunity than inactivated vaccines.

7) Institution of cooperative programs with wildlife conservation authorities for selectively reducing numbers of fox, skunk, and other wildlife hosts in areas of sylvatic rabies.

8) Preexposure immunization, with two 1.0-ml doses of non-nervous tissue vaccine 1 month apart and a third dose after 6–7 months, for individuals at high risk, e.g., veterinarians and wildlife conservation personnel in enzootic areas, staff of quarantine kennels, laboratory and field personnel working with rabies. Booster doses are given every 2–3 years if exposure continues. When feasible, serum should be tested 3–4 weeks after the third dose, for antirabies antibodies; if not present, ordinary postexposure prophylaxis (see 9A1 above) will be practiced. If an antibody response was demonstrated, one or five booster doses, depending on severity of the bite, will suffice.

B. Control of patient, contacts, and the immediate environment:

    1) Report to local health authority: Obligatory case report required in most states and countries, Class 2A (see Preface).

    2) Isolation: For duration of the illness.

    3) Concurrent disinfection: Of saliva and articles soiled therewith. Immediate attendants should be warned of the hazard of inoculation with saliva and should be provided with rubber gloves and protective gowns.

    4) Quarantine: None.

    5) Immunization of contacts: Contacts of a patient with rabies need not be vaccinated.

    6) Investigation of contacts and source of infection: Search for rabid animal and for persons and other animals bitten.

    7) Specific treatment: For clinical rabies, none.

C. Epidemic measures: Applicable only to animals: a sporadic disease in man.

    1) Establishment of area control under authority of state laws, public health regulations and local ordinances, in cooperation with appropriate wildlife conservation and livestock sanitary authorities.

    2) Widespread vaccination of dogs, preferably with an attenuated live vaccine, through officially sponsored intensified programs providing mass immunization at temporary and emergency stations. For protection of other domestic animals, vaccines at the proper level of attenuation for that animal species must be used.

    3) Strict enforcement of regulations requiring collection, detention and destruction of ownerless or stray dogs, and of unvaccinated dogs found off owner's premises.

    4) Encourage reduction in the dog population by castration, spaying, and drugs.

D. International measures:

    1) Strict compliance by common carriers and by travelers with national laws and regulations that institute quarantine or require vaccination of dogs.

    2) WHO Reference Centres (see Preface).

RAT-BITE FEVER

Two diseases are included under the general term of rat-bite fever; one is caused by *Streptobacillus moniliformis,* the other by *Spirillum minus.* Because they are similar in clinical and epidemiological behavior, and because it is seen occasionally in the U.S.A., *Streptobacillus moniliformis* is presented in detail. Variations manifested by *Spirillum minus* infection are noted under that disease.

A. STREPTOBACILLUS MONILIFORMIS DISEASE

1. Identification—Usually there is a history of rat bite within 10 days followed by primary edematous lesion with regional lymphadenitis, sharp febrile paroxysms, alternating afebrile intervals, and a morbilliform and petechial rash, polyarthritis and leucocytosis. The bite wound, although apparently healed, later breaks down to leave an ulcer that runs a chronic course, often painful and prolonged, and occasionally ending in a subcutaneous abscess. Fatality may reach 10% in untreated cases. Synonym: Haverhill fever.

Laboratory confirmation is by isolation of the organism by inoculation of material from primary lesion or lymph node, blood, joint fluid, or pus into appropriate bacteriological medium or into laboratory animals such as guinea pigs or mice. (One must be sure that the laboratory animals are not naturally infected.) Serum antibodies may be detected by agglutination test.

2. Occurrence—Distribution is worldwide; an uncommon disease in North and South America, in most European countries. Clinical reports show this to be the usual form of rat-bite fever in U.S.A.

3. Infectious agent—*Streptobacillus moniliformis (Streptothrix muris rattis, Haverhillia multiformis, Actinomyces muris).*

4. Reservoir—Reservoir is an infected rat, rarely other rodents (squirrel, weasel).

5. Mode of transmission—Infection is transmitted by secretions of mouth, nose, or conjunctival sac of an infected animal, most frequently introduced by biting. Sporadic cases without reference to bite have been recorded. Blood from an experimental laboratory animal has infected man. Actual contact with rats is not necessary; infection has occurred in persons working or living in rat-infested buildings. Some outbreaks have been traced to contaminated milk or milk products.

6. Incubation period—Three to 10 days, rarely longer.

7. Period of communicability—Not directly transmitted from man to man.

8. Susceptibility and resistance—No information.

9. Methods of Control—

A. Preventive measures:

1) Reduction of rat population.
2) Ratproofing of dwellings.

B. Control of patient, contacts, and the immediate environment:

1) *Report to local health authority:* Obligatory report of epidemics; no individual case report, Class 4 (Preface).

2) *Isolation:* None.

3) *Concurrent disinfection:* None.

4) *Quarantine:* None.

5) *Immunization of contacts:* None.

6) *Investigation of contacts and source of infection:* Not practicable.

7) *Specific treatment:* Tetracyclines or penicillin. Penicillin inhibits only the bacillary form and has no effect on the L_1 phase of *Streptobacillus*. Treatment should continue for 7 to 10 days.

C. *Epidemic measures:* Grouped cases presenting the typical symptoms require search for epidemiologic evidence of a relation to milk supply.

D. *International measures:* None.

B. SPIRILLUM MINUS DISEASE—SODOKU

A sporadic rat-bite fever, Sodoku, is caused by *Spirillum minus* (*Spirochaeta morsus muris*), is less frequent in U.S.A. than *Streptobacillus moniliformis* disease, but is the common form in Japan and the Far East. Incidence is no greater there than in western countries. Untreated case fatality is approximately 10%. Clinical *Spirillum minus* disease differs from *Streptobacillus* disease in the usual absence of arthritic symptoms, and a more plaque-like rash. The incubation period is generally longer, 1 to 3 weeks, and usually more than 7 days. Laboratory methods are essential for differentiation; animal inoculation is used for isolation of the spirillum.

RELAPSING FEVER

1. Identification—A systemic spirochetal disease in which periods of fever lasting 2 to 9 days alternate with afebrile periods of 2 to 4 days; the number of relapses varies from 2 to 10 or more. Each pyrexial period terminates by crisis and the total duration of the louse-borne disease averages 13 to 16 days; the tick-borne disease usually lasts longer. Transitory petechial rashes are common during the initial period of fever. The overall fatality rate in untreated cases is between 2 and 10%; it sometimes exceeds 50% in the epidemic louse-borne disease.

Diagnosis is by demonstration of the infectious agent in dark-field preparations of fresh blood or stained thick blood films, or by inoculation of laboratory rats or mice with 1 ml of blood taken during the pyrexial period and before crisis.

2. Occurrence—Characteristically epidemic where mode of spread is by lice, and endemic where ticks are the vector. Louse-borne relapsing fever occurs in limited localities in Asia, East Africa (Ethiopia and the Sudan), North and Central Africa, and South America. Epidemics are commonly incident to war, to famine, or to other situations where malnourished, overcrowded populations with poor personal hygiene favor multiplication and wide dissemination of the louse vector. The tick-borne endemic disease is widespread throughout tropical Africa; foci exist in Spain, northern Africa, Saudi Arabia, Iran, India, and parts of central Asia, as well as in North and South America. Louse-borne relapsing fever has not been reported in the U.S.A. for many years; human cases of tick-borne disease occur in limited localities of several western states.

3. Infectious agent—*Borrelia recurrentis,* a spirochete. Many different strains have been described, related to area of isolation and vector rather than to inherent biologic differences. Cross-protection occurs between louse- and tick-borne strains. Strains isolated during a relapse often show antigenic differences from those of an immediately preceding paroxysm.

4. Reservoir—Reservoir of louse-borne disease is man; immediate source of infection is an infective louse. Wild rodents are the natural reservoir of some tick-borne relapsing fevers, in the U.S.A. principally ground squirrels and prairie dogs; also ticks through transovarian transmission.

5. Mode of transmission—Epidemic relapsing fever is acquired by crushing an infective louse, *P. humanus humanus,* over the bite wound or over an abrasion of the skin. Man also is infected by the bite or coxal fluid of an infected argasid tick, principally *Ornithodoros turicata* and *Ornithodoros hermsi* in the U.S.A.; *Ornithodoros rudis* and *Ornithodoros talaje* in Central and South America; *Ornithodoros moubata* in tropical Africa; and *Ornithodoros tholozani* in the Near East and Middle East. The tick attacks, rapidly engorges, and promptly leaves the host. In Africa, certain ticks transmit spirochetes directly from man to man.

6. Incubation period—Five days to 15 days; usually 8.

7. Period of communicability—Not directly transmitted from man to man. The louse becomes infective 4 to 5 days after ingestion of blood from an infected person and remains so for life (20 to 40 days). Infected ticks can live without feeding for several years and remain infective.

8. Susceptibility and resistance—Susceptibility is general. Duration of immunity after clinical attack is unknown; probably less than 2 years.

9. Methods of control—

A. Preventive measures:

1) Louse control, by measures prescribed for Louse-borne typhus fever (see pp. 276–277).
2) Tick control, especially reduction of tick population in living quarters, by procedures prescribed for Rocky Mountain spotted fever (see p. 207).

B. Control of patient, contacts, and the immediate environment:

1) Report to local health authority: Obligatory report of louse-borne relapsing fever under International Sanitary and Health Regulations, Class 1 (see Preface). Tick-borne disease, in selected endemic areas, Class 3B (see Preface).

2) Isolation: None, provided the patient, his clothing, all household contacts, and the immediate environment have been deloused or freed from ticks.

3) Concurrent disinfection: None, if proper disinfestation has been carried out.

4) Quarantine: Exposed louse-infested susceptibles may be released after application of residual insecticide; otherwise, quarantine for 9 days.

5) Immunization of contacts: None.

6) Investigation of contacts and source of infection: For the individual tick-borne case, search for sources of infection; for louse-borne, unprofitable, calling for a community effort (see 9C following).

7) Specific treatment: Tetracyclines.

C. Epidemic measures: When reporting has been good and cases are few, application of insecticides with residual effect to contacts of all reported cases. Where infection is known to be widespread, systematic application of an effective residual insecticide to all persons in the community.

D. International measures:

1) Telegraphic notification by governments to WHO and to adjacent countries of the occurrence of an outbreak of louse-borne relapsing fever in an area previously free of the disease, regardless of source.

2) As of January 1, 1971, louse-borne relapsing fever ceases to be a quarantinable disease under international regulations, but the measures outlined in paragraph (1) above should be continued because it is now a *Disease under Surveillance by WHO,* in accordance with a Resolution of the 22nd World Health Assembly.

RESPIRATORY DISEASE, ACUTE VIRAL

Numerous acute respiratory illnesses of known and presumed viral etiology are grouped here under the general title of Acute Viral Respiratory Disease. Clinically they are of 2 forms: the more severe febrile illnesses, including pneumonias and croups, which are sometimes fatal, and the less severe nonfebrile common colds. Both clinical forms are undifferentiated in the sense that neither is regularly identified with a particular virus. The diseases caused by known viruses have important epidemiological attributes in common, such as reservoir and mode of spread. Their clinical characteristics cannot be distinguished from those of diseases of presumed but unidentified viral origin. Many of the viruses invade any part of the respiratory tract; others show a predilection for certain anatomical sites; few remain localized. Site may be influenced by epidemiological factors. Some predispose to bacterial complications, occasionally serious. High incidence and resulting disability with consequent economic loss make diseases of this group a major public health problem.

Several other nonbacterial infections of the respiratory tract are sufficiently uniform in their clinical and epidemiological manifestations and occur in such regular association with a specific infectious agent as to be recognized as disease entities. Psittacosis, influenza and herpangina are examples (pp. 186, 119 and 110, respectively). They are not included in the group as acute viral respiratory diseases.

A. ACUTE FEBRILE RESPIRATORY DISEASE

1. Identification—Viral diseases of the respiratory tract characterized by fever and one or more constitutional reactions such as chills or chilliness, headache or general aching, malaise, anorexia, and in infants occasional gastrointestinal disturbances. Localizing signs also occur at various sites in the respiratory tract, either alone or in combination, such as rhinitis, pharyngitis or tonsillitis, laryngitis, laryngotracheitis, bronchitis, bronchiolitis or pneumonitis, or pneumonia. Symptoms and signs usually subside in 2 to 5 days without complications; infection may, however, extend or be complicated by bacterial sinusitis, otitis media, pneumonitis or persistent bronchitis, depending on age, virus involved, prior experience with the same or related infectious agents, season of year and other environmental factors. Blood leucocytes and the respiratory bacterial flora are within normal limits except as modified by secondary infections. Commonly diagnosed clinical syndromes include upper respiratory infection (URI), and acute respiratory disease (ARD).

Specific diagnosis requires isolation of the virus from respiratory secretions in appropriate tissue or cell cultures and/or antibody studies of paired sera. Differentiation has minor usefulness in management of sporadic undifferentiated respiratory disease. In outbreaks or in continuing incidence at hyperendemic levels, it is important to identify cause in a representative sample of typical cases to determine whether effective specific control measures are available.

Practical management of acute respiratory disease depends on the differentiation of viral infections from disease entities for which specific measures are available, e.g., Q fever and streptococcal infection, by appropriate clinical and laboratory methods.

2. Occurrence—Worldwide, usually. Seasonal in temperate zones with greatest incidence during fall and winter. In large communities, some viral illnesses recur monthly with little seasonal pattern (e.g., parainfluenza types 1 and 3 and adenovirus type 1) ; others tend to occur in scattered outbreaks (e.g., respiratory syncytial, parainfluenza 2 and adenovirus 3 and 5). Annual incidence is high, particularly in children. During autumn, winter and spring, attack rates for preschool children may average 2% per week as compared with 1% for school children and 0.5% for adults. Incidence rate of disease depends upon proportion of susceptibles infected and the agent. Many pathogens may be prevalent in a community but one or another commonly predominates for a few weeks at a time. Under special host and environmental conditions, certain viral infections may disable ¼ of a population within a few weeks, e.g., outbreaks of adenovirus types 3, 4, or 7 in military recruits, and outbreaks of adenovirus type 3 (pharyngoconjunctival fever) in children attending summer camps.

3. Infectious agents—Although some are unidentified, 20 or more serotypes of myxovirus, adenovirus and picornavirus families are considered etiologic agents of acute febrile respiratory illnesses. Well established and common causes in infants and young children include adenovirus types 1, 3 and 5, parainfluenza types 1, 2 and 3, and respiratory syncytial viruses; each may cause pneumonia, severe bronchitis and pharyngitis or croup, but parainfluenza 1 is a predominant cause of croup and respiratory syncytial virus a predominant cause of pneumonia and bronchiolitis. In addition, poliovirus type 2, echovirus types 3, 11 and 20 and various other enteroviruses cause febrile respiratory illness in children under varying conditions. Coxsackie A2I (Coe virus) may cause febrile illness in adults and the Reo and ECHO viruses have an indefinite relationship. Adenovirus types 3, 14, 21, and particularly types 4 and 7 are common causes of acute respiratory disease in military recruits.

4. Reservoir—Reservoir is man. Many known viruses produce inapparent infection; adenoviruses may remain latent in tonsils and adenoids and be reactivated from time to time over a long period of years.

5. Mode of transmission—Mainly by direct oral contact or by droplet spread; indirectly by handkerchiefs, eating utensils or other articles freshly soiled by respiratory discharges of an infected person. Some viruses are discharged in the feces (enteroviruses and adenovirus) and these may be involved in transmission.

6. Incubation period—From a few days to a week or more.

7. Period of communicability—For the duration of active disease; little is known about subclinical or latent infections.

8. Susceptibility and resistance—Susceptibility is universal. Illness more frequent and severe in infants and children. Infection induces specific antibodies. Reinfection with respiratory syncytial and parainfluenza viruses is common, but illness from reinfection is generally milder or absent.

9. Methods of control—

A. Preventive measures:

1) Killed adenovirus and oral live attenuated adenovirus vaccines have proved effective against type-specific infections in military recruits. Not recommended for general use in civilian populations.
2) When possible, avoid crowding in living and sleeping quarters, especially in institutions, in barracks and on shipboard.
3) Education of the public in personal hygiene as in covering the mouth when coughing and sneezing and sanitary disposal of discharges from mouth and nose.

B. Control of patient, contacts, and the immediate environment:

1) *Report to local health authority:* Obligatory report of epidemics; no individual case report, Class 4 (see Preface).
2) *Isolation:* No established value. Infected persons should avoid direct and indirect exposure of others, particularly little children, feeble or aged persons, or patients with other illness. Such modified isolation as can be accomplished by rest in bed during the acute stage is advised.
3) *Concurrent disinfection:* Of eating and drinking utensils; sanitary disposal of nose and mouth discharges.
4) *Quarantine:* None.
5) *Immunization of contacts:* None.
6) *Investigation of contacts:* Unprofitable.
7) *Specific treatment:* None. Indiscriminate use of antibiotics is to be discouraged. These valuable therapeutic agents should be reserved for identified bacterial complications such as pneumonia, tracheobronchitis, otitis and sinusitis.

C. Epidemic measures: No effective measures known. Isolation may be helpful in institutions; procedures such as ultraviolet irradiation, aerosols and dust control have not proved useful. Avoid crowding. (See 9A2 above.)

D. International measures: WHO Reference Centres (see Preface).

B. THE COMMON COLD

1. Identification—Acute catarrhal infections of the upper respiratory tract characterized by coryza, lacrimation, irritated nasopharynx, chilliness and malaise lasting 2 to 7 days. Fever is uncommon in children and rare in adults. Probably never fatal; importance rests in many days of disability, industrial and school absenteeism, and predisposition to more serious bacterial complications such as sinusitis, otitis media, laryngitis, tracheitis and bronchitis. Blood leucocytes and bacterial flora of respiratory tract are within normal limits in the absence of complications.

Tissue culture of nasal secretions may demonstrate a known virus in 20–35% of cases. Specific clinical, epidemiologic and other manifestations aid differentiation from similar diseases due to toxic, allergic, physical or psychologic stimuli.

2. Occurrence—Worldwide distribution; endemic and epidemic. In temperate zones, incidence rises in fall, winter and spring. Many persons, except in small isolated communities, have 1 to 6 colds yearly. Incidence highest in children under 5 years; gradual decline with increasing age.

3. Infectious agents—55 or more rhinovirus types, several coronaviruses, and some unknown viruses. Many other serotypes of adenovirus, myxovirus and picornavirus families cause colds under varying conditions.

4. Reservoir—Reservoir is man.

5. Mode of transmission—Transmission presumably is by direct oral contact or by droplet spread; indirectly by articles freshly soiled by discharges of nose and throat of the infected person.

6. Incubation period—Between 12 and 72 hours, usually 24 hours.

7. Period of communicability—Nasal washings taken 24 hours before onset and for 5 days after onset have produced symptoms in experimentally infected volunteers.

8. Susceptibility and resistance—Susceptibility is universal. Inapparent and abortive infections occur; frequency of healthy carriers generally undetermined but known to be rare with some viral agents, notably rhinoviruses. The frequently repeated attacks may be due to transient homologous immunity, to the multiplicity of agents or to other causes. Artificial immunization is not available.

9. Methods of control—

1) Report to local health authority: Official report not ordinarily justifiable, Class 5 (see Preface).

2) Other control measures as for Acute Febrile Respiratory Disease 9A, B and C, p. 202.

RHEUMATIC FEVER

1. Identification—Rheumatic fever occurs as one of the sequelae in a small proportion of patients with Group A hemolytic streptococcal upper respiratory infection (1 to 3%). The streptococcal infection frequently is inapparent or clinically unrecognized but can almost always be identified by appropriate serum antibody tests.

The major clinical manifestations of rheumatic fever are carditis, polyarthritis, chorea, subcutaneous nodules and erythema marginatum. Fever, rapid pulse, epistaxis, pallor, weight loss, anorexia and abdominal and precordial pain are a second group of findings of lesser diagnostic significance. Mild and inapparent attacks occur, their relative frequency unknown; definite and even severe heart disease may develop in the absence of evident acute rheumatic fever.

Bacteriologic or serologic (chiefly antistreptolysin O) evidence of a preceding Group A streptococcal infection adds diagnostic weight to suggestive symptoms.

2. Occurrence—A frequent disease throughout the world; in U.S.A., most prevalent in Rocky Mountain region, New England, and North and Central Atlantic states; lowest in the south and southwest. Seasonal incidence is that of streptococcal infections, in U.S.A. predominant during late winter and early spring, and low during summer and early autumn. Reliable data on frequency in tropical areas are not available; the impression of a lesser prevalence than in temperate zones is not always supported. For unknown reasons, incidence and mortality of rheumatic fever in U.S.A. are declining.

3. Precipitating agent—Attacks usually follow Group A hemolytic streptococcal respiratory infections. However, rheumatic fever is not an infection in the usual sense but probably a sensitivity reaction induced by streptococci. No specific serotype of hemolytic streptococcus is regularly associated with the disease.

4. Reservoir—Usually man.

5. Mode of transmission of precipitating infection—See Hemolytic Streptococcal Disease (p. 239).

6. Incubation period—Not applicable. Symptoms appear about 2 to 3 weeks after Group A streptococcal infection.

7. Period of communicability—Not known to be communicable; the preceding streptococcal infection which induces rheumatic fever is communicable but usually has subsided by the time rheumatic fever develops.

8. Susceptibility and resistance—All ages are susceptible but rare prior to age 5 years; the greatest incidence is in children 6 to 12 years old. Has a natural tendency to recur with succeeding Group A streptococcal infections; no evidence that immunity develops although various antibodies to Group A streptococci or their extracellular products can be demonstrated.

9. Methods of control—

A. *Preventive measures:* Prevention is based on prevention cr proper therapy of Group A streptococcal infections (see Hemolytic Streptococcal Disease, pp. 240–241).

B. *Control of patient, contacts, and the immediate environment:*

1) *Report to local health authority:* In selected endemic areas (U.S.A.); in many states and countries not a reportable disease, Class 3B (see Preface). Areas of high incidence

will profit materially by encouraging individual case report over prescribed periods sufficient to acquire epidemiological data necessary for improved methods of control.

2) *Isolation:* None.

3) *Concurrent disinfection:* None.

4) *Quarantine:* None.

5) *Immunization of contacts:* Not applicable.

6) *Investigation of contacts:* None.

7) *Specific treatment:* Individuals known to have had rheu- matic fever or convalescent from that disease should receive chemoprophylaxis for long periods thereafter, possibly throughout life, at least until age 18 years, and past that age if necessary to give a period of 5 years from last at- tack. Patients with residual rheumatic heart disease are particularly in need of continued prophylaxis. Penicillin is the drug of choice and should be given orally on a daily basis, or intramuscularly as penicillin G benzathine (Bi- cillin) once monthly. Erythromycin or sulfonamides are alternative drugs. Prior to prophylaxis, proper treatment should be instituted to free the patient of Group A strepto- cocci (see Hemolytic Streptococcal Disease 9B7, p. 241) ; for this purpose, penicillin is the drug of choice, provided the patient is not allergic to it.

Salicylates are widely used in management of the acute phase of rheumatic fever, either acetylsalicylic acid or sodium salicylate, continued for duration of the active dis- ease. In severe cases, steroid therapy may be preferred and has been used with success. Patients must be pro- tected continuously from intercurrent infection, particularly with Group A hemolytic streptococci.

C. *Epidemic measures:* Epidemics of rheumatic fever occur only in association with epidemics of Group A streptococcal infec- tion. Proper therapy of recognized streptococcal infections will avert the subsequent development of rheumatic fever and thus prevent about half of the cases of rheumatic fever.

D. *International measures:* None.

RICKETTSIAL FEVERS, TICK-BORNE
(Spotted Fever Group)

The rickettsial diseases of the spotted fever group are clinically similar and are caused by closely related rickettsiae. They are trans- mitted by species of ixodid ticks, which are widely distributed throughout the world, and in different geographical areas. Similar control measures are applicable and the broad-spectrum antibiotics are effective therapeutically.

Complement-fixation tests using group-specific spotted fever antigens become positive in the 2nd week; the Weil-Felix reactions with Proteus OX-19 and Proteus OX-2 become positive less often. Definitive identification of a particular agent is essentially a research procedure; the need rarely arises because the diseases do not overlap in geographical distribution.

A. ROCKY MOUNTAIN SPOTTED FEVER

1. Identification—This prototype disease of the spotted fever group is characterized by sudden onset, with fever which ordinarily persists for 2 to 3 weeks, headache, chills, and conjunctival injection. A maculopapular rash, appearing on the extremities about the 3rd day, soon includes the palms and soles and spreads rapidly to most of the body; petechiae and hemorrhages are common. Fatality is about 20% in the absence of specific therapy; death is uncommon with prompt treatment. Synonyms: New World spotted fever, Tick-borne typhus fever.

2. Occurrence—Throughout most of the United States, during spring and summer. Most prevalent in South Atlantic states—less prevalent in Rocky Mountain region. Commonest in wooded suburban areas of the Piedmont Plateau. In western United States adult males are attacked most frequently, children in the East; the difference in infection relates to varied exposure to infected ticks. Fatality increases with age. Infection also occurs in western Canada, western and central Mexico, Panama, Colombia, and Brazil.

3. Infectious agent—*Rickettsia rickettsii.*

4. Reservoir—Infection in nature is maintained by transovarian and transstadial passage in ticks. The organisms can be transmitted to various rodents and other animals, which assists in maintaining the disease cycle.

5. Mode of transmission—Ordinarily by bite of an infected tick with several hours of attachment to allow "reactivation"; also contamination of skin with crushed tissues or feces of tick. In eastern and southern United States the common vector is the dog tick, *Dermacentor variabilis;* in northwestern United States, wood tick, *Dermacentor andersoni;* in southwestern United States, occasionally the Lone Star tick, *Amblyomma americanum.* The rabbit tick *Haemaphysalis leporispalustris* is infected in nature but usually does not bite man.

6. Incubation period—From 3 to about 10 days.

7. Period of communicability—Not directly transmitted from man to man. The tick remains infective for life, commonly as long as 18 months.

8. Susceptibility and resistance—Susceptibility is general. One attack probably confers immunity.

9. Methods of control—

A. *Preventive measures:*

1) Avoid tick-infested areas when feasible; remove ticks from the person promptly and carefully without crushing; protect hands when removing ticks from animals. Tick repellents of value are N, N-diethyl-m-toluamide and dimethylphthalate.

2) Measures designed to reduce tick populations are generally impractical. In selected land areas, direct application of chlordane, dieldrin, lindane, diazinon or benzene hexachloride gives excellent control of some vectors.

3) Vaccines containing killed *R. rickettsii* may result in lower fatality in cases not given specific therapy. Vaccination is generally limited to those persons at high risk such as persons frequenting highly endemic areas and laboratory workers exposed to the agent. Booster doses at yearly intervals are necessary.

4) Education of the public in mode of transmission by ticks and the means for personal protection.

B. *Control of patient, contacts, and the immediate environment:*

1) *Report to local health authority:* In selected areas (U.S.A.); in many countries not a reportable disease, Class 3B (see Preface).

2) *Isolation:* None.

3) *Concurrent disinfection:* Destroy all ticks on patients.

4) *Quarantine:* None.

5) *Immunization of contacts:* Unnecessary.

6) *Investigation of contacts and source of infection:* Not profitable except as a community measure; see 9C below.

7) *Specific treatment:* The tetracycline antibiotics or chloramphenicol in daily oral doses until patient is afebrile (usually 3 days) and for 1 or 2 additional days.

C. *Epidemic measures:* In hyperendemic areas particular attention should be paid to identification of the tick species involved and of infested areas, and to recommendations in 9 A1, 2, 4 above.

D. *International measures:* WHO Reference Centres (see Preface).

B. BOUTONNEUSE FEVER

1. Identification—A mild to moderately severe febrile illness of a few days to 2 weeks, characterized by a primary lesion at the site of a tick bite. The lesion (tache noire), usually present at onset of fever, is a small ulcer 2–5 mm in diameter with black center and red areola; regional lymph nodes are enlarged. A generalized maculopapular erythematous rash appears about the 4th or 5th day, usually involving palms and soles, and persists 6 to 7 days; with antibiotic treatment, fever lasts no more than 2 days. Fatality is less than 3% even without specific therapy. Synonyms: Marseilles fever, African tick typhus, Kenya tick typhus, India tick typhus.

2. **Occurrence**—Widely distributed throughout the African continent, in India and in those parts of Europe and the Middle East adjacent to the Mediterranean, Black and Caspian Seas. In more temperate areas, highest incidence is during warmer months, when ticks are numerous; in tropical areas throughout the year. Outbreaks may occur when groups of susceptibles are brought into an endemic area.

3. **Infectious agent**—*Rickettsia conori.*

4. **Reservoir**—As in Rocky Mountain Spotted Fever, preceding.

5. **Mode of transmission**—In the Mediterranean area, by bite of infected *Rhipicephalus sanguineus* infesting dogs. In South Africa, ticks infected in nature and presumed to be vectors include *Haemaphysalis leachi, Amblyomma hebraeum, Rhipicephalus appendiculatus, Boophilus decloratus,* and *Hyalomma aegyptium.*

6. **Incubation period**—Usually 5 to 7 days.

7, 8, 9. **Period of communicability, Susceptibility and resistance, and Methods of control**—As in Rocky Mountain Spotted Fever, preceding, except that vaccine is not employed.

C. QUEENSLAND TICK TYPHUS

1. **Identification**—Clinically similar to Boutonneuse fever, except that primary lesion is uncommon.

2. **Occurrence**—Queensland, Australia.

3. **Infectious agent**—*Rickettsia australis.*

4. **Reservoir**—As in Rocky Mountain Spotted Fever, preceding.

5. **Mode of transmission**—As in Rocky Mountain Spotted Fever, preceding. *Ixodes holocyclus* infesting small marsupials and wild rodents is probably the major vector.

6. **Incubation period**—About 7 to 10 days.

7, 8, 9. **Period of communicability, Susceptibility and resistance Methods of control**—As in Boutonneuse fever (see above).

D. NORTH ASIAN TICK-BORNE RICKETTSIOSIS

1. **Identification**—Clinically similar to Boutonneuse fever. Synonym: Siberian tick typhus.

2. **Occurrence**—Asiatic USSR and the Mongolian Peoples Republic.

3. **Infectious agent**—*Rickettsia siberica.*

4. **Reservoir**—As in Rocky Mountain Spotted Fever, preceding.

5. **Mode of transmission**—By the bite of ticks of the genera *Dermacentor* and *Haemaphysalis,* which infest certain wild rodents.

6. Incubation period—Two to 7 days.

7, 8, 9. Period of communicability, Susceptibility and resistance and **Methods of control**—As in Boutonneuse fever, preceding.

RICKETTSIALPOX

1. Identification—Rickettsialpox is characterized by initial skin lesion, chills, fever, varicelliform rash, and a mild to severe course; even without specific therapy, fatality is less than 1%. The initial lesion is a firm red papule appearing about a week in advance of fever, most commonly on covered parts of the body; becomes vesicular, then covered by a scab, and after about 3 weeks leaves a small pigmented scar. Fever, often preceded by chills, is remittent, with peaks of 39.4 C to 40.6 C (103 F to 105 F) and usually lasts less than 1 week. Headache, muscular pain, and general malaise are frequent. The secondary rash is manifest 3 to 4 days after onset of fever; has no characteristic distribution; seldom on palms or soles; progresses through papular and papulovesicular stages, lasting less than a week and leaving no scars; local lymphadenopathy in region of the initial lesion. Synonym: Vesicular rickettsiosis.

Specific diagnosis is by complement-fixation test, positive between the 2nd and 3rd week of the disease.

2. Occurrence—In the U.S.A. cases occur annually in New York City, principally among residents of apartment houses where mouse, mite and rickettsia maintain a natural cycle of infection; a few cases have been recognized in Boston, Hartford, Philadelphia, and Cleveland. The vector occurs in foci from the Atlantic Coast to Arizona and Utah. Disease also occurs in the USSR in the same pattern as in the U.S.A., but commensal rats are also involved in the natural cycle. In Equatorial and South Africa, cases clinically and serologically consistent with rickettsialpox are contracted in the bushveld, suggesting involvement of a wild rodent and various mites. *Rickettsia akari* has been recovered from a field mouse in Korea, although the disease in man is unrecognized there.

3. Infectious agent—*Rickettsia akari,* a member of the spotted fever group of rickettsiae (see pp. 205–209 preceding).

4. Reservoir—The infected house mouse *(Mus musculus),* and possibly the vector mite, *Allodermanyssus sanguineus,* in which transovarian passage of rickettsiae occurs.

5. Mode of transmission—From mouse to mouse and from mouse to man by bite of an infective rodent mite, *A. sanguineus.*

6. Incubation period—Probably 10 to 24 days.

7. Period of communicability—Not directly transmitted from man to man. Duration of infectivity of mouse for mite, and of mite for mouse or man, is unknown.

8. Susceptibility and resistance—Susceptibility appears general. Duration of immunity after attack is unknown.

9. Methods of control—

    A. Preventive measures: Rodent and mite control by elimination of mice and mouse harborages, including proper care and firing of incinerators in dwellings and application of residual miticides (dieldrin and others) to infested areas. Commercial vaccine is neither available nor currently needed.

    B. Control of patient, contacts, and the immediate environment:

        1) Report to local health authority: In selected endemic areas (U.S.A.) ; in most states and countries not reportable, Class 3B (see Preface).

        2) Isolation: None.

        3) Concurrent disinfection: None.

        4) Quarantine: None.

        5) Immunization of contacts: None.

        6) Investigation of contacts and source of infection: Search for mice in dwelling and, if feasible, undertake isolation of rickettsiae from rodents and mites.

        7) Specific treatment: The tetracycline antibiotics and chloramphenicol are equally effective.

    C. Epidemic measures: When groups of cases occur in the same or adjacent dwellings, apply preventive measures listed under 9A above. Observe all residents and treat promptly if disease develops.

    D. International measures: WHO Reference Centres (see Preface).

RUBELLA

1. Identification—A mild febrile infectious disease with a characteristic diffuse punctate and macular rash sometimes resembling that of measles, scarlet fever or both ; few or no constitutional symptoms in children but adults may experience a 1–5 day prodrome characterized by low-grade fever, headache, malaise, mild coryza and conjunctivitis. Postauricular, suboccipital or postcervical lymphadenopathy is common but not pathognomonic ; occasionally adenopathy is generalized. As many as 20–50% of infections may occur without evident rash. Leukopenia is common and thrombocytopenia occurs but only rarely results in hemorrhagic manifestations. Arthritis complicates a significant percentage of infections among adults, particularly among females. Encephalitis is a rare complication. Synonym: German measles.

Congenital Rubella Syndrome occurs among 20–25% of infants born to women who had acquired rubella during the first trimester of pregnancy, with decreasing frequency thereafter. This syndrome includes cataracts, microphthalmia, microcephaly, mental retardation, deafness, patent ductus arteriosus with other cardiac defects, thrombocytopenic purpura, hepatosplenomegaly with jaundice, and radiographically distinctive bone defects. Moderate and severe cases of congenital rubella syndrome are immediately recognizable at birth; mild cases having only slight cardiac involvement or partial deafness may not be detected for months or years after birth. These congenital malformations and even fetal death may occur following both clinically manifest and inapparent rubella infection in the pregnant woman in the first trimester.

Differentiation of rubella from rubeola (pp. 145–149), scarlet fever (pp. 237–242) and a number of mild infections of similar nature is often required (see paragraphs on erythema infectiosum and exanthem subitum below).

In addition, macular and maculopapular rashes occur irregularly in 10 to 15% of patients with infectious mononucleosis; also observed in infections with echoviruses (Types 2, 4, 6, 9, 14, 16), most commonly with ECHO 9, and usually in association with meningeal reaction, fever to 104 F, headache, sore throat and gastroenteritis. Similar rashes occasionally are associated with Coxsackie A–16, A–9, and B–5 infections.

Diagnosis of rubella, especially in pregnant women, should be confirmed by virus isolation from throat swabs or blood in tissue culture, or by demonstration of an antibody response by hemagglutination, complement fixation, or neutralization test with acute and convalescent sera. Recent infection can be confirmed by demonstration of specific IgM antibodies for several weeks after infection.

2. Occurrence—Worldwide in distribution, essentially a universal infection except in remote and isolated communities. Both endemic and epidemic, most prevalent in winter and spring. Extensive epidemics occur occasionally, as in U.S.A. in 1935 and 1964 and Australia in 1940. Primarily a disease of childhood but occurring at somewhat greater frequency among adolescents and adults than measles or chickenpox. Epidemics and outbreaks are common in institutions, colleges and military populations.

3. Infectious agent—The virus of rubella.

4. Reservoir—Reservoir is man.

5. Mode of transmission—Nasopharyngeal secretions of infected persons are infectious; virus is also recoverable from blood, urine, and feces of infected persons. Infants with congenital rubella syndrome, with or without obvious damage from their prenatal infection, excrete the virus and serve as sources of infection to their contacts. Infection is by droplet spread or direct contact with patients, or presumably by indirect contact with articles freshly soiled with discharges from nose and throat, and possibly blood, urine or feces. Airborne transmission may occur.

6. Incubation period—From 14 to 21 days; usually 18 days.

7. Period of communicability—For about 1 week before and at least 4 days after onset of rash. Highly communicable. Infants with congenital rubella syndrome may shed virus for months after birth; the period of shedding is extremely variable.

8. Susceptibility and resistance—Susceptibility is general among young children. In the U.S.A. and some other highly urbanized countries, approximately 85% of adults possess rubella antibody, but studies in Japan, Jamaica, Trinidad and Hawaii reveal that, overall, about 60% of adults were immune—in some countries less than in others, and less in rural than in urban populations. With rare exceptions, one attack of confirmed rubella confers permanent immunity.

9. Methods of control—Efforts to control rubella are prompted primarily by the hazard of significant congenital defects in offspring of women who acquire the disease during pregnancy. Therefore, no attempt should be made to protect female children in good health against exposure to disease before puberty. The immune status of an individual can be determined by the hemagglutination-inhibition test.

A. *Preventive measures:*

1) A single dose of live attenuated rubella virus vaccine has been demonstrated to protect 90–95% of susceptibles against natural exposure. Virus is shed from the nasopharynx 7–18 days after parenteral injection, but no transmission of infection to susceptible contacts has been clearly documented. Because of the induced transient viremia and the unknown teratogenicity of the attenuated virus, administration to a pregnant or potentially pregnant woman *must* be avoided. Administration to all prepubertal children over 1 year of age to increase the immunity of the population to the point where virus transmission cannot take place is the objective of the program in the U.S.A.

2) Immune serum globulin (human) has been used to protect contacts of rubella, with highly variable results. Unconfirmed reports suggest that lots with high levels of specific antibody protect the fetus of exposed pregnant women when given early in the incubation period.

3) Rubella in the early stages of pregnancy is now legally recognized as an indication for therapeutic abortion in many states of the U.S.A. and in many other countries.

B. *Control of patient, contacts, and the immediate environment:*

1) *Report to local health authority:* Case report obligatory (U.S.A.); Class 3B (see Preface).

2) *Isolation:* Impractical for the usual mild childhood or ado-

lescent case unless contacts include nonimmune pregnant women. Susceptible married nurses and other female attendants should avoid exposure to infants with congenital rubella syndrome.

3) Concurrent disinfection: None.

4) Quarantine: None.

5) Immunization of contacts: Immune serum globulin might be considered in the case of susceptible pregnant women exposed to rubella (see 9A2). Susceptible female attendants of patients with possible congenital rubella syndrome should be immunized, provided they are not pregnant and will not become pregnant for at least 2 months.

6) Investigation of contacts: Of no practical value except to clarify diagnosis or to identify adult female contacts in the first trimester of pregnancy. Where facilities exist, and time permits (see 9A2 above), such pregnant contacts should be serologically tested for susceptibility.

7) Specific treatment: None.

C. Epidemic measures: None.

D. International measures: None.

ERYTHEMA INFECTIOSUM : A mild, nonfebrile erythematous eruption occurring in epidemics among children. Characterized clinically by a malar flush and reddening of the skin which occurs, fades and recurs; exaggerated by exposure to sunlight, and unaccompanied by constitutional symptoms. Outbreaks are now recognized more frequently; nonfatal.

EXANTHEM SUBITUM (Roseola infantum) : An acute illness with sudden onset, usually in children under 4 years of age, commonly at about 1 year. A sudden, intermittent fever, sometimes 105 F or 106 F, lasts 3 to 5 days. A typical maculopapular rash on the trunk and later on the rest of the body ordinarily follows lysis of the fever. The rash fades rapidly. Incidence is greatest in the spring. The incubation period is about 10 days, with a range of 7 to 18 days; only mildly communicable. Many inapparent and unrecognized infections seemingly occur among older children. Isolation of an infectious agent has been reported but not confirmed.

SALMONELLOSIS

1. Identification—The commonest clinical manifestation of *Salmonella* infections is acute gastroenteritis, an acute infectious disease with sudden onset of abdominal pain, diarrhea, nausea and vomiting. Dehydration, especially among infants, may be severe. Fever is nearly always present. Anorexia and looseness of the bowels often persist for several days. Occasionally the clinical course is that of an enteric fever or of septicemia with or without focal infection. Although every *Salmonella* strain is potentially capable of producing any of these three clinical syndromes, the more severe illnesses are more likely to be associated with some bacterial serotypes and certain host factors. A *Salmonella* infection may begin as acute gastroenteritis and develop into enteric fever or septicemia. The infectious agent may localize in any tissue of the body, producing abscesses and causing arthritis, cholecystitis, endocarditis, meningitis, pericarditis, pneumonia or pyelonephritis. Deaths are uncommon except in the very young or very old, or in debilitated persons.

In cases of enteric fever and septicemia, *Salmonella* may be recovered on usual enteric media from feces and from the blood during the acute stages of illness, but with increasing difficulty from feces as convalescence progresses in cases of gastroenteritis.

2. Occurrence—A worldwide common disease, more extensively reported in North American and European countries, often classified with food poisoning (pp. 89–94) because of the predominant source of infection. The proportion of cases that are recognized is small and is largely dependent on diligence and effort in the field investigation. Small outbreaks in the general population are the more usual manifestation of *Salmonella* gastroenteritis. Large outbreaks in hospitals, institutions for children, restaurants and nursing homes are not infrequent, arising from food contaminated at its source or cross-contaminated during food processing, or due to spread from an undetected carrier. Outbreaks in which cases occur over a long period, particularly among young children, suggest person-to-person spread.

3. Infectious agents—Numerous serotypes of *Salmonella* are pathogenic for both animals and man. Host-adapted human strains (see Typhoid and Paratyphoid Fevers, pp. 271, 166) are excluded. The types most common in the period 1963–1968 in U.S.A. were *S. typhimurium, S. heidelberg, S. newport, S. infantis, S. enteritidis, S. derby,* and *S. st. paul;* there is much variation from country to country. In most countries maintaining *Salmonella* surveillance, *S. typhimurium* is most commonly reported. Serological types that may be involved approximate 1200.

4. Reservoir—Domestic and wild animals, including pet animals such as turtles and chicks; also man—patients and convalescent carriers, especially mild and unrecognized cases; rare chronic carriers.

5. Mode of transmission—By ingestion of the organisms; in a food contaminated by infected feces of man or animal; in whole eggs and egg products (frozen and dried whole egg, egg albumin and egg yolk, especially duck eggs) ; in meat and meat products; in poultry (especially turkey) ; and in pharmaceuticals of animal origin. Infection is disseminated by animal feeds and fertilizers prepared from contaminated meat scraps, tankage, fish meal and bones.

Epidemics of *Salmonella* infection are usually traced to foods such as commercially processed meat pies, poultry or poultry products (especially turkey), raw sausages, lightly cooked foods containing eggs or egg products; unpasteurized milk or dairy products; to foods contaminated with rodent feces or by an infected food handler; or to utensils, working surfaces or tables previously used for contaminated foods such as poultry products. Sporadic cases may be related to ingestion of contaminated food or direct contact with an infected person. Hospital epidemics tend to be protracted, with organisms persisting in the environment; person-to-person transmission via the hands of personnel is considered the major mode of spread, and infection by inhalation has been considered a possibility. In 1966, a severe epidemic of *S. typhimurium* diarrhea occurring in Riverside, California, and affecting more than 15,000 cases, resulted from contamination of the unchlorinated public deep water supply.

6. Incubation period—Six to 48 hours, usually about 12 to 24 hours.

7. Period of communicability—Throughout course of infection. Extremely variable—usually 3 days to 3 weeks; a temporary carrier state occasionally continues for months, especially in young babies. Chronic carriers (over 1 year) are rare.

8. Susceptibility and resistance—Susceptibility is general and is usually increased by gastrointestinal surgery, neoplastic disease, and other debilitating conditions. Severity of the disease is related to serotype of the organism, the number of organisms ingested, and host factors. Inapparent infections are frequent. There is no active or passive immunization.

9. Methods of control—

A. Preventive measures:

1) Thorough cooking of all foodstuffs derived from animal sources, particularly turkeys and other fowl, egg products, and meat dishes. Avoid recontamination within kitchen after cooking is completed. Avoid raw eggs, as in egg drinks, and the use of dirty or cracked eggs; pasteurize egg products. Refrigerate prepared foods during storage before use.

2) Education of food handlers and housewives in the necessity of refrigerating foods, washing hands before and after food preparation, maintaining a sanitary kitchen, and protecting prepared food against rodent or insect contamination.

3) Recognition, control and prevention of *Salmonella* infections among domestic animals and pets. Chicks, ducklings and turtles are particularly dangerous.

4) Meat and poultry inspection, with adequate supervision of abattoirs and butcher shops.

5) Adequate cooking or heat treatment and protection of prepared animal feeds (meat meal, bone meal, fish meal and others) against contamination by *Salmonella*.

B. Control of patient, contacts, and the immediate environment:

1) *Report to local health authority:* Obligatory case report, Class 2B (see Preface).

2) *Isolation:* Exclusion of infected persons from food handling, patient care, or occupations involving care of young children and the elderly until cultures of feces are free from *Salmonella* for 3 successive days.

3) *Concurrent disinfection:* Of feces and of articles soiled therewith. In communities with a modern and adequate sewage disposal system, feces can be discharged directly into sewers without preliminary disinfection. Terminal cleaning.

4) *Quarantine:* None. Family contacts should not be employed as food handlers during period of contact.

5) *Immunization of contacts:* None.

6) *Investigation of contacts:* Culture all family contacts. Search for unrecognized mild cases and carriers, including those convalescing.

7) *Specific treatment:* None indicated except supportive measures. Use of antibiotics may result in prolongation of the carrier state or in development of resistant strains. However, with continued fever or septicemia, a short course of chloramphenicol or ampicillin therapy should be given.

C. Epidemic measures: See Staphylococcal Food Poisoning 9C, p. 93.

D. International measures: WHO Reference Centres (see Preface).

SCABIES

1. Identification—An infectious disease of the skin caused by a mite whose penetration is visible as papules or vesicles, or as tiny linear burrows containing the mites and their eggs. Lesions are prominent around finger webs, anterior surfaces of wrists and elbows, anterior axillary folds, belt line, thighs, and external genitalia in men; nipples, abdomen, and lower portion of buttocks in women. Itching is intense, especially at night, but complications are few except as lesions become secondarily infected by scratching.

Diagnosis may be established by locating the female mite in its burrow and identifying it microscopically.

2. Occurrence—Widespread and a common disease during time of war, poverty, or social upheaval. Uncommon in communities where bathing is common practice. It is endemic in many underdeveloped countries and in certain social groups in affluent countries.

3. **Infectious agent**—*Sarcoptes scabiei,* a mite.

4. **Reservoir**—Reservoir is man; *Sarcoptes* of animals can live on man but do not reproduce in the skin.

5. **Mode of transmission**—Transfer of parasites is by direct contact and to a limited extent from undergarments or soiled bedclothes freshly contaminated by infected persons. The disease is frequently acquired during sexual contact.

6. **Incubation period**—Several days or even weeks before itching is noticed.

7. **Period of communicability**—Until mites and eggs are destroyed by treatment, ordinarily after 1 or occasionally 2 courses of treatment a week apart.

8. **Susceptibility and resistance**—No known resistance.

9. **Methods of control**—

A. *Preventive measures:* Education on the need for maintaining cleanliness of person, garments and bedclothes.

B. *Control of patient, contacts, and the immediate environment:*

1) *Report to local health authority:* Official report not ordinarily justifiable, Class 5 (see Preface).
2) *Isolation:* Exclude infected children from school until treated adequately.
3) *Concurrent disinfection:* Proper laundering of underwear, sheets, and occasionally of blankets.
4) *Quarantine:* None.
5) *Immunization of contacts:* None.
6) *Investigation of contacts:* Search for unreported or unrecognized cases among companions or household members. Single infections in a family are uncommon.
7) *Specific treatment:* When multiple areas are infected, a bath followed by application of 1% gamma benzene hexachloride (Kwell), or of crotamiton (Eurax), an emulsion of benzyl benzoate ointment, to the whole body. The following day a cleansing bath is taken and a change made to fresh clothing and bedclothes. Itching may persist for days and is not to be regarded as a sign of superinfection; this is important, for overtreatment is common. In perhaps 5% of cases a second course of treatment is necessary after an interval of 7 to 10 days.

C. *Epidemic measures:*

1) Treatments are undertaken on a coordinated mass basis.
2) Case-finding efforts are extended to screen whole families, military units or institutions.
3) Soap and facilities for mass bathing and laundering are essential.
4) Health education of infected persons and others at risk,

as well as treatment. Cooperation of civilian or military authorities, often both, is needed.

D. International measures: None.

SCHISTOSOMIASIS

1. Identification—A blood fluke (trematode) disease with adult male and female worms living in veins of the host. Eggs deposited there produce minute granulomata and scars in organs where they lodge. Symptomatology is related to the life cycle of the parasite; *Schistosoma mansoni* and *Schistosoma japonicum* give rise primarily to intestinal, and *Schistosoma haematobium* to urinary, manifestations. The complications that arise from chronic infection are the important consideration; liver involvement and portal hypertension in the intestinal form, obstruction and superimposed infection in the urinary disease. Synonym: Bilharziasis.

Diagnosis depends on the demonstration of ova in the stool or urine; skin and serological tests are helpful.

2. Occurrence—*S. mansoni* occurs in Africa, the Arabian peninsula, northeastern and eastern South America and the Caribbean area. *S. haematobium* occurs in Africa, the Middle East, and a small focus in India. *S. japonicum* occurs in the Orient (China, Japan, Philippines, Celebes, Laos and Thailand). In some endemic areas more than half of the population is affected. None of these species is indigenous to North America.

The larvae of certain other schistosomes of birds and rodents may penetrate the human skin causing a dermatitis known as swimmer's itch. This is prevalent among bathers in lakes in many parts of the world including North America; also in certain coastal sea water beaches. These schistosomes do not mature in man.

3. Infectious agents—*Schistosoma mansoni, Schistosoma haematobium* and *Schistosoma japonicum.*

4. Reservoir—Man is the principal reservoir of both *S. haematobium* and *S. mansoni,* although primates and other animals are naturally infected with both species. Dogs, cats, pigs, cattle, water buffalo, horses, field mice and wild rats are epidemiologically important animal hosts of *S. japonicum.* Persistence of the disease depends on the presence of an appropriate snail as intermediate host; i.e., members of the genera *Biomphalaria* for *S. mansoni, Bulinus* for *S. haematobium,* and *Oncomelania* for *S. japonicum.*

5. Mode of transmission—Infection is acquired from water contaminated with larval forms (cercariae) derived from snails. The eggs of *S. haematobium* leave the mammalian body mainly with urine, those of *S. mansoni* and *S. japonicum* with feces. The egg hatches in water and the liberated larva or miracidium enters a suitable freshwater snail host. Free-swimming larvae, cercariae, emerge from the snail after several weeks and penetrate human skin, usually while the person is working, swimming, or wading in water; they enter the bloodstream, are carried to blood vessels of the lung, migrate to the liver, develop to maturity, and then migrate to veins of the abdominal cavity. Adult forms of *S. mansoni* and *S. japonicum* usually remain in mesenteric veins; those of *S. haematobium* usually migrate through anastomoses into the pelvic veins. Eggs are deposited in venules and escape into the lumen of bowel or urinary bladder, or lodge in other organs.

6. Incubation period—Systemic manifestations usually begin when worms are reaching maturity, 4 to 6 weeks after infection. Eggs usually are found in feces or urine a week or two after onset of symptoms.

7. Period of communicability—As long as eggs are discharged in urine or feces of infected persons, usually 1 to 2 years, but it may be 25 years or longer. Infected snails may give off cercariae for several months.

8. Susceptibility and resistance—Susceptibility is universal; whether or not resistance develops as a result of infection is controversial.

9. Methods of control—

A. Preventive measures:

1) Disposal of feces and urine so that eggs will not reach bodies of fresh water containing snail intermediate host. Control of animals infected with *S. japonicum* is desirable but usually not practical.
2) Improved irrigation and agricultural practices; drainage and reclamation of swamps.
3) Treatment of snail breeding places with molluscicides.
4) Provision of water for drinking, bathing and washing clothes from sources free from cercariae.
5) Provision of cercaria-repellent or protective clothing against cercariae for persons required to enter contaminated water.
6) Education of people in endemic areas regarding mode of transmission and methods of protection.
7) Mass treatment of infected persons in endemic areas may help to reduce transmission through lessened severity and duration of the disease; in the past has not materially reduced prevalence.

B. Control of patient, contacts, and the immediate environment:

1) *Report to local health authority:* In selected endemic areas; in many countries not a reportable disease, Class 3C (see Preface).
2) *Isolation:* None.

3) *Concurrent disinfection:* Sanitary disposal of feces and urine.

4) *Quarantine:* None.

5) *Immunization of contacts:* None.

6) *Investigation of contacts:* Examine contacts for infection from a common source. Search for source is a community effort, see 9C.

7) *Specific treatment:* For *S. mansoni* and *S. haematobium,* stibophen (Fuadin) intramuscularly is used; tartar emetic (potassium or sodium antimony tartrate) is more effective but must be given intravenously. For *S. japonicum,* tartar emetic intravenously is essential, as Fuadin frequently fails. Toxic side effects occur. Lucanthone (for *S. haematobium* and *S. mansoni*) and niridazole, recently introduced, are given orally, but their effectiveness is counteracted by toxicity. Hycanthone methane sulfonate (Etrenol), available from NCDC, Atlanta, Ga., on an investigational basis, has promise for the treatment of infections due to *S. mansoni* and *S. haematobium.*

C. *Epidemic measures:* In areas of high incidence, determine areas with high snail density and treat with molluscicides. Schistosomes have a high snail host specificity; expert aid is needed to determine which snails to control. Prohibit entering contaminated water. Provide clean water, examine population for infection, and treat diseased persons.

D. *International measures:* WHO Reference Centres (see Preface).

SHIGELLOSIS

1. Identification—An acute bacterial disease of the intestine characterized by diarrhea, accompanied by fever and often vomiting, cramps and tenesmus. In severe cases the stools may contain blood, mucus and pus. Under usual circumstances in temperate climates the disease is self-limited, complications are rare, mild cases and inapparent infections are numerous, and fatality is less than 1%. In epidemics in tropical areas with much overcrowding and poor sanitation, fatality is greater, sometimes as high as 10 to 20% for hospitalized patients. Synonym : Bacillary dysentery.

Bacteriological diagnosis is by isolation of *Shigella* from feces, or preferably from rectal swabs.

2. Occurrence—In all parts of the world : arctic, temperate, and tropical; two-thirds of cases are children under 10 years of age. In tropical and subtropical populations of less developed countries where malnutrition is common, dysentery is a frequent and serious disease, occurring at all ages and causing many deaths, particularly of older infants, children in the first years of life, and elderly debilitated persons. Outbreaks are frequent in jails, institutions for children, and mental hospitals. A recurring problem of armies under field conditions and an important component of the acute endemic gastroenteritis of tropical populations (see p. 76). In U.S.A., moderately endemic in the lower socioeconomic areas and on Indian reservations; with occasional epidemics, mainly in the warmer seasons.

3. Infectious agents—There are currently 30 serotypes of the genus *Shigella* (dysentery bacillus), which are divided into four main groups: Group A, *S. dysenteriae;* B, *S. flexneri;* C, *S. boydii;* D, *S. sonnei;* with serotypes of each group. More than one serotype is commonly present in a community, and cases not infrequently show mixed infection with other intestinal pathogens. Within the U.S.A. during 1963–1966, 37.1% of isolations were *S. sonnei* and 25.4% *S. flexneri 2.*

4. Reservoir—Reservoir is man; domestic animals may harbor and disseminate organisms.

5. Mode of transmission—Through fecal-oral transmission from an infected person; indirectly, by objects soiled with such feces; by eating contaminated foods or drinking contaminated water or milk; by flies; also by direct contact.

6. Incubation period—One to 7 days, usually less than 4 days.

7. Period of communicability—During acute infection and until the infectious agent is no longer present in feces, usually within a few weeks. In rare instances the carrier state may persist for a year or two.

8. Susceptibility and resistance—Susceptibility general, but the disease more common and more severe in children than in adults. The extent of type-specific immunity after attack is unknown. Repeated attacks are common.

9. Methods of control—

A. Preventive measures:

1) Sanitary disposal of human feces.
2) Education of the public in the hygiene of breast feeding; scrupulous cleanliness in preparation, handling and refrigeration of food for children; boiling of milk and water for infant feeding and continuous supervision of diet.
3) Protection and purification of water supplies (see Typhoid Fever 9A1, p. 272).
4) Pasteurization of milk and dairy products or boiling of milk (see Typhoid Fever 9A4, also p. 272).
5) Sanitary supervision of processing, preparation and serving of all foods, particularly moist foods and those eaten raw; special attention to provision and use of hand-washing facilities. Protection of foods against contamination by flies.

6) Fly control and control of fly breeding (see Typhoid Fever, 9A3, p. 272).

B. Control of patient, contacts, and the immediate environment:

1) *Report to local health authority:* Case report obligatory in most states and countries, Class 2B (see Preface). Recognition and report of epidemics has more than usual importance in schools and institutions.

2) *Isolation:* During acute illness. Rigid personal precautions by attendants.

3) *Concurrent disinfection:* Of feces and of articles contaminated therewith. In communities with a modern and adequate sewage disposal system, feces can be discharged directly into the sewer without preliminary disinfection. Terminal cleaning.

4) *Quarantine:* Contacts should not be employed as food handlers during period of contact and not before three cultures of feces at daily intervals are negative.

5) *Immunization of contacts:* No satisfactory method presently available.

6) *Investigation of contacts:* Search for unrecognized mild cases and convalescent carriers among contacts. For sporadic cases, this is time-consuming and gives meager results.

7) *Specific treatment:* Fluid and electrolyte replacement is the important consideration. An antimicrobial drug to which the infectious agent is sensitive may be used.

C. Epidemic measures:

1) Groups of cases of acute diarrheal disorder are always reported at once to the local health authority, even in the absence of specific identification of the disease.

2) Investigation of food, water and milk supplies, general sanitation, and search for unrecognized mild cases and carriers.

3) Prophylactic administration of antibiotics is not indicated.

D. International measures: WHO Reference Centres (see Preface).

SMALLPOX

1. Identification—A viral systemic disease generally demonstrating a characteristic exanthem. Onset is sudden, with fever, malaise, headache, severe backache, prostration and occasionally abdominal pain. The 2 to 4 day pre-eruptive illness frequently resembles influenza.

The temperature falls and a deep-seated rash appears. This rash passes through successive stages of macules, papules, vesicles, pustules and finally scabs, which fall off at the end of the 3rd-4th week; fever frequently intensifies after the rash has evolved to the pustular stage. The lesions become evident first on the face and subsequently on the body and extremities. They are more abundant on the face and extremities than on the trunk (centrifugal distribution) and are more densely concentrated over irritated areas, prominences and extensor surfaces. Most frequently confused with varicella (chickenpox), smallpox can usually be identified by the clear-cut prodromal illness, by the centrifugal distribution of the rash, by the appearance of all lesions more or less simultaneously, by the similarity of appearance of all lesions in a given area, and by the more deeply seated lesions. In previously vaccinated persons, the rash may be significantly modified to the extent that only a few highly atypical lesions are seen; generally the prodromal illness is not modified.

Two types of smallpox are recognized: *variola minor* (alastrim) and *variola major* (classical smallpox). An intermediate form may be present in Africa. In variola major, the case fatality rate among the unvaccinated is 40–50% or more. Death normally occurs between the 5th and 7th day, occasionally as late as the 2nd week. Approximately 3% of variola major cases experience a fulminating disease characterized by a severe prodrome, prostration and bleeding into the skin and mucous membranes. Such hemorrhagic cases are rapidly fatal; the usual rash does not appear and the disease may be confused with severe acute leukemia, meningococcemia or idiopathic thrombocytopenic purpura. A "flat" variety is observed in 5% of cases; in this type, the focal lesions are slow to appear, the vesicles tend to project only slightly above the surrounding skin and are soft and velvety to the touch. In the few patients with this type who survive, the lesions resolve without pustulation.

Outbreaks of variola minor are normally associated with a case fatality rate of 2% or less; although the rash is similar to that observed in variola major, the patient generally experiences less severe systemic symptoms, and cases of "hemorrhagic" and "flat" varieties are rarely observed.

Laboratory confirmation is by isolation of the virus on chorioallantoic membrane or tissue culture from scrapings of lesions, from vesicular or pustular fluid, from crusts, and often from the blood during the febrile pre-eruptive period. A rapid provisional diagnosis is often possible by special stains of thin slides of material from macular or vesicular lesions: virus particles may be seen and multinucleated giant cells of chickenpox are absent. Material from cutaneous lesions may also be used for a rapid presumptive test employing electron microscopy, for the precipitation-in-gel technique, or for complement-fixation tests to detect poxvirus group antigen.

2. Occurrence—Smallpox is a continuing threat to all countries and is introduced to smallpox-free countries by international travelers. As of 1969, smallpox (alastrim) was endemic in Brazil, in some Asian countries, specifically Afghanistan, India, Pakistan, Nepal and Indonesia (classical), and in most African countries south of the Sahara (both types). Under a global smallpox eradication program, the extent of the endemic regions is decreasing. The last outbreak in the U.S.A. occurred in 1949 in the Rio Grande Valley. In 1962 a boy from Brazil, who traveled through New York City, developed smallpox (alastrim) in Toronto, Canada; no transmission from this case occurred.

3. Infectious agent—Variola virus.

4. Reservoir—The only reservoir is man.

5. Mode of transmission—Transmission normally occurs through close contact with respiratory discharges of patients and the lesions of skin and mucous membranes, or materials which they recently contaminated. Household, hospital and school contacts are especially at risk. Transmission to laundry workers through bedding and other linens has been frequently observed. Virus may persist for several years in separated scabs but does not appear to be particularly infectious in this form. Inapparent infections are rare and are rarely implicated in further disease transmission.

6. Incubation period—From 8 to 17 days; commonly 10 to 12 days to onset of illness and 2 to 4 days more to onset of rash.

7. Period of communicability—From the development of the earliest lesions to disappearance of all scabs, about 3 weeks. Most communicable during first week.

8. Susceptibility and resistance—Susceptibility is universal. Permanent immunity usually follows recovery; second attacks are rare.

9. Methods of control—

A. Preventive measures:

1) Effective vaccination, before exposure, prevents the disease. Immunity gradually wanes but virtually complete protection is afforded by revaccination with fully potent vaccine every 3 to 5 years.
2) Many nations have been kept free of endemic disease for long periods by an alert surveillance and outbreak control program and by vigilance at airports, ports and border-crossing points.
3) In smallpox-free countries, routine primary vaccination is recommended at 3 to 18 months of age with revaccination every 5–10 years. In the U.S.A. and Britain, primary vaccination is recommended during the 2nd year of life. In countries in which smallpox is endemic or in those countries geographically proximate to endemic areas, primary vaccination as soon after birth as possible is advised, with revaccination at 1 year and repeated revaccination every 3 to 5 years. Vaccination is required within 3 years for international travelers under the provisions of the International Health Regulations. WHO. It is particularly im-

portant also for those at special risk such as transport workers in contact with international travelers, hospital employees (including physicians, nurses, attendants, laboratory and laundry workers), and morticians and others handling the dead. Those working in communicable disease wards which might admit smallpox patients should be revaccinated annually.

4) Vaccination is accomplished by inserting potent smallpox vaccine into the superficial layers of the skin. The use of vaccine fully potent at the moment of insertion is the most important (and most neglected) part of the vaccination procedure. Freeze-dried vaccine, which is reconstituted at the time of use, is now generally available; its use assures adequate potency particularly in tropical areas. Glycerinated vaccine maintains its potency for at least 6 months if kept below freezing at all times before use; if stored below 10C (50F), it should maintain its potency for at least 14 days. It deteriorates rapidly at ambient temperatures and therefore only freeze-dried vaccine may be used in WHO eradication programs. The preferred site for vaccination is the outer aspect of the upper arm over the insertion of the deltoid muscle. No cleansing of the skin is needed unless the vaccination site is obviously dirty, in which case it should be gently wiped with a cloth or cotton moistened with water, and permitted to dry. The vaccination techniques of multiple pressure, multiple puncture and jet injection give the highest percentage of successful vaccinations. In the *multiple pressure technique,* a small drop of vaccine is placed on the skin and a series of pressures is made with the side of a sharp needle held tangentially to the skin into the smallest possible area—about ⅛ inch (3 mm) in diameter. The strokes are completed in 5 to 6 seconds with an up-and-down motion perpendicular to the skin. In smallpox-free countries, 6–10 strokes are normally used for primary vaccination and 30 for revaccination; in others, 30 strokes are used for both primary and revaccination. Following vaccination, a trace of blood appearing in some pressure points within 30 seconds is evidence that vaccination has been performed with sufficient vigor. In the *multiple puncture technique,* a forked (bifurcated) needle is used. The needle is dipped into the vaccine and touched to the surface of the skin. The needle is held perpendicular to the skin and 15 punctures are made in an up-and-down manner within the smallest possible area—about ⅛ inch (3 mm) in diameter. For primary vaccination in smallpox-free areas, only 2 or 3 strokes are employed. A trace of blood should be observed at the vaccination site. Vaccination by *jet injection* requires an injector which deposits intradermally about 0.1 ml of a

purified, less concentrated vaccine prepared especially for this purpose.

No dressing should be applied at the time of vaccination; if the lesion should ooze later, a loose nonocclusive dressing protects the clothing. Vaccination is repeated as above 1 week later (6–8 days) unless a "major reaction" is present, evidence that an immunizing vaccinal infection had occurred. A "major reaction" is one which, one week after vaccination, presents a vesicular or pustular lesion, or an area of definite induration or discoloration surrounding the scab or ulcer remaining at the point of vaccine insertion. All other responses are termed "equivocal reactions" and the individual should be revaccinated, using vaccine of known potency and more vigorous technique. Primary vaccinations should ultimately develop a Jennerian vesicle, a major reaction. Revaccinations, except in often vaccinated and highly immune groups, should produce major reactions in 80–90% of subjects. Persons with a high level of immunity often exhibit a hypersensitivity reaction in the first 2 to 3 days, with erythema and the appearance of papules or vesicles resulting in a scab which may still be present at 1 week. Such a reaction may be induced either by potent or inactivated vaccine and thus immunity cannot be assumed. For this reason, all persons showing equivocal (or doubtful) reactions should be revaccinated with potent vaccine and proper technique.

Complications and undesirable sequelae of vaccination are unusual. Most are rare and the majority are prevented by observing the contraindications below and by using fewer insertions in those without immunity. Major complications are (1) encephalitis, rare in U.S.A. but somewhat more frequent in some parts of Europe; (2) progressive vaccinia (vaccinia necrosum), exceptionally rare, occurring in individuals with immunological defects either of a congenital nature or as a consequence of tumors of the reticuloendothelial system or of therapy with immunosuppressive drugs, corticosteroids or radiation; (3) eczema vaccinatum with vaccinial lesions appearing at the site of past or present eczematous lesions; (4) generalized of vaccina to mucous membranes or to abraded skin; 10 days on various parts of the body; (5) autoinoculation of vaccinia to mucous membranes or to abraded skin; (6) secondary infections, caused by tetanus and staphylococcal organisms, from contamination of the vaccination site. Vaccinia immune globulin * (VIG), 0.3–0.6 ml/kg, is indicated in the treatment of eczema vaccinatum and progressive vaccinia; it is considered to be of no value in

---

* In the United Kingdom, human antivaccinial immunoglobulin.

postvaccinal encephalitis; and the other specific complications are self-limited and do not usually warrant its use. It may be obtained in the U.S.A. within a few hours by contacting one of the designated consultants listed by the Regional Blood Centers of the American Red Cross, or commercially. Methisazone (Marboran) has also been reported to be of benefit in treatment of these conditions.

5) Contraindications to vaccination:

In endemic areas, the risk of acquiring fatal smallpox far exceeds the danger of vaccination complications. In general, serious acute illness is the only recognized contraindication to vaccination.

In smallpox-free countries, the following are additional contraindications to vaccination: (a) eczema and other forms of chronic dermatitis in the individual to be vaccinated or in a household contact; (b) leukemia; lymphoma; other reticuloendothelial malignancies; (c) dysgammaglobulinemia; (d) patients receiving immunosuppressive drugs such as steroids or antimetabolites or ionizing radiation; (e) pregnancy. In the face of any such contraindication, an individual requiring vaccination because of potential exposure in an endemic area should be given vaccinia immune globulin (VIG), 0.3 ml per kg, at the same time as vaccination. In the U.S.A., VIG may be obtained commercially or as noted in 9A4 above.

6) Contact with cattle, especially dairy cows, should be avoided when an oozing vaccinial lesion is present, since cattle are susceptible and can spread infection.

B. Control of patient, contacts, and the immediate environment:

1) *Report immediately by telephone or telegraph to local health authorities:* Case reports required by International Sanitary and Health Regulations, Class 1 (see Preface).

2) *Isolation:* Until all scabs have disappeared, preferably under hospital conditions in screened rooms. Strict precautions; infection can be carried outside the hospital by various materials contaminated by the patient, especially on clothing and linen.

3) *Concurrent disinfection:* Deposit oral and nasal discharges in a paper container and burn. Bedclothes and other fabrics should be sterilized by boiling or autoclaving. Terminal disinfection: The floors, walls and other hard surfaces should be sprayed or mopped with disinfecting agents known to kill poxviruses and allowed to remain for 4 hours before washing with water. Compounds found to be of value include phenolic and quaternary ammonium compounds, formalin and chlorine preparations. When fumigation is practiced, spaces can be disinfected by exposure to moist formalin vapor for 6 hours, or to ethylene

oxide. When chemical disinfectants are not available, simpler methods may be used such as boiling of bedclothes and linen and copious washing of hard surfaces with soap and water and allowing them to stand for 48 hours. Exposure to ultraviolet or sunlight over several hours is also effective if surfaces are fully exposed.

4) *Quarantine:* All persons living in the same house with the smallpox patient as well as face-to-face contacts should be promptly vaccinated with known potent vaccine and placed under daily surveillance for 17 days after last contact with the smallpox patient. Quarantine should be substituted for surveillance of intimate contacts whose co-operation is uncertain. At the first sign of fever or other illness, the individual should be isolated. Unvaccinated individuals (as determined by absence of vaccination scar) who have been in intimate contact with the patient should be placed under quarantine for the period when disease might appear, i.e., from 10 days after the first, to 16 days after the last contact.

5) *Immunization of contacts:* All contacts, both intimate and casual, should be vigorously and promptly vaccinated at two sites, employing a known potent vaccine. Previously vaccinated contacts exposed 7 or more days before, as well as all unvaccinated contacts, should receive vaccinia immune globulin if available, 0.3 ml/kg (see 9A4 above). Methisazone (Marboran) has been shown to afford protection when given early in the incubation period.

6) *Investigation of contacts and source of infection:* Prompt investigation to determine the source of infection is of the greatest importance. Many outbreaks in smallpox-free areas are diagnosed only after the 3rd or 4th generation of cases. Since inapparent cases of smallpox are rare and do not appear to transmit infection, the source of infection should always be determined. Persons with supposed "chickenpox," or those who have recently experienced pustular or hemorrhagic disease (especially fatal cases), should be considered as the possible source of infection.

7) *Specific treatment:* None.

C. Epidemic measures:

1) Isolation of patients, vaccination of contacts, laboratory confirmation of diagnosis and investigation of source of infection (see 9B above).

2) In smallpox-free areas, vaccination of an entire community should be used *only* when steps taken above do not appear successful. In endemic areas and countries geographically proximate, the occurrence of an outbreak may provide excellent motivation for participation in an area-wide mass vaccination program.

3) Immediate publicity, stating frankly and clearly the situation and control measures taken, can often avert panic on the part of the population. At best, however, in normally smallpox-free areas, an increased demand for vaccination can be anticipated and special provision should be made to supply the needs of physicians and clinics without disrupting the identification, vaccination and surveillance of contacts.

D. International measures:

1) Telegraphic notification by governments to WHO and to adjacent countries of first imported, first transferred, or first nonimported case of smallpox in an area previously free of the disease.

2) Measures applicable to international travelers are specified in International Health Regulations,* WHO, Geneva. For entry into other countries international travelers must possess an international certificate of vaccination. The validity of this certificate extends for 3 years, beginning 8 days after a successful primary vaccination was performed, or for a revaccination, on the date of that revaccination. This must be dated, be signed by a physician, and bear a stamp authorized by the national health authority. In the U.S.A., validation of vaccination can be obtained from most health departments. For individuals for whom vaccination is normally contraindicated, vaccination may be performed while administering VIG at the same time at another site (see 9A4 above). Alternately, a statement signed by a physician may be presented stating that vaccination is contraindicated. Under the International Health Regulations, health authorities are requested to take such a statement into consideration when deciding whether or not the traveler should be admitted to the country, placed under surveillance or quarantined; however, some countries do not waive the requirement and will place the traveler in quarantine.

3) WHO initiated a 10-year global smallpox eradication program in 1967. WHO Reference Centres (see Preface).

---

* These will come into force on January 1, 1971. Until that date, the *International Sanitary Regulations,* 3rd edition (Geneva: WHO, 1966), are applicable.

SPOROTRICHOSIS

1. Identification—A fungus disease, usually of the skin, beginning as a nodule. As the nodule grows, lymphatics draining the area become firm and cord-like, forming a series of nodules which in turn may soften and ulcerate. Arthritis, pneumonitis and other visceral infections are rare. A fatal result is uncommon.

Laboratory confirmation is through cultivation of the fungus, rarely by direct smear and then only with selective fungus stains.

2. Occurrence—Reported from all parts of the world, in males more frequently than in females, and in adults more than in children; often an occupational disease of farmers, gardeners and horticulturists. No differences in racial susceptibility. The disease is characteristically sporadic, and relatively uncommon. An epidemic among gold miners in South Africa involved some 3,000 persons; fungus was growing on mine timbers. Many animals are susceptible, including horses, mules, dogs, cats, rats and wild animals.

3. Infectious agent—*Sporothrix schenckii (Sporotrichum schenckii),* a dimorphic fungus.

4. Reservoir—Reservoir is soil, vegetation, wood.

5. Mode of transmission—Introduction of fungus through skin following pricks by thorns or barbs, the handling of sphagnum moss, by slivers from wood or lumber, or through skin lesions of persons handling contaminated dressings of patients. Transmission by inhalation of spores is rare.

6. Incubation period—The lymphatic form may develop 3 weeks to 3 months after injury.

7. Period of communicability—Rarely transmitted from man to man. Contamination of environment presumably for duration of active lesions.

8. Susceptibility and resistance—Man probably is highly susceptible.

9. Methods of control—

> **A. Preventive measures:** Treatment of lumber with fungicides in industries where disease occurs.
>
> **B. Control of patient, contacts, and the immediate environment:**
>
> 1) *Report to local health authority:* Official report ordinarily not justifiable, Class 5 (see Preface).
> 2) *Isolation:* None.
> 3) *Concurrent disinfection:* Of discharges and dressings. Terminal cleaning.
> 4) *Quarantine:* None.
> 5) *Immunization of contacts:* None.
> 6) *Investigation of contacts and source of infection:* Not profitable.
> 7) *Specific treatment:* Iodides are effective in lymphocutane-

ous infection; in other forms, amphotericin B (Fungizone) is more effective.

C. *Epidemic measures:* In the South African epidemic, mine timbers were sprayed with a mixture of zinc sulfate and triolith. This and other sanitary measures controlled the epidemic.

D. *International measures:* None.

STAPHYLOCOCCAL DISEASE

Staphylococci produce a variety of syndromes with clinical manifestations that range from a single pustule or impetigo to septicemia and death. A lesion or lesions containing pus is the primary clinical finding, abscess formation the typical pathology. Few among the many strains of staphylococci are associated with disease. The most useful index of pathogenicity is an ability to coagulate plasma (coagulase); almost all virulent strains are coagulase-positive. Other ways of identifying a virulent strain include phage-typing and tests for antibiotic sensitivity.

Staphylococcal disease has distinctly different clinical and epidemiological patterns when seen in the general community, in the hospital nursery or among hospitalized patients. Each will therefore be presented separately. Staphylococcal food poisoning, an intoxication and not an infection, is discussed separately (pp. 90–92); attention here is to staphylococcal infections, local and general.

A. STAPHYLOCOCCAL DISEASE IN THE COMMUNITY

1. Identification—The common skin lesions are impetigo, boils, carbuncles, abscesses and infected lacerations. The basic lesion of impetigo is described in Section B; the others are localized and discrete. Constitutional symptoms are unusual; if lesions extend or are widespread, fever, malaise, headache or anorexia may develop. Usually lesions are uncomplicated, but may lead to pneumonitis, lung abscess, osteomyelitis, septicemia, pyarthrosis, meningitis, and brain abscess. In addition to primary lesions of the skin, staphylococcal conjunctivitis, osteomyelitis, and pneumonia following influenza and other viral respiratory disease are relatively frequent.

2. Occurrence—Worldwide in distribution. Maximal incidence is in areas where personal hygiene (especially the use of soap and water) is neglected and people are crowded. Common among children, especially in warm weather. Occurs sporadically and as small epidemics in families and summer camps, with various members developing recurrent illness due to the same staphylococcal strain.

3. Infectious agent—Various strains of coagulase-positive staphylococci (*Staphylococcus aureus*); may be characterized by phage type, antibiotic resistance or serological agglutination. Epidemics are caused by relatively few strains and these are usually resistant to plain penicillin. Presently, in U.S.A. phage group 52/52A/80/81 is most common.

4. Reservoir—Man.

5. Mode of transmission—The major site of colonization is the anterior nares; 30 to 40% of normal persons may shed coagulase-positive staphylococci in their nasal secretions. A person with a draining sinus or any purulent discharge is a source of epidemic spread. Transmission is by contact with a person who has either a purulent lesion or who is an asymptomatic nasal carrier of a pathogenic strain. Some carriers are more effective disseminators of disease than others. The role of contaminated toys or other objects is undetermined. Airborne spread may be important.

6. Incubation period—Variable and indefinite. Commonly 4 to 10 days.

7. Period of communicability—As long as purulent lesions continue to drain or the carrier state persists. Autoinfection may continue for the period of nasal colonization or duration of active lesions.

8. Susceptibility and resistance—Immune mechanisms not well understood. Susceptibility is greatest among the newborn and the chronically ill. Elderly and debilitated persons, as well as those with diabetes mellitus, cystic fibrosis, agammaglobulinemia, agranulocytosis and neoplastic disease are particularly susceptible to staphylococcal disease. Use of steroids and antimetabolites has also increased susceptibility.

9. Methods of control—

A. *Preventive measures:*

1) Public health education in personal hygiene, especially the importance of avoiding common use of toilet articles.
2) Prompt treatment of initial case in children and families.

B. *Control of patient, contacts, and the immediate environment:*

1) *Report to local health authority:* Obligatory report of outbreaks in schools, summer camps or other population groups; also any recognized concentration of cases in the community. No individual case report, Class 4 (see Preface).
2) *Isolation:* Not practical in most communities; infected persons should avoid contact with infants and debilitated persons.
3) *Concurrent disinfection:* Place dressings from open lesions and discharges in paper bag and burn or dispose in other practical manner.

4) Quarantine: None.

5) Immunization of contacts: None.

6) Investigation of contacts: Search for draining lesions or determine nasopharyngeal carrier status of the pathogenic strain among family members.

7) Specific treatment: In localized skin infections, systemic antibiotics are not indicated unless infection spreads significantly or complications ensue. For serious staphylococcal infections, employ penicillinase-resistant penicillin or, when allergy to penicillins is present, use semisynthetic cephalosporin or vancomycin. Use penicillin or other antibiotics only if tests show organisms to be sensitive; for serious systemic infection, prompt maximal parenteral treatment is essential.

C. Epidemic measures:

1) Search for persons with draining lesions and for nasal carriers of the epidemic strain; remove from group and treat with local application of an appropriate antibiotic (i.e., bacitracin). Institute strict personal hygiene. Treat all persons with clinical disease.

2) An unusual or abrupt increase in prevalence of staphylococcal infections in the community suggests the possibility of an unrecognized hospital epidemic.

D. International measures: WHO Reference Centres (see Preface).

B. STAPHYLOCOCCAL DISEASE IN HOSPITAL NURSERIES

1. Identification—Impetigo of the newborn (pemphigus neonatorum) and other purulent skin manifestations are the most frequent nursery-acquired staphylococcal diseases; the characteristic skin lesions develop secondary to colonization of nose or umbilicus, conjunctiva, circumcision site or rectum of infants with a pathogenic strain. (Colonization of these sites with usual strains of staphylococci is a normal occurrence in infants and does not produce disease.) Lesions may be distributed anywhere on the body but most commonly in diaper and intertriginous areas; lesions are initially vesicular, rapidly turning seropurulent, surrounded by an erythematous base. Rupture of pustules favors peripheral spread. Usually uncomplicated; but furunculosis, breast abscess, staphylococcal pneumonia, septicemia, meningitis, osteomyelitis, brain abscess or any form of more serious disease may occur.

2. Occurrence—Worldwide distribution. Problems occur mainly in hospitals, are promoted by laxity in aseptic techniques and exaggerated by development of antibiotic-resistant strains of the infectious agent.

3. Infectious agent, 4. Reservoir, 5. Mode of transmission, 6. Incubation period, 7. Period of communicability—Same as for Staphylococcal Disease in the Community (A above).

8. Susceptibility and resistance—Susceptibility among the new-born appears to be general. Infants remain at risk of disease for duration of colonization with pathogenic strains.

9. Methods of control—

A. Preventive measures:

1) Use of aseptic techniques and adequate hand washing in nurseries.

2) The use of hexachlorophene washes immediately after delivery, with repetition on arrival in the nursery and daily washes thereafter, has been reported to be successful in reducing nasal and umbilical colonization. Direct particular attention to removal of vernix from body folds and from base of the umbilicus.

3) A rotational system in the nursery whereby one unit (A) is filled and subsequent babies admitted to a second nursery (B) while the initial unit (A) discharges infants and is cleaned before new admissions. If facilities are present for rooming-in of baby with mother, this reduces risk.

4) Surveillance and supervision through an active Hospital Infections Control Committee, including a regular system of reporting, investigating and reviewing all hospital-acquired infections. Illness developing after discharge from hospital also should be recorded and investigated.

5) The value of bacterial interference is under investigation, whereby the newborn is exposed to a nonvirulent strain; colonization with this strain prevents colonization by virulent staphylococcal strains.

B. Control of patient, contacts, and the immediate environment:

1) *Report to local health authority:* Obligatory report of epidemics; no individual case report, Class 4 (see Preface).

2) *Isolation:* Without delay, all known or suspect cases in the nursery. Do not permit hospital personnel with minor staphylococcal lesions (pustules, boils, abscesses, paronychia, conjunctivitis, severe acne, otitis externa or infected lacerations) to work in the nursery.

3) *Concurrent disinfection, 4) Quarantine, and 5) Immunization of contacts:* Same as A. Staphylococcal Disease in the Community.

6) *Investigation of contacts and source of infection:* See epidemic measures given below.

7) *Specific treatment:* For localized impetiginous lesions, remove crusts, treat with bacitracin ointment or wash with 3% hexachlorophene solution 4 to 6 times daily. Systemic antibiotics are not indicated unless disease is progressing, with constitutional signs of fever, severe malaise or secondary complications. For serious infections, treat as in Section A preceding, paragraph 9B7.

C. *Epidemic measures:*

1) The occurrence of 2 or more concurrent cases of impetigo related to a nursery or a single case of breast abscess in a nursing mother or infant is presumptive evidence of an epidemic and warrants investigation. Culture all lesions and determine antibiotic resistance and phage type of epidemic strain.

2) In a nursery outbreak, institute group isolation and quarantine of cases and contacts until all have been discharged. Before admitting new patients, wash cribs, beds, isolettes and other furniture with phenolic or iodinated detergents. Autoclave instruments and basins and sterilize mattresses, bedding and diapers.

3) Examine all nurses, aides and attendants, including physicians, for draining lesions anywhere on the body. Culture noses of all persons in contact with nursery. Exclude and treat all carriers of the epidemic strain until cultures are negative.

4) Investigate adequacy of nursing procedures; emphasize strict aseptic technique. Personnel assigned to isolation and quarantine nurseries must not work with normal newborns.

C. STAPHYLOCOCCAL DISEASE IN MEDICAL AND SURGICAL WARDS OF HOSPITALS

1. Identification—Lesions vary from a simple furuncle or stitch abscess to an extensively infected bedsore, surgical wound or septic phlebitis, a chronic osteomyelitis or even to a fulminant pneumonia, endocarditis or septicemia. Postoperative staphylococcal disease is a constant threat to the convalescence of the hospitalized surgical patient. Wide and sometimes injudicious use of antibiotic therapy has increased the number of antibiotic-resistant staphylococci, and its use often promotes false security, with resultant relaxation of aseptic techniques. In over 90% of hospital-acquired staphyloccocal disease, the infecting organisms are resistant to penicillin or other commonly used antibiotics. The increasing complexity of surgical operations, with greater organ exposure and more prolonged anesthesia, promotes easier entry of staphylococci. Staphylococcal enteritis is a serious complication in antibiotic-treated patients.

Verification depends on isolation of *Staphylococcus aureus* associated with a clinical illness compatible with the bacteriologic findings.

2. Occurrence—Worldwide distribution. Staphylococcal infection has become recognized as a major form of acquired sepsis in the general wards of hospitals, though recently it appears to be giving place to infection with gram-negative organisms. At times, attack rates assume epidemic proportions. Spread to the community may occur when persons infected in the hospital are discharged.

3. Infectious agent, 4. Reservoir, 5. Mode of transmission, 6. In-

cubation period, 7. **Period of communicability**—Same as A. Staphylococcal Disease in the Community.

8. Susceptibility and resistance—Susceptibility is general, but greatest in chronically ill or debilitated patients, those receiving systemic steroid or antimetabolite therapy, and those undergoing major and prolonged surgical operations. The widespread use of parenteral injections and continuous intravenous therapy with indwelling plastic cannulae has opened new portals of entry to infectious agents.

9. Methods of control—

A. Preventive measures:

1) Strictly enforced aseptic techniques coordinated through a Hospital Infections Control Committee.
2) Education of hospital medical staff to use common antibiotics for simple infections and reserve certain antibiotics for staphylococcal infections (e.g., oxacillin, methicillin, vancomycin).

B. Control of patient, contacts, and the immediate environment:

1) *Report to local health authority:* Obligatory report of epidemics; no individual case report, Class 4 (see Preface).
2) *Isolation:* Whenever a moderate abundance of staphylococci is known or suspected to be present in sputum or draining pus, the patient should be isolated promptly. Isolation is not required when wound drainage is scanty, provided that an occlusive dressing and care in changing dressings prevent contamination of the environment.
3) *Concurrent disinfection:* Collect and burn dressings; autoclave bedclothing, towels and linens prior to laundering. Terminal cleaning.
4) *Quarantine:* None.
5) *Immunization of contacts:* None.
6) *Investigation of contacts and source of infection:* Not practical for sporadic cases (see 9C below).
7) *Specific treatment:* Appropriate antibiotics as determined by bacteriologic sensitivity tests.

C. Epidemic measures:

1) The occurrence of 2 or more cases in epidemiologic association is sufficient to suspect epidemic spread and to initiate investigation.
2) Search for additional cases due to same strain among ward patients and those recently discharged. Investigate all cases for common factor of exposure. Examine attendants, including physicians, for infected lesions. Culture all related personnel to determine asymptomatic nasopharyngeal carriers of the epidemic strain; remove infected persons from further contact with patients until free of infection.

3) Review and enforce rigid aseptic techniques. Provide strict isolation for each patient with purulent lesions, where practical; in large outbreaks, group isolation may be unavoidable.

D. International measures: WHO Reference Centres (see Preface).

STREPTOCOCCAL DISEASE, HEMOLYTIC

Scarlet Fever, Streptococcal Sore Throat and Other Related Infections

Group A hemolytic streptococci cause a wide variety of diseases differentiated clinically according to their portal of entry and tissue of localization; also by the presence or absence of a scarlatinal rash. The more important conditions are streptococcal sore throat and scarlet fever (streptococcal tonsillitis, streptococcal pharyngitis), erysipelas and puerperal fever. Other diseases include cellulitis, lymphadenitis, mastoiditis, otitis media, peritonitis, septicemia, impetigo contagiosa and various skin and wound infections. Those characterized by purulent exudates are most likely to spread infection, but others, such as septicemia, are also important because of frequent association with upper respiratory streptococcal infection. Insofar as these clinical categories are caused by Group A streptococci, they are different manifestations of the same infectious agent. They constitute an epidemiologic entity and similar principles of control hold generally for the group.

1. Identification—*Scarlet fever* is a streptococcal sore throat, with rash, which occurs if the infectious agent produces erythrogenic toxin and the patient is not immune to this toxin. If the organism is not a good toxin producer, or if the patient is immune to the toxin, *streptococcal sore throat* results. The distinguishing characteristics of scarlet fever are fever, sore throat, exudative tonsillitis or pharyngitis, tender cervical adenopathy, leucocytosis, enanthem, strawberry tongue and rash (exanthem). Injection and edema of the pharynx involve the faucial pillars and soft palate, often extending to the hard palate; petechiae are sometimes seen against the background of diffuse redness. Tonsils, if present, often show the exudate of acute follicular tonsillitis. The rash is usually a fine erythema, commonly punctate, blanching on pressure, and appearing most often on the neck, chest, in folds of axilla, elbow and groin, and on inner surfaces of the thighs. Typically, rash does not involve the face except in Negroes, but there is flushing of the cheeks and circumoral pallor. High fever, nausea and vomiting accompany severe infections. During convalescence, a desquamation of the skin is seen at tips of fingers and toes, less often over wide areas of trunk and limbs, including palms and soles. Scarlet fever and streptococcal sore throat may be accompanied or followed by suppurative sequelae such as otitis media and peritonsillar abscess, and may be followed at an interval of 1 to 5 weeks by the nonsuppurative complications—acute rheumatic fever and acute glomerulonephritis.

Scarlet fever occasionally occurs in patients with other types of streptococcal infections, such as infected wounds and puerperal infections. Severity of the disease has been decreasing in the U.S.A. for many years; the fatality is low, about 1 death for each 300 to 400 reported cases. The fatality in some parts of the world is as high as 3%.

Erysipelas is an acute infectious disease characterized by fever, constitutional symptoms, leucocytosis and a red, tender edematous spreading lesion of the skin, often with a definite raised border. The central point of origin tends to clear as the periphery extends. Face and legs are common sites. Recurrences are frequent. The disease may be especially severe, with bacteremia, in patients suffering from debilitating disease. Fatality varies greatly with the part of body affected and any associated disease; rates of 1 to 2% are now common in hospital practice. Erysipelas due to Group A streptococci is to be distinguished from erysipeloid, caused by *Erysipelothrix rhusiopathiae,* a localized cutaneous infection primarily an occupational disease of persons handling animals, meat, poultry and fish.

Streptococcal puerperal fever is an acute infectious disease, usually febrile, accompanied by local and general symptoms and signs of bacterial invasion of the genital tract—and sometimes of blood—of the postpartum or postabortum patient. Fatality for streptococcal puerperal fever is low when adequately treated. A goodly proportion of puerperal infections are of other origin than hemolytic streptococci. They are clinically similar but differentiated bacteriologically and epidemiologically. The infectious agents include a variety of bacteria: nonhemolytic streptococci, anaerobic streptococci, *Staphylococcus aureus, Escherichia coli, Clostridium perfringens, Bacteroides* sp., and others. Group A streptococci are of primary importance in postpartum infections; the anaerobic organisms, colon bacilli, *Bacteroides* sp., and staphylococci in postabortion infections. Treatment is by appropriate antibiotics. Epidemiologic characteristics and methods of control are those of Group A streptococcal infections.

Laboratory diagnosis of hemolytic streptococcal disease is based on colonial morphology and production of clear or beta hemolysis on blood agar. However, a few Group A strains produce little or no beta hemolysis, and these are likely to be nephritogenic. Identification as Group A is suggested by bacitracin sensitivity and established by precipitin reactions with specific antisera. Immunofluorescent techniques are also available for rapid identification. A rise in serum antibody titer (antistreptolysin O, antihyaluronidase or other tests) occurs from acute to convalescent phase of the illness.

2. Occurrence—*Scarlet fever* and *streptococcal sore throat* are common in temperate zones, well recognized in semitropical areas and relatively rare in tropical climates. Inapparent infections are as common or more common in the tropics than in temperate zones. In the U.S.A., epidemiological behavior may be endemic, epidemic, or sporadic. Epidemic occurrence is more frequent in certain geographic areas, such as New England, the Great Lakes region, and the Rocky Mountain area. Group A streptococcal infection due to M-types 2, 4, 12, 25 and 49 have frequently been associated with the development of acute glomerulonephritis; acute rheumatic fever may occur as a nonsuppurative complication following infection with almost any Group A serotype. Milk and milk products have been associated most frequently with food-borne outbreaks; recently, opened (and "stuffed") hard-boiled eggs have become more frequently implicated. Apart from food-borne epidemics, which may occur in any season, highest incidence is during late winter and spring. The 3 to 12 year age group is most affected; no sex or racial differences in susceptibility have been defined; military and school populations are frequently affected.

For *erysipelas,* geographic and seasonal distributions are similar to those for scarlet fever and streptococcal sore throat. Common after 20 years of age, with highest attack rates at 40 to 60 years, and frequent in infants. Occurrence is sporadic, even during epidemics of streptococcal infection.

Reliable morbidity data do not exist for *puerperal fever.* In U.S.A. and the Western world generally, morbidity has declined more than 80% in the past 20 years, with fatality rates declining precipitously since the advent of antibiotic drugs. Now chiefly a sporadic disease, although epidemics may occur in institutions where aseptic techniques are faulty.

All clinical forms may be associated in a single epidemic of Group A infection.

3. Infectious agent—*Streptococcus pyogenes,* Group A streptococci of at least 40 serologically distinct types which vary greatly in geographic and time distributions. In scarlet fever, two immunologically different types of erythrogenic toxin (A and B) have been demonstrated. Hemolytic streptococci of Groups B, C, D and G have been identified occasionally; mixed infections with other bacteria are common.

4. Reservoir—Reservoir is man; acutely ill or convalescent patients and carriers.

5. Mode of transmission—Respiratory transmission is by direct or intimate contact with patient or carrier, rarely by indirect contact with objects handled or by spread of droplet nuclei. Dried streptococci reaching the air via contaminated floor dust, lint from bedclothing, handkerchiefs, etc., are viable but noninfectious. Nasal carriers are particularly liable to transmit disease. Casual contact rarely leads to infection.

Explosive outbreaks of streptococcal sore throat may follow ingestion of contaminated milk or other food.

6. Incubation period—Short, usually 1 to 3 days, rarely longer.

7. Period of communicability—In uncomplicated cases, mainly during clinical illness and for approximately 10 days. Thereafter, in untreated patients, communicability decreases progressively, becoming of low order in 2 to 3 weeks, although the carrier state may persist for months. Persons with untreated complications resulting in purulent discharges may spread infection for weeks or months. Adequate treatment with penicillin will eliminate the probability of transmission in most patients or carriers within 24 hours, but some streptococci may persist longer.

8. Susceptibility and resistance—Susceptibility to *scarlet fever* is general, although many persons develop either antitoxic or type-specific antibacterial immunity, or both, through inapparent infection. Antibacterial immunity develops only against the specific M-type of Group A streptococcus that induces the patient's disease or inapparent infection and lasts for years. Immunity against erythrogenic toxin, hence to rash, develops within a week of the onset of scarlet fever and is usually permanent. Second attacks of scarlet fever with a rash are rare but may occur because of the 2 immunological forms of toxin; or because early antibiotic therapy of the first attack interfered with the formation of antitoxin. Repeated attacks of sore throat or other streptococcal disease due to a different type of streptococcus are relatively frequent. Both active and passive immunization against erythrogenic toxin are possible but not practical. Passive immunity occurs in newborns with transplacental maternal antibodies; active immunization with M-protein extracts produces bactericidal activity in man, but such immunization is not practical at present.

One attack of erysipelas appears to predispose to subsequent attacks; recurrences may be due to streptococcal infection or to hypersensitivity.

9. Methods of control—

A. *Preventive measures:*

1) Provision of laboratory facilities for isolation of hemolytic streptococci and identification of serologic group and type.
2) Education of the public in modes of transmission; in the relationship of streptococcal infection to heart disease; and in the necessity for completing the course of antibiotic therapy prescribed for the streptococcal infection.
3) Boiling or pasteurization of milk; exclusion of infected persons from handling milk or other food likely to be contaminated. Milk from any cow with evidence of mastitis should be excluded from sale or use. Foods such as deviled eggs should be prepared just prior to serving or be adequately refrigerated at 41 F or lower. All food handlers should be questioned daily about respiratory illness or skin lesions and those with symptoms excluded from work.

4) Strict asepsis in obstetrical procedures, with special attention to possible contamination from mouth and nose of attendants, as well as by hands and instruments. Protection of patient during labor and postpartum from attendants, visitors and other patients with respiratory or skin infection.

5) Specific chemoprophylaxis orally with an acid-resistant penicillin, or by monthly injections of a long-acting penicillin, for persons to whom recurrent streptococcal infection constitutes a special risk, such as individuals who have had rheumatic fever (pp. 203–205) or chorea or recurrent erysipelas. Persons who do not tolerate penicillin may be given erythromycin.

B. Control of patient, contacts, and the immediate environment:

1) *Report to local health authority:* Obligatory report of epidemics; no individual case report, Class 4 (see Preface).

2) *Isolation:* In order of preference, in a single room, cubicle, or small ward; in uncomplicated cases until clinical recovery or no less than 7 days from onset. Isolation may be terminated after 24 hours' treatment with penicillin or other effective antibiotics, provided therapy is continued for 10 days.

3) *Concurrent disinfection:* Of purulent discharges and all articles soiled therewith. Terminal cleaning.

4) *Quarantine:* None.

5) *Immunization of contacts:* None.

6) *Investigation of contacts:* Search for and treat carriers.

7) *Specific treatment:* Penicillin. Several forms are acceptable for treatment: (1) benzathine penicillin G (Bicillin); (2) procaine penicillin G in aluminum monostearate in oil; (3) procaine penicillin G as an aqueous suspension; (4) of the oral penicillins, phenoxymethyl penicillin (penicillin V) because of better absorption. A buffered soluble salt of penicillin G or potassium penicillin G should be used to supplement benzathine penicillin. Therapy should be started as early as possible and continued for at least 10 days irrespective of the mildness of the infection. Such treatment ameliorates the acute illness, reduces frequency of suppurative complications, prevents the development of the majority of cases of acute rheumatic fever (and to a lesser extent cases of acute glomerulonephritis), and prevents further spread of the organism. Sulfonamides are not effective in eliminating the streptococcus from the throat and in preventing nonsuppurative complications. Many strains are resistant to the tetracyclines—hence rheumatic fever may occur after therapy with these drugs. Erythromycin is preferred as an alternate for penicillin-

sensitive patients when *in vitro* sensitivity tests confirm that the organism is sensitive to this antibiotic.

C. *Epidemic measures:*

1) Determine the source and manner of spread, as person-to-person, by milk, or food-borne. Outbreaks can often be traced to an individual with a persistent streptococcal infection through identification of the serologic type of streptococcus.

2) With limited population groups or under special circumstances, penicillin prophylaxis may be given to household or other intimate contacts, to those known to have been exposed to contaminated milk or other food, or to the entire population group (see 9A5).

3) Prompt investigation of any unusual grouping of cases as to the possibility of contaminated milk, with exclusion of suspected milk supply from sale or use until pasteurized. Contamination of milk or food can be determined by bacteriological methods.

D. *International measures:* WHO Reference Centres (see Preface).

STRONGYLOIDIASIS

1. Identification—A helminthic disease of the duodenum and upper jejunum. Clinical manifestations include dermatitis as larvae of the parasite penetrate the skin; cough and rales, or even pneumonitis when they pass through the lungs; abdominal symptoms when the adult females lodge in the mucosa of the intestine. Symptoms may be mild or severe, depending upon intensity of infection; in order of frequency, pain, usually epigastric and often suggesting peptic ulcer, nausea, weight loss, vomiting, diarrhea, weakness and constipation. Urticaria may occur, especially with reinfection. Rarely, internal autoinfection with increasing worm burden may lead to wasting and death. Eosinophilia is usually moderate.

Diagnosis is by identifying motile larvae in freshly passed feces, or motile larvae in fluids obtained by duodenal intubation. Held at room temperature for 24 hours or longer, feces may show developing stages of the parasite, including filariform or infective larvae and free-living nonparasitic male and female adults.

2. Occurrence—Geographic distribution closely parallels that of hookworm disease (see p. 5), but indigenous cases occur far beyond the usual confines of that disease. Prevalence in endemic areas is not accurately known.

3. Infectious agent—*Strongyloides stercoralis,* a nematode.

4. Reservoir—Reservoir is an infected person, or possibly dogs.

5. Mode of transmission—Infective (filariform) larvae in moist soil contaminated with feces penetrate the skin, usually of the foot, and are carried to the lungs. They penetrate capillary walls, enter alveoli, ascend the trachea to the epiglottis, and descend the digestive tract to reach upper part of the small intestine, where development of the adult parasitic female is completed. The female, generally held to be parthenogenetic, lives embedded in mucosa of the intestine, where eggs are deposited, promptly hatch and liberate noninfective rhabditiform larvae which migrate into the lumen of the intestine, leave the host with feces, and develop either into infective filariform larvae, which reinfect the host, or into free-living adults. The free-living fertilized females produce eggs which soon hatch, liberating rhabditiform larvae, which become filariform larvae.

6. Incubation period—From penetration of skin by filariform larvae until rhabditiform larvae appear in feces is about 17 days; incubation period, until symptoms appear, is indefinite and variable.

7. Period of communicability—As long as living worms remain in the intestine, up to 35 years.

8. Susceptibility and resistance—Susceptibility to infection is universal. Acquired immunity demonstrated in laboratory animals but not man.

9. Methods of control—

A. Preventive measures:

1) As for Hookworm Disease (see p. 5 herein). Sanitary disposal of human excreta, particularly the use of sanitary privies in rural areas.
2) Rigid attention to hygienic habits, particularly the wearing of shoes.
3) Treat infected dogs with cyanine dyes. Destroy stray dogs.

B. Control of patient, contacts, and the immediate environment:

1) *Report to local health authority:* Official report ordinarily not justifiable, Class 5 (see Preface).
2) *Isolation:* None.
3) *Concurrent disinfection:* Sanitary disposal of excreta.
4) *Quarantine:* None.
5) *Immunization of contacts:* None.
6) *Investigation of contacts:* Family members for evidence of infection.
7) *Specific treatment:* Thiabendazole (Mintezol), pyrvinium pamoate (Povan).

C. Epidemic measures: Not applicable, a sporadic disease.

D. International measures: None.

SYPHILIS

Two distinctive forms are recognized. That form which is venereally spread is of worldwide occurrence. The other, believed by many to be a closely related but different disease, is often referred to as endemic syphilis or bejel. This is of nonvenereal spread and confined to parts of the world where economic, social and climatic conditions favor its development; does not occur in U.S.A.

I. VENEREAL SYPHILIS

1. Identification—An acute and chronic relapsing treponematosis characterized clinically by a primary lesion, a secondary eruption involving skin and mucous membranes, long periods of latency, and late lesions of skin, bone, viscera, and central nervous and cardiovascular systems. The primary lesion appears after about 3 weeks as a papule; after erosion, it presents a variety of forms, the most distinctive although not the most frequent being an indurated chancre; invasion of blood precedes the initial lesion, and a firm nonfluctuant, painless satellite bubo commonly follows. Infection without chancre is fairly frequent. During next 4 to 6 weeks, even without specific treatment the chancre begins to involute and a generalized secondary eruption appears, often accompanied by mild constitutional symptoms. Secondary manifestations disappear spontaneously within weeks to as long as 12 months, with subsequent clinical latency of weeks to years, often interrupted in early years by recurrence of infectious lesions of skin and mucous membrane or developing lesions of eye and central nervous system; in later years (5 to 20) by destructive noninfectious lesions of skin, viscera, bone, and mucosal surfaces. Latency sometimes continues through life; sometimes spontaneous recovery occurs; in other instances, and unpredictably, late disabling manifestations occur in cardiovascular, central nervous system or other systems. Actual fatality rates cannot be accurately estimated, but prenatal infection is frequently fatal, before birth or in infancy. Early acquired syphilis does not result in death or serious disability but the late manifestations shorten life, impair health, and limit occupational efficiency. Synonym: Lues.

Primary and secondary syphilis are confirmed by dark-field or phase-contrast examination of exudates of lesions (if no antibiotic has been administered), and in all instances by serologic tests for syphilis through examination of blood and spinal fluid. Tests with nontreponemal antigens may be supplemented by treponemal immobilization, agglutination, or fluorescent antibody tests to aid in exclusion of biologic false-positive reactions. The dark-field examination is indispensable in seronegative primary syphilis.

2. Occurrence—One of the more frequent and widespread communicable diseases, primarily involving young persons between 15 and 30 years of age. Considerable differences in racial incidence are related more to social than to biologic factors. More prevalent in urban than rural areas and in males than females. Since 1957, early venereal syphilis has increased significantly throughout much of the world.

3. **Infectious agent**—*Treponema pallidum,* a spirochete.

4. **Reservoir**—Man is the only reservoir.

5. **Mode of transmission**—By direct contact in heterosexual or homosexual activity, with exudates from obvious or concealed moist early lesions of skin and mucous membrane, body fluids and secretions (saliva, semen, blood, vaginal discharges) of infected persons during infectious periods. Rarely by kissing, fondling of children. Indirect contact with contaminated articles has practically no significance. Prenatal infection may occur after fourth month of pregnancy through placental transfer; transmission occurs occasionally through blood transfusion.

6. **Incubation period**—Ten days to 10 weeks, usually 3 weeks.

7. **Period of communicability**—Variable and indefinite; during primary and secondary stages, also mucocutaneous recurrence, intermittently during 2 to 4 years. Extent of communicability through sexual activity during latency period (2 to 4 years) not established; possible inapparent lesions make this stage potentially infectious. Adequate penicillin treatment in its infectious stages usually ends infectivity within 24 hours.

8. **Susceptibility and resistance**—Susceptibility is universal, with no natural immunity. Infection leads to gradually developing resistance against the homologous strain of *Treponema* and to some extent against heterologous strains; immunity may be overcome by large reinfecting dose or fail to develop because of treatment in primary or secondary stage. Superinfection may produce lesions simulating those of the currently existing stage; in late latency, superinfection has special significance by its ability to produce benign late lesions of skin and mucous membrane.

9. **Methods of control**—

    A. *Preventive measures:* The following are applicable to all venereal diseases: syphilis, chancroid, lymphogranuloma venereum, granuloma inguinale, and gonorrhea.

        1) General health promotional measures, health and sex education, preparation for marriage, premarital and prenatal examinations, including blood serology as part of general physical examination; improvement of social and economic conditions, including provision of recreational facilities.

        2) Protection of community by control of commercialized prostitution and discouragement of clandestine sexual promiscuity, in cooperation with social and law enforcement agencies; by teaching methods of personal prophylaxis applicable before, during and after exposure; by repeated prenatal serologic examination of pregnant women.

        3) Provision of facilities for early diagnosis and treatment;

encouragement of their use through education of the public about symptoms of the venereal diseases and modes of spread, and through making these services available irrespective of economic status. Intensive case-finding programs, to include interview of patients and tracing of contacts; repeated mass serologic examination of special groups with known high incidence of venereal disease.

4) Emphasis on control of patients with venereal disease in a transmissible stage should not preclude search for persons past that stage to prevent relapse, congenital syphilis, and disability due to late manifestations.

B. Control of patient, contacts, and the immediate environment:

1) *Report to local health authority:* Case report of early infectious syphilis is required in all states, and variously in other countries, Class 2A (see Preface); report of positive serology and dark-field examinations by laboratories in some states.

2) *Isolation:* None. To avoid reinfection, patients should refrain from sexual intercourse with previous partners not under treatment.

3) *Concurrent disinfection:* None in adequately treated cases; care in disposal of discharges from open lesions and articles soiled therewith.

4) *Quarantine:* None.

5) *Immunization of contacts:* Not applicable.

6) *Investigation of contacts:* Interview of patients and tracing of contacts are fundamental features of a program for control of venereal disease. Trained interviewers obtain best results. The stage of disease determines criteria for contact-tracing: (a) for primary syphilis, all sexual contacts of preceding 3 months; (b) for secondary syphilis, those of preceding 6 months; (c) for early latent syphilis, those of preceding year, provided time of primary and secondary lesions is not established; (d) for late and late latent syphilis, marital partners and children of infected mothers; (e) for congenital syphilis, all members of immediate family.

7) *Specific treatment:* Long-acting penicillin (PAM, benzathine penicillin, or equivalent preparation); in general, large amounts initially on day of diagnosis, to assure reasonably effective therapy should the patient fail to return. Erythromycin, tetracycline antibiotics or chloramphenicol may be used in penicillin-sensitive persons. Such patients require extended post-treatment observation and follow-up checks of serological reactions.

C. Epidemic measures: Intensification of measures outlined under 9A and 9B, preceding.

D. *International measures:*

1) Appropriate examination of groups of adolescents and young adults moving from areas of high prevalence of treponemal infections.
2) Adherence to agreements among nations (e.g., Brussels Agreement) as to records, provision of diagnostic and treatment facilities, and contact interviewing at seaports for foreign merchant seamen.
3) Provision for rapid international exchange of information on contacts.
4) WHO Reference Centres (see Preface).

II. NONVENEREAL SYPHILIS

1. Identification—A disease of limited geographical distribution, acute nature, and characterized clinically by an eruption of skin and mucous membrane, usually without evident initial primary sore. Mucous patches of the mouth are often the first lesions, soon followed by moist papules in folds of skin and by drier lesions of trunk and extremities. Other early skin lesions are macular or papular, often hypertrophic, and frequently circinate, resembling those of venereal syphilis. Plantar and palmar hyperkeratoses occur frequently, often with painful fissuring; patchy depigmentation and hyperpigmentation of the skin and alopecia are common. Inflammatory or destructive lesions of skin, long bones, and nasopharynx are late manifestations. Unlike venereal syphilis, nervous and cardiovascular systems are rarely involved. Case fatality is negligible. Synonyms: Bejel, Dichuchwa, Njovera.

Organisms demonstrable in lesions by dark-field examination; serologic tests for syphilis are reactive in the early stages and remain so for many years of latency, gradually tending toward reversal; response to treatment as in venereal syphilis.

2. Occurrence—A common disease in localized areas where poor economic and social conditions prevail, with primitive sanitary and dwelling arrangements. Present in the Balkans and in eastern Mediterranean countries. Numerous foci in Africa, particularly in arid regions.

3. Infectious agent—*Treponema pallidum,* a spirochete.

4. Reservoir—Reservoir is man.

5. Mode of transmission—Direct or indirect contact with infectious early lesions of skin and mucous membranes is favored by common use of eating and drinking utensils and generally unsatisfactory hygienic conditions. Congenital transmission is rare.

6. Incubation period—Two weeks to 3 months, usually about 6 weeks.

7. Period of communicability—During moist eruptions of skin and until mucous patches disappear; sometimes several weeks or months.

8. Susceptibility and resistance—Similar to venereal syphilis.

9. **Methods of control—**

    A. *Preventive measures:* Those of the nonvenereal treponematoses. See Yaws, 9A (pp. 285–286).

    B. *Control of patient, contacts, and the immediate environment:*

        1) *Report to local health authority:* In selected endemic areas; in most countries not a reportable disease; Class 3B (see Preface).

        2) See Yaws 9B (p. 286) for items 2–7, applicable to all nonvenereal treponematoses.

    C. *Epidemic measures:* Intensification of preventive and control activities.

    D. *International measures:* See Venereal Syphilis 9D4 (preceding); and Yaws 9D (p. 286).

TAENIASIS AND CYSTICERCOSIS

    1. Identification—An infection with the adult stage of the beef tapeworm *(Taenia saginata)* or the adult or larval stage of the pork tapeworm *(T. solium)*. The larval infection, cysticercosis, is a severe somatic disease involving many different organs and tissues in which encystment occurs. Clinical manifestations of infection with the adult worm (taeniasis) are variable and may include nervousness, insomnia, anorexia, loss of weight, abdominal pain, and digestive disturbances. Some infections are asymptomatic. A nonfatal disease. Synonym: Beef or Pork tapeworm disease.

    Infection with an adult tapeworm is diagnosed by identification of proglottids (segments) of the worm or of eggs in feces on adhesive cellulose tape swab. Specific diagnosis is through morphological features of gravid proglottids; obtaining the scolex or head confirms the identification and assures elimination of the worm.

    If eggs of the pork tapeworm are swallowed by man, they hatch in the small intestine and larval forms (cysticerci) develop in the subcutaneous tissues, striated muscles and other regions of the body. Consequences may be grave when larvae localize in heart, eye or central nervous system. Autoinfection with cystocercosis may result from regurgitation of eggs into the stomach of persons harboring an adult worm. Subcutaneous or visceral cysticercosis is recognized by excision of the larva and microscopic examination. In the presence of somatic cysticercosis, cerebral symptoms strongly suggest cerebral involvement—a chronic disease of relatively high fatality.

    Taenia eggs must be differentiated from eggs of *Hymenolepis nana,* which are relatively common, especially in children, and *Hymenolepis diminuta* and *Dipylidium caninum,* which are rare.

2. Occurrence—Cosmopolitan distribution; particularly frequent wherever beef or pork is eaten raw or lightly cooked. Incidence is highest in East Africa, Tibet, Mexico, Peru and eastern Europe. Where *Taenia saginata* and *Taenia solium* coexist, *T. saginata* is by far the commoner. Infection with *T. solium* is rare in the U.S.A. and Canada.

3. Infectious agents—*Taenia saginata,* the beef tapeworm of man, intestinal infection with adult worm only; *Taenia solium,* the pork tapeworm of man, intestinal infection with adult worm and somatic infection with the larvae, *Cysticercus cellulosae.*

4. Reservoir—Reservoir is an infected person discharging eggs of the parasite in feces.

5. Mode of transmission—For *Taenia saginata,* by ingestion of raw or inadequately cooked beef containing the infective larva—a cysticercus. For *Taenia solium* (1) by ingestion of raw or inadequately cooked pork containing the infective larva (cysticercus) and subsequent development of the adult worm in the intestine; or (2) by direct hand-to-mouth transfer of eggs in feces of an infected person or indirectly through ingestion of food or water contaminated with eggs, resulting in somatic cysticercosis.

6. Incubation period—From 8 to 10 weeks.

7. Period of communicability—The eggs of *T. saginata* are not directly transmitted from man to man but those of *T. solium* may be; eggs of both species are disseminated in the environment as long as man harbors the worm in the intestine, sometimes 30 to 40 years; they may remain viable for months.

8. Susceptibility and resistance—Man is universally susceptible. No apparent resistance follows infection.

9. Methods of control—

A. *Preventive measures:*

1) Health education of the public to prevent soil and water contamination with human feces in rural areas; to avoid use of sewage effluents for pasture irrigation; and to assure thorough cooking of beef and pork.
2) Adequate inspection of the carcasses of cattle and swine will detect most infected meat; cysticerci in beef may be few. Condemn carcasses of infected animals.
3) Do not allow swine access to latrines or to human feces.
4) Immediate treatment of persons harboring adult *T. solium* is essential to prevent human cysticercosis.

B. *Control of patient, contacts, and the immediate environment:*

1) Report to local health authority: Selectively reportable, Class 3C (see Preface).
2) Isolation: None; patients with *T. solium* infection should be excluded from preparation and serving of food.

3) *Concurrent disinfection:* Sanitary disposal of feces; for *T. solium* rigid sanitation with washing of hands after defecating and before eating.

4) *Quarantine:* None.

5) *Immunization of contacts:* None.

6) *Investigation of contacts:* Usually not profitable.

7) *Specific treatment:* For intestinal infection: quinacrine hydrochloride (Atabrine). For *T. saginata;* niclosamide (Yomesan) available in the U.S.A. from the National Communicable Disease Center, Atlanta, Ga. No specific chemotherapy for cysticercosis—surgical excision only satisfactory treatment.

C. Epidemic measures: None.

D. International measures: None.

TETANUS

1. Identification—An acute disease induced by toxin of the tetanus bacillus growing anaerobically at the site of an injury; characterized by painful muscular contractions, primarily of masseter and neck muscles, secondarily of trunk; rigidity is sometimes confined to the region of injury. History of injury or apparent portal of entry is sometimes lacking. Fatality varies from 35 to 70%, according to age, therapy, length of incubation, and geographic area. Synonym: Lockjaw.

Laboratory confirmation is of little help because of low recovery rate of the organism from the site of infection and the usual absence of antibody response.

2. Occurrence—Worldwide and at all ages; sporadically, never in epidemics. In U.S.A. and most industrial countries, relatively uncommon. Relatively more common in agricultural regions and in underdeveloped areas where contact with animal excreta is more likely and immunization is generally insufficient; a hazard of the use of drugs parenterally by addicts. An important cause of death in many countries of Asia, Africa and South America, especially in rural tropical areas and as tetanus neonatorum.

3. Infectious agent—*Clostridium tetani,* the tetanus bacillus.

4. Reservoir—Intestinal canal of animals, especially horses, in which the organism is a harmless normal inhabitant; also man.

5. Mode of transmission—Tetanus spores introduced into the body during injury, usually a puncture wound contaminated with soil, street dust or animal and human feces, but also through burns and trivial or unnoticed wounds. Presence of necrotic tissue favors growth of the anaerobic pathogen. Tetanus neonatorum usually occurs through infection of the unhealed umbilicus. The majority of cases follow injuries considered too trivial for medical consultation.

6. Incubation period—Commonly 4 days to 3 weeks, dependent on character, extent and location of wound; average 10 days. Majority within 14 days, but may be prolonged.

7. Period of communicability—Not directly transmitted from man to man.

8. Susceptibility and resistance—Susceptibility is general. Prolonged active immunity is induced by tetanus toxoid; transient passive immunity follows injection of tetanus immune globulin (human) or tetanus antitoxin. Recovery from tetanus does not imply immunity; second attacks occur.

9. Methods of control—

A. Preventive measures:

1) Education about the value of routine immunization with tetanus toxoid, the kinds of injury liable to be complicated by tetanus, and the need after injury for either a booster injection if previously actively immunized, or passive protection by tetanus immune globulin (human) or tetanus antitoxin if not immunized.

2) Active immunization with tetanus toxoid gives solid protection. The initial inoculation is preferably given in infancy or early childhood, together with diphtheria toxoid and pertussis vaccine (see Diphtheria 9A, pp. 78–79).

Tetanus toxoid is recommended for universal use but is especially important for workers in contact with soil or domestic animals and for military forces, policemen, firemen and others with greater than usual risk of traumatic injury. Pregnant women should be actively immunized where tetanus neonatorum is prevalent. In U.S.A., active immunization is by 2 initial doses of alum-precipitated (adult type) toxoid not less than 4 weeks apart, followed by a reinforcing injection about 8 to 12 months later; and thereafter, in the absence of injury, by booster doses at intervals of 10 years; can be given at any age.

3) For a person actively immunized against tetanus before contracting an injury with danger of tetanus, a single booster injection of tetanus toxoid administered promptly on the day of injury; reactions are infrequent but have been observed, especially after too frequent boosters. This procedure has a great advantage over passive immunization with tetanus immune globulin (human) or tetanus antitoxin (equine or bovine). It obviates the risk of serum reactions and provides protection against injuries considered too trivial to warrant medical attention.

4) Where there has been no previous active immunization (including recovered cases) and if the patient is seen on the day of injury and there are no compound fractures, gunshot wounds or other wounds not readily debrided,

passive protection by injection of 250 units of tetanus immune globulin (human) or 5,000 units of equine or bovine tetanus antitoxin. The human tetanus immune globulin is preferred because of the absence of serum reactions. If delay is greater, or such complications exist, the dose should be at least doubled. Protection from tetanus immune globulin lasts about 21 days; from tetanus antitoxin about 10 days or even less. Active immunization should be started at this time by giving the first dose (9A2) at a different site from that selected for the immune globulin or antitoxin.

5) Under all circumstances, removal of foreign matter from wounds by thorough cleansing, with debridement of necrotic tissue when present.

6) Licensing of midwives, with professional supervision and education as to methods, equipment and techniques of asepsis in childbirth.

7) Health education of mothers, relatives and attendants in the practice of strict asepsis of the umbilical stump of newborn infants. Important in many lesser developed areas where ashes, poultices or other contaminated substances are traditionally applied to the cord.

B. Control of patient, contacts, and the immediate environment:

1) *Report to local health authority:* Case report required in most states and countries, Class 2A (see Preface).

2) *Isolation:* None.

3) *Concurrent disinfection:* None.

4) *Quarantine:* None.

5) *Immunization of contacts:* None.

6) *Investigation of contacts and source of infection:* Case investigation to determine circumstances of injury. In tetanus neonatorum, rigid inquiry into the competence and licensure of attendants-at-birth and into methods of umbilical care employed by the family.

7) *Specific treatment:* Tetanus immune globulin (human) in large doses intramuscularly. Tetanus antitoxin in a single large dose should be given intravenously with appropriate precautions; penicillin in large doses intramuscularly. Maintain an adequate airway; employ sedation as indicated. Actively immunize recovered patients.

C. Epidemic measures: In the uncommon hospital outbreaks, thorough search for inadequacies in sterilization.

D. International measures: Active immunization against tetanus is advised for international travelers.

TOXOPLASMOSIS

1. Identification—A systemic protozoan disease. Early prenatal infection may lead to death of the fetus; or later infection to chorioretinitis, brain damage with intracerebral calcification, fever, jaundice, rash, hepatomegaly and splenomegaly; xanthochromic spinal fluid and convulsions are evident at birth or shortly thereafter. Postnatal infections are usually mild and may go undetected; rarely may be acute, with fever, lymphadenopathy and lymphocytosis persisting for days or weeks; even more rarely severe, with generalized muscle involvement, cerebral manifestations, and death. Adult chorioretinitis is more frequently associated with chronic infection.

Diagnosis is by demonstration of the agent in body tissues or fluids during life or at necropsy, or in laboratory-reared albino mice inoculated with extracts of such materials. Isolation should be supported by clinical and serologic evidence. Methylene blue dye test, complement fixation, hemagglutination, fluorescence inhibition and demonstration of gamma M (19S) antibodies in infants, as well as patterns of titer changes on sequential sera, are other laboratory aids.

2. Occurrence—Distribution worldwide in animals and man. Infection in man is common but clinical disease exceptional.

3. Infectious agent—*Toxoplasma gondii*, a protozoan.

4. Reservoir—Rodents, dogs, cats, swine, cattle, sheep, goats, chickens, and other mammals and birds.

5. Mode of transmission—Unclear for postnatal infections but consumption of raw or undercooked infected meat implicated. Congenital infection apparently occurs through the placenta of women experiencing a primary infection. Infection is also possible during delivery. No proven arthropod vector, although laboratory-infected ticks have transmitted infection to experimental animals, and experimental and natural transmission of *T. gondii* by cat feces with and without nematode (*Toxocara cati*) eggs has been reported.

6. Incubation period—Unknown; 10 to 13 days in one common-source outbreak.

7. Period of communicability—Probably not directly transmitted from man to man except during gestation. In animals, probably during acute stage, possibly longer.

8. Susceptibility and resistance—Susceptibility is general. Duration and degree of immunity are unknown.

9. Methods of control—

> **A. Preventive measures:** No known specific preventive measures. Suggested measure is thorough cooking of meat foods.

> **B. Control of patient, contacts, and the immediate environment:**

> *1) Report to local health authority:* Not ordinarily required; desirable, to facilitate research, Class 3C (see Preface).

    2) Isolation: None.
    3) Concurrent disinfection: None.
    4) Quarantine: None.
    5) Immunization of contacts: None.
    6) Investigation of contacts: In congenital cases, determine antibodies in mother and other members of family; in acquired cases, determine contact with infected animals and history of bites by arthropods.
    7) Specific treatment: In experimental infections of animals, sulfonamides have prophylactic value; when administered early may have therapeutic effect. Pyrimethamine (Daraprim) combined with triple sulfonamides is the preferred treatment in man; results in the treatment of acute disease are more favorable than the treatment of chronic forms. Duration of treatment should approximate 4 weeks.

C. Epidemic measures: Not applicable—a sporadic disease.

D. International measures: None.

TRACHOMA

    1. Identification—A specific communicable keratoconjunctivitis of insidious or abrupt onset; if untreated, of long or even lifetime duration. It is characterized by conjunctival inflammation with follicles and papillary hyperplasia, usually followed by vascular invasion of the cornea (pannus) and in its later stages by cicatrization which may lead to gross deformity of the eyelids, progressive visual disability and blindness. Associated bacterial infections, common in many areas, increase communicability and severity, and modify clinical behavior.

    Laboratory diagnosis is by demonstration of intracytoplasmic inclusion bodies in scrapings of epithelial cells, by isolation of the agent in chick embryo yolk sac, and by demonstration of characteristic cytological changes in expressed follicular material. The agent has not been clearly differentiated from that of inclusion conjunctivitis (see p. 63), although the 2 diseases are dissimilar epidemiologically.

    A number of forms of follicular conjunctivitis of bacterial or viral origin may resemble trachoma and require differentiation.

    2. Occurrence—Worldwide, in tropical, subtropical, temperate and cold climates, but with unequal and varying distributions, marked by differences in age of onset, clinical evolution, frequency of spontaneous cure, frequency of disabling sequelae and response to treatment. Trachoma is widespread in the Middle East, in Asia, along the Mediterranean littoral and in parts of Africa and South America; in U.S.A., among Indians and Mexican immigrants of the Southwest. High prevalence is generally associated with poor hygiene, poverty, and crowded living conditions, particularly in dry, dusty regions. Nomadic persons generally have a less severe form than stationary populations.

3. Infectious agent—The filterable agent of trachoma, a bedsonia (chlamydia).

4. Reservoir—Man.

5. Mode of transmission—By direct contact with ocular discharges and possibly mucoid or purulent discharges of nasal mucous membranes of infected persons, or materials soiled therewith. Genital localization of the agent has been demonstrated. Flies, especially *Musca sorbens,* may contribute to spread of the disease, but transmission occurs in their absence. Communicability is relatively low.

6. Incubation period—Five to 12 days in volunteer studies.

7. Period of communicability—While active lesions are present in conjunctivae and adnexal mucous membranes. The concentration of the agent in the tissues is greatly reduced with cicatrization but increases again with reactivation, and infective discharges recur.

8. Susceptibility and resistance—Susceptibility is general; affects children more frequently than adults, particularly persons of unclean habits and those whose eyes are irritated by exposure to sun, wind and sand. No demonstrable immunity results from an attack of the disease.

9. Methods of control—

A. Preventive measures:

1) Provision of adequate case-finding and treatment facilities, with emphasis on preschool children.
2) Health education of the public in the need for personal hygiene, especially the risk in common use of toilet articles.
3) Improved basic sanitation, including availability of soap and water.
4) Conduct epidemiological investigations to determine important factors in occurrence of the disease in each specific situation.
5) Experimental vaccines are under trial but their efficacy has not been established.

B. Control of patient, contacts, and the immediate environment:

1) Report to local health authority: Case report required in some states and countries of low endemicity, Class 2B (see Preface).
2) Isolation: Not practical in most areas where the disease occurs.

3) *Concurrent disinfection:* Of eye discharges and contaminated articles.
4) *Quarantine:* None.
5) *Immunization of contacts:* None.
6) *Investigation of contacts:* Members of family, playmates and schoolmates.
7) *Specific treatment:* Oral sulfonamides or topical tetracyclines are effective in acute disease; these therapeutic agents are far less effective in chronic cases.

C. *Epidemic measures:* In regions of hyperendemic prevalence, mass treatment campaigns have been successful in reducing severity and frequency, when associated with health education of the people in personal hygiene and effort toward an improved sanitary environment.

D. *International measures:* WHO Reference Centres (see Preface).

TRICHINOSIS

1. Identification—A disease caused by migration through the body of larvae of *Trichinella spiralis* and their encystment in muscles. Clinical disease in man is markedly irregular. Sudden appearance of edema of upper eyelids is a common, early and characteristic sign, usually noted about the 11th day; sometimes followed by subconjunctival, subungual and retinal hemorrhage, pain and photophobia. Gastrointestinal symptoms, such as diarrhea, may precede ocular manifestations. Muscle soreness and pain, skin lesions, thirst, profuse sweating, chills, weakness, prostration and rapidly increasing eosinophilia may shortly follow ocular signs. Fever is usual, remittent, and terminates by lysis in 1 to 3 weeks; sometimes as high as 40 C (104 F) for several days. Respiratory and neurological symptoms may appear in the 3rd to 6th week, myocardial failure between the 4th and 8th weeks. Usually a mild febrile disease, but can range from inapparent infection to a fulminating, fatal disease. Synonyms: Trichiniasis, Trichinellosis.

Increasing blood eosinophilia and skin tests, flocculation and complement-fixation tests may aid in diagnosis. Biopsy of skeletal muscle frequently provides conclusive evidence.

2. Occurrence—Worldwide but variable in incidence, depending on practices in eating and preparing pork, and the extent to which the disease is recognized and reported. Necropsy surveys reveal former wide prevalence in U.S.A., now only 4%; cases usually sporadic, outbreaks localized.

3. Infectious agent—Larva (trichina) of *Trichinella spiralis,* an intestinal roundworm.

4. Reservoir—Swine and many wild animals, including fox, wolf, bear, polar bear, marine mammals and rats, are reservoirs of infection.

5. Mode of transmission—Eating of raw or insufficiently cooked flesh of animals containing viable encysted trichinae, chiefly pork and pork products, and beef products such as hamburger adulterated either intentionally or inadvertently with pork. In the small intestine, larvae develop into mature adults and mate. Gravid female worms then pass larvae, which penetrate the intestinal wall, enter the lymphatics, and are disseminated via the bloodstream throughout the body. The larvae encyst in striated skeletal muscle.

6. Incubation period—About 9 days after ingestion of infective meat; varies between 2 and 28 days.

7. Period of communicability—Not transmitted directly from man to man. Animal hosts remain infective for months, and meat from such animals for appreciable periods unless treated to kill the larvae.

8. Susceptibility and resistance—Susceptibility universal. Infection is not known to result in acquired immunity.

9. Methods of Control—

A. Preventive measures:

1) Regulations to assure adequate processing of pork products. In the U.S.A., pork inspection is considered to be impractical and costly while affording a false sense of security. Pork must be ground in a separate grinder, or the grinder thoroughly cleaned, before processing other meats.

2) Adoption of suitable laws and regulations insuring cooking of garbage and offal before feeding to swine. Incineration or burial of garbage may be cheaper than feeding to swine.

3) Education on the need to cook all fresh pork and pork products at a temperature and time sufficient to allow all parts to reach at least 65.6 C (150 F), which allows a good margin of safety, or until meat changes from pink to grey, unless established that these meat products have been processed either by heating, curing or refrigeration adequate to kill trichinae.

4) Low temperatures maintained throughout pork are effective in killing trichinae, −27 C (−16 F) for 36 hours or higher temperatures for longer periods of time.

B. Control of patient, contacts, and the immediate environment:

1) *Report to local health authority:* Case report desirably required in most states and countries, Class 2B (see Preface.)

2) *Isolation:* None.

3) *Concurrent disinfection:* None.
4) *Quarantine:* None.
5) *Immunization of contacts:* None.
6) *Investigation of contacts:* Other family members and persons who have consumed suspected meat, for evidence of infection.
7) *Specific treatment:* Thiabendazole has been used experimentally with encouraging results but full efficacy and safety remain to be determined. Corticosteroids are indicated in severe cases.

C. **Epidemic measures:** Institute epidemiologic study to determine the common food involved. Confiscate remainder of food and correct faulty practices.

D. **International measures:** None.

TRICHOMONIASIS

1. **Identification**—A common nonfatal chronic disease of the genitourinary tract characterized in women by vaginitis, frequently with small petechial or punctate hemorrhagic lesions, and a profuse, thin, foamy, yellowish discharge of foul odor. In men, the infectious agent lives in prostate, urethra, or seminal vesicles, rarely producing symptoms or demonstrable lesions. Infection is frequently asymptomatic.

Diagnosis is through identification of the motile parasite, either by microscopic examination of discharges, or by culture.

2. **Occurrence**—Geographically widespread, and a frequent disease of all continents and all peoples, primarily of adults, with highest incidence among young girls and women aged 16 to 35 years. In sampled areas of U.S.A., the prevalence among females has been as high as 50%.

3. **Infectious agent**—*Trichomonas vaginalis,* a protozoan.

4. **Reservoir**—Reservoir is man.

5. **Mode of transmission**—By contact with vaginal and urethral discharges of infected persons during sexual intercourse; during birth; and possibly by contact with contaminated articles.

6. **Incubation period**—Four to 20 days, average 7 days.

7. **Period of communicability**—For the duration of the infection.

8. **Susceptibility and resistance**—Susceptibility to infection general and high, but clinical disease is mainly in females.

9. **Methods of control—**

   A. *Preventive measures:* Avoidance of sexual intercourse with known infected individuals.

   B. *Control of patient, contacts, and the immediate environment:*

   1) *Report to local health authority:* Official report not ordinarily justifiable, Class 5 (see Preface).
   2) *Isolation:* None; avoid sexual relations during period of infection and treatment.
   3) *Concurrent disinfection:* None; the organism cannot withstand drying.
   4) *Quarantine:* None.
   5) *Immunization of contacts:* None.
   6) *Investigation of contacts:* Sexual partner, particularly if infection is recurrent.
   7) *Specific treatment:* Metronidazole (Flagyl) by mouth is effective in both male and female patients. Most infected females respond to a variety of chemotherapeutic agents used locally in conjunction with a maintained vaginal acidity and cleanliness. Concurrent treatment of sexual partner to prevent reinfection.

   C. *Epidemic measures:* None.

   D. *International measures:* None.

TRICHURIASIS

1. Identification—A nematode infection of the large intestine, often asymptomatic and detected only by examination of feces. Heavy infections result in intermittent abdominal discomfort, diarrhea, loss of weight and anemia. Synonyms: Trichocephaliasis, Whipworm disease.
Diagnosis is by demonstration of eggs of parasite in feces.

2. Occurrence—Cosmopolitan, especially in warm, moist regions.

3. Infectious agent—*Trichuris trichiura* (*Trichocephalus trichiurus*), a nematode; the human whipworm.

4. Reservoir—An infected person discharging eggs in feces.

5. Mode of transmission—Indirect; eggs passed in feces require about 3 weeks for embryonation in soil. Ingestion of soil containing fully embryonated eggs is followed by hatching and attachment of the developing worm to the mucosa of cecum and proximal colon. About 90 days are required from ingestion to passage of eggs.

6. Incubation period—Long and indefinite.

7. Period of communicability—As long as eggs are in feces; several years.

8. Susceptibility and resistance—Susceptibility is universal.

9. Methods of control—

A. Preventive measures:

1) Provision of adequate facilities for disposal of feces.
2) Education of all members of the family, particularly children, in the use of toilet facilities. Encouragement of satisfactory hygienic habits, especially in the practice of washing the hands before handling food.

B. Control of patient, contacts and the immediate environment:

1) *Report to local health authority:* Official report not ordinarily justifiable, Class 5 (see Preface). School health authorities should be advised of unusual frequency in school populations.
2) *Isolation:* None.
3) *Concurrent disinfection:* None; sanitary disposal of feces.
4) *Quarantine:* None.
5) *Immunization of contacts:* None.
6) *Investigation of contacts:* Examine feces of all members of family group, especially children and playmates.
7) *Specific treatment:* Thiabendazole (Mintezol) should be used first. If not sufficiently effective, 0.2% hexylresorcinol enemata may be necessary. Most light infections require no treatment.

C. Epidemic measures: Not applicable.

D. International measures: None.

TRYPANOSOMIASIS, AFRICAN

1. Identification—In early stages, fever, intense headache, insomnia, lymph node enlargement (especially posterior cervical), anemia, local edema and rash; later, wasting, somnolence, and signs referable to the central nervous system. May run a protracted course of several years, or death may follow within a few months; highly fatal. Synonym: African sleeping sickness.

Diagnosis in early stages is by finding trypanosomes in lymph from punctured nodes; less readily in peripheral blood. In late stages trypanosomes may be found in cerebrospinal fluid. Inoculation of laboratory rats or mice, or culture on appropriate media is sometimes useful.

2. Occurrence—The disease is confined to tropical Africa between 15 N and 20 S latitude, corresponding to distribution of the tsetse fly; in some endemic regions up to 30% of persons have been infected. Epidemics occur when the disease is introduced into nonimmune populations. Where *Glossina palpalis* is the principal vector, infection occurs mainly along streams (Gambia, Liberia, Sierra Leone, Ghana, Congo, Sudan, Uganda); where the vector is *Glossina morsitans,* over wider dry savannas (Zambia, Rhodesia, Mozambique, Malawi and Tanzania).

3. Infectious agents—*Trypanosoma gambiense* and *Trypanosoma rhodesiense,* hemoflagellates. Criteria for species differentiation are not absolute; isolates from cases of virulent, rapidly progressive disease are considered to be *T. rhodesiense.*

4. Reservoir—Man is a main reservoir of *T. gambiense.* Wild game, especially bushbuck and antelopes, and domestic cattle are chief animal reservoirs of *T. rhodesiense.*

5. Mode of transmission—By bite of an infective *Glossina,* the tsetse fly; direct mechanical transmission by blood on proboscis is presumably possible. Six species are mainly concerned in nature: *Glossina palpalis, G. tachinoides, G. morsitans, G. pallidipes, G. swynnertoni,* and *G. fuscipes.* The tsetse fly, whether male or female, is infected by ingested blood of an infected person or animal that contains trypanosomes. The parasite multiplies in the fly for 18 days or longer according to temperature and other factors, until infective forms develop in the salivary glands. Once infected, a tsetse fly remains infective for life (up to 3 months); infection is not passed from generation to generation in flies; congenital transmission can occur in man. Not directly transmissible from man to man.

6. Incubation period—Usually 2 to 3 weeks. May be as short as 7 days.

7. Period of communicability—To the tsetse fly, as long as the parasite is present in the blood of the infected person; extremely variable in untreated cases, but communicable in late as well as early stages of the disease.

8. Susceptibility and resistance—Susceptibility is general. Spontaneous recovery in cases without symptoms of central nervous system involvement has been reported rarely; also in a few untreated advanced cases with nervous system disease. Inapparent infection with *T. gambiense* has occurred.

9. Methods of control—

A. Preventive measures:

1) Selection of appropriate methods of prevention must be based on knowledge of the local ecology of infection. Thus, in a given geographic area, priority may be given to one or more of the following:

a) Destruction of vector tsetse fly habitats by selective

brush clearing along certain water courses or around villages.

b) Reduction of fly population by appropriate use of insecticides (5% DDT or 3% dieldrin).

c) Removal of people from fly-infested areas and congregation into larger settlements.

d) Reduction of parasite population by survey of human population for infection and treatment of positive persons.

e) Informing people of personal measures to protect against tsetse fly-bite.

f) Prophylactic medication with pentamidine isethionate*; a single 250-mg adult dose intramuscularly protects for 3 to 6 months against *T. gambiense* only. This is not generally recommended for the casual visitor to an endemic area.

B. Control of patient, contacts, and the immediate environment:

1) *Report to local health authority:* In selected endemic areas obtain records of prevalence and encourage control measures; not a reportable disease in most countries, Class 3B (see Preface).

2) *Isolation:* Prevent tsetse fly from feeding on patients with trypanosomes in blood; isolation is not practicable. In some countries legal restrictions are placed on movement of untreated patients.

3) *Concurrent disinfection:* None.

4) *Quarantine:* None.

5) *Immunization of contacts:* None.

6) *Investigation of contacts:* None.

7) *Specific treatment:* Early in course of infection suramin* or pentamidine* is used; the former is drug of choice for *T. rhodesiense* infections, while the latter is preferred for *T. gambiense* infections. Melarsoprol* (Mel B) has been used effectively for treatment of late cases of either form.

C. Epidemic measures: Mass survey and treatment, with tsetse fly control, is urgent. If epidemics recur in an area despite control measures, it may be necessary to move villages to a safer district. Other measures as in 9A.

D. International measures: Promote cooperative efforts of governments in endemic areas. WHO Reference Centres (see Preface).

---

* Available in the U.S.A. from the National Communicable Disease Center, Atlanta, Ga., on an investigational basis.

TRYPANOSOMIASIS, AMERICAN

1. Identification—Acute stages are generally seen in children; chronic manifestations generally appear later in life. Acute disease is characterized by variable fever, malaise, lymphadenopathy and hepatosplenomegaly. An inflammatory response at the site of infection (chagoma) may occur lasting up to 8 weeks. Unilateral bipalpebral edema (Romaña's sign) is characteristic and occurs in a significant percentage of acute cases. Life-threatening or fatal manifestations include myocarditis and meningoencephalitis. Chronic sequelae include myocardial damage with cardiac dilatation and disturbance of rhythm, and intestinal involvement with megacolon and megaesophagus. Many infected persons have no clinical manifestations. Synonym: Chagas' disease.

Diagnosis in acute phase is established by demonstration of the organism in blood (or, rarely, in lymph node or skeletal muscle) by direct examination, by culture, by inoculation into rats or mice, or by xenodiagnosis (feeding uninfected triatomid bugs on the patient and finding the parasite in the bug's feces several weeks later). Parasitemia is most intense during febrile episodes early in the course of infection. In chronic phase xenodiagnosis may be positive but other methods will rarely reveal parasites. Positive serologic tests, especially CF tests, are helpful but standardized methods have not yet been developed.

2. Occurrence—The disease is confined to the Western Hemisphere, with wide geographic distribution in rural Mexico and Central and South America; in some areas highly endemic. Two human infections have been reported recently in U.S.A. (Texas), but serologic studies suggest asymptomatic cases may occur. *Trypanosoma cruzi* has been found in small mammals in Alabama, Arizona, California, Florida, Georgia, Louisiana, Maryland, New Mexico, Texas and Utah.

3. Infectious agent—*Trypanosoma cruzi*, a hemoflagellate.

4. Reservoir—Reservoirs include infected persons and many domestic and wild animals such as dog, cat, pig, guinea pig, bat, house rat, wood rat, fox, opossum and armadillo.

5. Mode of transmission—By fecal material from infectious vectors: blood-sucking species of *Reduviidae* (cone-nosed bugs), especially *Triatoma, Rhodnius* and *Panstrongylus*. Infection is through contamination of conjunctiva, mucous membranes, and abrasions or wounds of the skin by fresh infected bug feces. Transmission may occur by blood transfusion and organisms also may pass through the placenta to cause congenital infection. Many known accidental laboratory infections.

6. Incubation Period—About 5 to 14 days after bite of insect vector; but 30–40 days if infected by blood transfusion.

7. Period of communicability—Not directly transmitted from man to man. Organisms are present regularly in the blood during the acute period and usually persist in very small numbers throughout life in symptomatic and asymptomatic persons. The vector becomes infective

8 to 10 days after biting an infective host and remains infective for life (as long as 2 years).

8. Susceptibility and resistance—All ages are susceptible, but in younger persons the disease is said to be more severe.

9. Methods of control—

A. Preventive measures:

1) Systematic attack upon vectors through use of effective insecticides with residual action.
2) Construction or repair of dwellings to eliminate hiding places for the insect vector and shelter for the domestic and wild reservoirs.
3) Elimination of infected domestic animals and destruction of wild hosts in known endemic areas.
4) Use of bed nets in houses infested by the vector.
5) Health education of the public as to mode of spread and methods of prevention.
6) In endemic areas, screen blood donors by complement-fixation or other suitable test to prevent infection by transfusion. Addition of gentian violet (25 ml of 0.5% solution per 500 ml of blood 24 hours before use) will prevent transmission.

B. Control of patient, contacts, and the immediate environment:

1) *Report to local health authority:* In selected endemic areas ; not a reportable disease in most countries, Class 3B (see Preface).
2) *Isolation:* None.
3) *Concurrent disinfection:* None.
4) *Quarantine:* None.
5) *Immunization of contacts:* None.
6) *Investigation of contacts and source of infection:* Search bedding and rooms for the vector, and investigate domestic and wild animals for evidence of infection. Other members of the family should be examined.
7) *Specific treatment:* No drug has recognized value. A nitrofurfurylidine derivative, Bayer 2502, is available from the National Communicable Disease Center on an investigational basis.

C. Epidemic measures: In areas of high incidence, field surveys to determine distribution and frequency of vectors and animal hosts.

D. International measures: None.

TUBERCULOSIS

1. Identification—A chronic bacterial disease and an important cause of death in many parts of the world. Primary infection usually goes unnoticed clinically; tuberculin sensitivity appears within a few weeks; lesions commonly become inactive, leaving no residual changes except pulmonary or tracheobronchial lymph node calcifications. May progress, however, to pulmonary tuberculosis, pleurisy or lymphohematogenous dissemination of bacilli to produce miliary, meningeal or other extrapulmonary involvement. Serious outcome of primary infection is more frequent in infants than in older persons.

Pulmonary tuberculosis generally arises as reactivation of a latent focus and has a chronic, variable and often asymptomatic course, with exacerbations and remissions, and is capable of arrest or relapse at any stage. Three stages (minimal, moderately advanced, and far advanced) are distinguished according to extent of lung involvement; activity is determined by presence of tubercle bacilli in sputum, or by progression or retrogression as detected in serial x-rays. Abnormal x-ray densities indicative of pulmonary infiltration, cavitation, or fibrosis commonly occur in advance of clinical manifestations. Cough, fatigue, fever, weight loss, hoarseness, chest pain and hemoptysis may occur but often are absent until advanced stages.

Diagnosis by x-ray is confirmed by demonstration of tubercle bacilli in sputum or gastric washings, by stained smear, and by culture on suitable media.

The tuberculin test with 5 TU (tuberculin units) is positive except in critically ill persons and during certain intercurrent diseases (e.g., measles).

Extrapulmonary tuberculosis is much less common than pulmonary; includes meningitis, miliary tuberculosis, and involvement of bones and joints, eyes, lymph nodes, kidneys, intestines, larynx, skin or peritoneum. Diagnosis is by recovery of tubercle bacilli from lesions or exudates.

2. Occurrence—Present in all parts of the world; numerous countries have shown a downward trend of mortality for many years. Mortality rates range from below 5 to over 100 deaths per 100,000 population per year. In 1967, the reported incidence of new cases in U.S.A. was 23.1 per 100,000 population. The mortality rate, 3.3, increased with age; was higher in males than in females; and much higher in nonwhites than in whites. Prevalence of pulmonary tuberculosis is low under 20 years and rises with age; highest in males over 50. Epidemics have been reported among children in crowded classrooms or other groups congregated in enclosed spaces. Most tuberculosis, especially in low-incidence areas, arises from old latent foci remaining from the initial infection, i.e., it is endogenous.

Prevalence of infection, as manifested by tuberculin test, increases with age; usually higher in cities than in rural areas. Rapid decline in recent decades; in U.S.A., only 3% of males aged 17 to 20 years now react positively to 5TU of PPD (purified protein derivative).

Bovine type in man is now rare in the U.S.A. and many other countries; still a problem in some.

3. Infectious agent—*Mycobacterium tuberculosis,* the human tubercle bacillus, and *M. bovis* in cattle, swine and other animals. Predominantly, the human type causes pulmonary tuberculosis and the bovine type, extrapulmonary. So-called atypical mycobacteria occasionally produce disease indistinguishable from pulmonary tuberculosis except by culture of the organisms and, less reliably, by skin testing with several antigens.

4. Reservoir—Reservoir is primarily man; in some areas, also diseased cattle.

5. Mode of transmission—Contact with bacilli in pulmonary secretions or sputum of infected persons. Prolonged household exposure to an active case usually leads to infection of contacts and frequently to active disease. Airborne route is the predominant mode of spread. Indirect contact through contaminated articles or dust is not important; direct invasion through mucous membranes or breaks in the skin is extremely rare. Bovine tuberculosis results from exposure to tuberculous cows, usually by ingestion of unpasteurized milk or dairy products and sometimes is airborne among farmers and animal handlers.

6. Incubation period—From infection to demonstrable primary lesion, about 4 to 6 weeks; to progressive pulmonary or extrapulmonary tuberculosis may be years; the first 6 to 12 months after infection is the most hazardous period.

7. Period of communicability—As long as infectious tubercle bacilli are being discharged. Some untreated or inadequately treated patients may be intermittently sputum-positive for years. The degree of communicability depends on numbers of bacilli discharged and opportunities for their aerosolization by coughing, sneezing, singing, etc. Antimicrobial therapy generally terminates communicability within a few weeks. Extrapulmonary tuberculosis is not directly communicable.

8. Susceptibility and resistance—Susceptibility is general; highest in children under 3 years, lowest in later childhood, then again high in adolescents and young adults; undernourished, neglected and fatigued persons or those with silicosis or diabetes, and alcoholics are especially susceptible. Relapse of long latent infection, particularly in older persons, accounts for a large proportion of active cases.

9. Methods of control—

A. *Preventive measures:*

1) Correction of such social conditions as overcrowding and poverty, which increase the risk of becoming infected; health education of the public in the importance, mode of spread and methods of control of the disease.

2) Availability of medical, laboratory and x-ray facilities for examination of patients, contacts and suspects, and for

early treatment of cases; beds for those needing hospitalization.

3) Public health nursing service for home supervision of patients and to encourage and arrange for examination of contacts.

4) Preventive treatment, defined as prevention of active disease by administration of isoniazid in therapeutic dosage for 1 year, has been shown to be effective for household associates of active cases, and for other populations in which risk of tuberculosis is unusually great, e.g., persons who, during the previous year, converted from tuberculin-negative to tuberculin-positive, and optimally for all tuberculin-positive persons, particularly those under excessive risk due to age, underlying disease, or prolonged corticosteroid therapy. A course of isoniazid will reduce the risk of relapse in arrested cases never previously treated with effective antibacterial drugs. (For purposes of this recommendation, tuberculin positivity is a response of 10 mm or greater induration 48 to 72 hours after a properly applied Mantoux test, using 5 TU of PPD-S.)

5) BCG vaccination of uninfected (tuberculin-negative) persons induces tuberculin sensitivity in over 90% of individuals and confers good protection. Controlled trials have provided evidence that this protection may persist for at least 12 years. Where risk of infection is low, as presently it is in most parts of the U.S.A., mass vaccination has little role. In some parts of the world, vaccine is used routinely as part of the program of control. Vaccine may be used for newborn infants and also for household contacts of active cases, as well as for persons demonstrably at high risk of infection.

6) Elimination of tuberculosis among dairy cattle by tuberculin testing and slaughter of reactors; pasteurization of milk.

7) Measures to prevent inhalation of dangerous concentrations of silica dust in industrial plants and mines.

8) Routine x-ray examination of groups that have a high prevalence of tuberculosis, such as patients in general and mental hospitals and impoverished segments of the population; also those who constitute a special hazard to others if infected, such as school personnel. When feasible, initial screening by tuberculin test may be substituted, with x-ray examination restricted to reactors.

9) Periodic x-ray screening of tuberculin-positive populations.

10) Tuberculin-testing surveys, as at school entrance and at 14 years of age, employing 5 TU of PPD intracutaneously, are helpful in identifying foci of infection. Periodic retesting of tuberculin-negative persons, with preventive treatment of those whose reaction converts to positive, and a search for their source of infection are of value.

B. Control of patient, contacts, and the immediate environment:

1) *Report to local health authority:* Obligatory case report in most states and countries, Class 2B (see Preface). Health departments should maintain a current register of active cases.

2) *Isolation:* Control of infectivity is best achieved by prompt specific drug therapy, which usually reduces infectiousness rapidly and produces sputum conversion within a few months. Hospital treatment is desirable for patients with severe illness and those whose medical or social circumstances make it undesirable to treat them at home. For those who are treated at home, public health nursing supervision, including instruction in personal hygiene, especially in the need to cover the mouth and nose when coughing and sneezing, and in the careful handling and disposal of sputum; compulsory isolation only of patients with infectious tuberculosis who do not observe necessary precautions.

3) *Concurrent disinfection:* Of sputum and articles soiled therewith, including handkerchiefs, cloth or paper napkins, and eating utensils. Disinfection of air by bactericidal agents (e.g., ultraviolet light) and ventilation. Ordinary hygienic precautions suffice when patient is on specific therapy. Terminal cleaning.

4) *Quarantine:* None.

5) *Immunization of contacts:* Preventive treatment of contacts (see 9A4 preceding) is indicated. BCG vaccination of tuberculin negative household contacts may be warranted under special circumstances. (See Section 9A5).

6) *Investigation of contacts:* Tuberculin testing of all members of the household and intimate extrahousehold contacts (or all, if feasible) with x-ray examination of reactors. If negative, monthly skin tests should be performed for 3 months. Annual retest of tuberculin-negative persons. Preventive treatment of converters (see 9A4) with intensive study of the contacts is indicated.

7) *Specific treatment:* Although most primary infections heal without treatment, when they are recognized in an active or inactive stage, antimicrobial therapy is indicated to reduce the risk of progressive disease or later reactivation.

Patients with active pulmonary tuberculosis should be given prompt treatment with an appropriate combination of antimicrobial drugs continued for no less than 18 months. Current accepted regimens include 2 or 3 of the following: isoniazid (INH), paraaminosalicylic acid (PAS), streptomycin (SM) and ethambutol. Initial cultures of tubercle bacilli should be examined for drug susceptibility, with the test repeated in 3 months if sputum fails to become negative or reverts to positive after a series of negatives or if clinical response is poor. Drug resistance necessitates a change in regimen; at least two effective drugs should be included. Thoracic surgery, chiefly pulmonary resection, is used in selected cases.

In extrapulmonary tuberculosis, antimicrobial therapy is combined with other specific measures, often surgical, suited to the form and type of disease.

C. *Epidemic measures:* Alertness to recognize aggregations of new infections resulting from contact with an unrecognized infectious case and intensive search for the source of infection.

D. *International measures:* X-ray screening of individuals prior to emigration.

WHO Reference Centres (see Preface).

TULAREMIA

1. Identification—An infectious disease of wild animals and man; onset begins with chills and fever, the patient usually prostrated and confined to bed. An ulcer commonly appears at site of original infection; the regional lymph nodes become swollen and tender and often suppurate. Fatality in untreated cases is about 5%; with treatment, negligible.

Diagnosis is by inoculation of laboratory animals with material from lesions or with sputum, by recovery of infectious agent on glucose cystine blood agar, and by development of an agglutination reaction with patient's serum.

2. Occurrence—Throughout North America; in many parts of continental Europe, USSR, and in Japan. Occurs in U.S.A. every month of the year but especially in autumn during rabbit hunting season.

3. Infectious agent—*Francisella tularensis (Pasteurella tularensis, Bacterium tularense).*

4. Reservoir—Numerous wild animals, especially rabbits, muskrats, and some domestic animals; also wood ticks.

5. Mode of transmission—Inoculation of skin or conjunctival sac with blood or tissue while handling infected animals, as in skinning, dressing, or performing necropsies; or by fluids from infected flies, ticks or other animals. By mechanical transmission through the bite of arthropods including a species of deer fly, *Chrysops discalis;* in Sweden, the mosquito *Aedes cinereus.* By bite of reservoir wood ticks, *Dermacentor andersoni;* dog ticks, *Dermacentor variabilis;* Lone Star ticks, *Amblyomma americanum;* rabbit ticks, *Haemaphysalis leporis-*

palustris. By ingestion of insufficiently cooked rabbit meat and drinking of contaminated water. Rarely from bites of coyotes, skunks, hogs, cats, and dogs whose mouths presumably are contaminated from eating infected rabbits. Laboratory infections are common and frequently appear as a primary pneumonia.

6. Incubation period—One to 10 days, usually 3 days.

7. Period of communicability—Not directly transmitted from man to man. The infectious agent may be found in the blood during the first 2 weeks of disease, and in lesions up to a month from onset, sometimes longer. Flies are infective for 14 days, ticks throughout lifetime (about 2 years). Rabbits kept constantly frozen at −15 C (5 F) may remain infective more than 3 years.

8. Susceptibility and resistance—All ages are susceptible; permanent immunity follows recovery. Through abrasions and contact with contaminated material, an immune person may acquire a local tularemic papule harboring virulent organisms but causing no constitutional reaction.

9. Methods of control—

A. Preventive measures:

1) Education of the public to avoid bites of flies, mosquitoes and ticks or the handling of such arthropods when working in endemic areas; and to avoid drinking raw water where infection prevails among wild animals.

2) Use of rubber gloves when dressing wild rabbits or conducting laboratory experiments. Thorough cooking of the meat of wild rabbits.

3) Prohibition of interstate or interarea shipment of infected animals or their carcasses.

4) Killed vaccines are of limited value. Live vaccines are used extensively in USSR and to a limited extent in the U.S.A. Administration of a viable vaccine, intradermally by the multiple-puncture method, has very materially reduced the incidence of laboratory-acquired disease. If necessary, this vaccine can be obtained from the National Communicable Disease Center, Atlanta, Ga.

B. Control of patient, contacts, and the immediate environment:

1) Report to local health authority: In selected endemic areas (U.S.A.); in many countries, not a reportable disease, Class 3B (see Preface).

2) Isolation: None.

3) Concurrent disinfection: Of discharges from ulcer, lymph nodes, or conjunctival sac.

4) Quarantine: None.

5) Immunization of contacts: Not indicated.

6) Investigation of contacts: Important in each case, with search for the origin of infection.

7) *Specific treatment:* Streptomycin is the drug of choice; the tetracyclines and chloramphenicol are effective when continued until temperature is normal for 4–5 days. Fully virulent streptomycin-resistant organisms have been described.

C. Epidemic measures: Search for sources of infection related to arthropods, to animal hosts, and to water. Control measures as indicated in 9A above.

D. International measures: None.

TYPHOID FEVER

1. Identification—A systemic infectious disease characterized by continued fever, malaise, anorexia, slow pulse, involvement of lymphoid tissues, especially ulceration of Peyer's patches, enlargement of spleen, rose spots on trunk, and constipation more commonly than diarrhea. Many mild and atypical infections. A usual fatality rate of 10% is reduced by antibiotic therapy to 2–3% or less. Synonyms: Enteric fever, Typhus abdominalis.

Typhoid bacilli are found in blood early in the disease and in feces or urine after 1st week. The agglutination reaction becomes positive during 2nd week.

2. Occurrence—Widespread throughout the world, and a common disease in many countries of the Far East, Middle East, eastern Europe, Central and South America, and Africa. In U.S.A., steadily falling in incidence, particularly in urban areas.

3. Infectious agent—*Salmonella typhi,* the typhoid bacillus. About 50 types can be distinguished by Vi-phage.

4. Reservoir—Reservoir is man; patients and carriers. Family contacts may be transient carriers; in most parts of the world fecal are more common than urinary carriers. The carrier state is most common among persons infected during middle age, especially females; fecal carriers frequently have a typhoid cholecystitis. Urinary carriers are seen frequently in areas where *Schistosoma haematobium* infections occur.

5. Mode of transmission—Direct or indirect contact with feces or urine of a patient or carrier. Principal vehicles of spread are contaminated water and food. Improperly cooked starchy foods and pastries in which the bacilli multiply are common offenders. Raw fruits and vegetables are important vehicles in some parts of the world; milk, milk products and shellfish in others; contamination is usually by hands of carrier or missed case. Under some conditions flies are important vectors. One outbreak was traced to imported canned meats.

6. Incubation period—Variable; average 2 weeks, usual range 1 to 3 weeks.

7. Period of communicability—As long as typhoid bacilli appear in excreta; usually from 1st week throughout convalescence, thereafter variable. About 10% of patients will discharge bacilli 3 months after onset; 2 to 5% become permanent carriers.

8. Susceptibility and resistance—Susceptibility is general, although many adults acquire immunity through unrecognized infections; attack rates decline with age after the second or third decades. A high degree of resistance usually follows recovery.

9. Methods of control—

A. Preventive measures:

1) Protection, purification and chlorination of public water supplies; construction of safe private supplies. For individual or small group protection and while traveling or in the field, water is preferably boiled; or chlorine (Halazone) or iodine (Globaline) disinfecting tablets can be added directly to water, their number depending on turbidity and amount of water to be treated.

2) Sanitary disposal of human excreta.

3) Fly control by screening, spraying with residual insecticides and use of insecticidal baits and traps. Control of fly breeding by provisions for adequate garbage collection; elimination of open garbage dumps and substitution of landfill operations; provision for proper disposal of feces.

4) Boiling or pasteurization of milk and dairy products, including cheese. Sanitary supervision of commercial milk production, transport, processing, and delivery. Proper storage and refrigeration in stores and homes.

5) Limiting the collection and marketing of shellfish to supplies from approved sources.

6) Sanitary supervision of processing, preparation and serving of foods in public eating places, especially foods eaten raw; special attention to the provision and use of handwashing facilities.

7) Discovery and supervision of typhoid carriers. If carrier state lasts 1 year, carriers may be released from supervision and restriction of occupation (see par. 8 below) only after 6 consecutive negative cultures of authenticated specimens of feces and urine taken 1 month apart (cf. 9B2 following). Prolonged antibiotic therapy may end the carrier state; for fecal carriers, cholecystectomy is highly effective.

8) Instruction of convalescents and chronic carriers in personal hygiene, particularly as to sanitary disposal of ex-

creta, hand washing after defecation and before eating, and exclusion from occupation as food handlers.

9) Health education of the general public, and particularly of food handlers, concerning sources of infection and modes of transmission.

10) Immunization with a vaccine of high antigenicity, given in a primary series of 2 injections spaced by several weeks; in Britain, a third injection is given 6 to 12 months later. Current practice is to vaccinate persons subject to unusual exposure through occupation or travel, those living in areas of high endemic incidence, and institutional populations where maintenance of good sanitation is difficult. Periodic single reinforcing injections are desirable, commonly once in 3 years.

B. Control of patient, contacts and the immediate environment:

1) *Report to local health authority:* Obligatory case report in most states and countries, Class 2A (see Preface).

2) *Isolation:* In flyproof room. Hospital care desirable for patients who cannot command adequate sanitary environment and nursing care at home. Release from supervision by local health authority should be based on no less than 3 negative cultures of feces and urine taken at least 24 hours apart not earlier than 1 month after onset; and if any one of this series is positive, no less than 3 negative cultures at intervals of 1 month and within the 12 months following onset (cf. 9A8 above).

3) *Concurrent disinfection:* Of feces and urine and articles soiled therewith. In communities with modern and adequate sewage disposal systems, feces and urine can be disposed of directly into sewer without preliminary disinfection. Terminal cleaning.

4) *Quarantine:* Family contacts should not be employed as food handlers during period of contact or until repeated negative feces and urine cultures are obtained.

5) *Immunization of contacts:* Administration of typhoid vaccine to family, household and nursing contacts who have been or may be exposed to cases or carriers is of dubious value.

6) *Investigation of contacts and sources of infection:* Actual or probable source of infection of every case should be determined by search for common and individual sources, unreported cases and carriers, or contaminated food, water, milk or shellfish. Presence of Vi agglutinins in blood of suspected carriers is suggestive of the carrier state. Phage typing of organisms from patients and carriers and identification of the same type suggest the chain of transmission.

7) *Specific treatment:* Chloramphenicol; an initial oral loading

dose is followed by oral doses every 6 hours until temperature is normal—then in smaller doses for total of 14 days;
use with caution because of side effects. Ampicillin is
effective but the response is slower and less predictable.

C. Epidemic measures:

1) Intensive search for case or carrier who is source of infection.
2) Exclusion of suspected food.
3) Boiling of milk or pasteurization or exclusion of milk supplies or other foods suspected on epidemiologic evidence,
until safety is assured.
4) Chlorination, under competent supervision, of suspected
water supply or its exclusion from use. All drinking water
must be chlorinated or boiled before use.

D. International measures:

1) Inoculation with typhoid vaccine is advised for international travelers to endemic areas. Not a legal requirement
of any country.
2) WHO Reference Centres (see Preface).

TYPHUS FEVER, ENDEMIC FLEA-BORNE

1. Identification—The clinical course resembles that of epidemic
louse-borne typhus (see Preface) but tends to be milder. Fatality for
all ages is about 2%; fatality increases with age. Synonym: Murine
typhus.

Absence of louse infestation, seasonal distribution, and sporadic
occurrence of the disease help to differentiate from epidemic typhus.
The complement-fixation reaction with group-specific typhus antigen
becomes positive, usually in the 2nd week. The Weil-Felix reaction
with Proteus OX-19 also becomes positive, but is less helpful because
it may be positive in other diseases. Differentiation from louse-borne
typhus is by serologic tests using washed rickettsial antigens.

2. Occurrence—Worldwide in areas where men and rats occupy
the same buildings. Formerly, several thousand cases occurred yearly
in U.S.A. concentrated in the southeastern states; the current level is
less than 100 cases. Seasonal peak in late summer and autumn. Cases
tend to be scattered, with no connection to each other.

3. Infectious agent—*Rickettsia typhi (Rickettsia mooseri).*

4. Reservoir—Infection is maintained in nature by a rat-flea-rat
cycle. Rats are the reservoir, commonly *Rattus rattus* and *Rattus
norvegicus;* infection in rats is inapparent.

5. Mode of transmission—Infective rat fleas (usually *Xenopsylla cheopis*) defecate rickettsiae after sucking blood, and contaminate the bite site and other fresh skin wounds. An occasional case may follow inhalation of dried infective flea feces.

6. Incubation period—From 1 to 2 weeks, commonly 12 days.

7. Period of communicability—Not directly transmitted from man to man. Once infected, fleas remain so for life (up to 1 year).

8. Susceptibility and resistance—Susceptibility is general. One attack confers immunity.

9. Methods of control—

A. Preventive measures:

1) Application of insecticide powders with residual action to rat runs, burrows and harborages.
2) Rodent control measures should be delayed until flea populations have been reduced by insecticides, to avoid temporary increase in cases. (See Plague, 9B5, p. 172).

B. Control of patient, contacts, and the immediate environment:

1) *Report to local health authority:* Case report obligatory in most states and countries, Class 2B (see Preface).
2) *Isolation:* None.
3) *Concurrent disinfection:* None.
4) *Quarantine:* None.
5) *Immunisation of contacts:* None.
6) *Investigation of contacts and source of infection:* Search for rodents around premises or home of patient.
7) *Specific treatment:* As for epidemic typhus; see Typhus, Epidemic Louse-borne, 9B7 following.

C. Epidemic measures: In endemic areas with numerous cases, widespread use of DDT has markedly reduced the flea index of rats and incidence of infection in rats and man.

D. International measures: WHO Reference Centres (see Preface).

TYPHUS FEVER, EPIDEMIC LOUSE-BORNE

1. Identification—Onset is variable, often sudden and marked by headache, chills, prostration, fever and general pains; a macular eruption appears on 5th or 6th day, toxemia is usually pronounced, and the disease terminates by rapid lysis after about 2 weeks of fever. In the absence of specific therapy, fatality varies from 10 to 40%, and increases with age. Mild infections may occur with or without eruption, especially in vaccinated persons. The disease may recrudesce years after the primary attack (Brill-Zinsser disease); this differs from the first attack in that it need not be associated with lousiness and is milder, with fewer complications and lower fatality. Synonyms: Typhus exanthematicus, Classical typhus fever.

The complement-fixation reaction with group-specific typhus antigen becomes positive, usually in the 2nd week. The Weil-Felix reaction with Proteus OX-19 also becomes positive, but is less helpful because it may be positive in other diseases.

2. Occurrence—In most colder areas where people live under unhygienic conditions and are louse-infested, as in war and famine. Endemic centers exist in mountainous regions of Mexico, Central and South America, the Balkans and eastern Europe, Africa and numerous countries of Asia. A few cases of Brill-Zinsser disease occur annually in U.S.A., where the last outbreak of louse-borne typhus occurred in 1921.

3. Infectious agent—*Rickettsia prowazeki.*

4. Reservoir—Man is the reservoir and is responsible for maintaining the infection during interepidemic periods.

5. Mode of transmission—The body louse, *P. humanus humanus,* is infected by feeding on the blood of a patient with febrile typhus fever. Patients with recrudescent typhus (Brill-Zinsser disease) can infect lice and probably serve as foci for new outbreaks in louse-infested communities. Infected lice excrete rickettsiae in their feces and usually defecate at time of feeding. Man is infected by rubbing feces or crushed lice into the wound made by the bite or into superficial abrasions. Inhalation of dried infective louse feces as dust from dirty clothes may account for some infections.

6. Incubation period—From 1 to 2 weeks, commonly 12 days.

7. Period of communicability—The disease is not directly transmitted from man to man. Patients are infective for lice during the febrile illness and possibly for 2 or 3 days after the temperature returns to normal. The living louse is infective as soon as it begins to pass rickettsiae in feces (within 2 to 6 days after the infected blood meal); earlier if crushed. The louse is regularly killed within 2 weeks by the infection. Rickettsiae may remain viable in the dead louse for weeks.

8. Susceptibility and resistance—Susceptibility is general. The disease in children and in vaccinated adults is mild and may go unrecognized. One attack usually confers permanent immunity.

9. Methods of control—

A. Preventive measures:

1) Immunization of susceptible persons or groups of persons entering typhus areas, particularly military or labor forces, or of residents at unusual risk. The usual vaccine con-

tains rickettsiae grown in yolk sac of developing chick embryo, inactivated by formalin and extracted with ether or other suitable solvents. It is administered in 2 doses at an interval of not less than 7 days. A booster dose repeated at yearly intervals is indicated where typhus is a hazard. In vaccinated persons, the course of the disease is modified, and fatality lowered. A live vaccine prepared from the attenuated Strain E of *R. prowazeki* is under evaluation.

2) Application by hand or power blower of residual insecticide powder (10% DDT or 1% lindane) at appropriate intervals to clothes and persons of populations living under conditions favoring lousiness. Lice are known to become resistant to DDT, in which case 1% Malathion or other effective lousicide should be substituted.

3) Improvement of living conditions with provision for frequent bathing and washing of clothes.

4) Individual prophylaxis of persons subject to unusual risk through insecticide applied at appropriate intervals to clothing by dusting or impregnation.

B. Control of patient, contacts, and the immediate environment:

1) *Report to local health authority:* Case report universally required by International Sanitary and Health Regulations, Class 1 (see Preface).

2) *Isolation:* Not required after proper delousing of patient, clothing, living quarters and household contacts.

3) *Concurrent disinfection:* Appropriate insecticide powder applied to clothing and bedding of patient and contacts; treatment of hair for louse eggs (nits) with effective chemical agents. Lice tend to leave abnormally hot or cold bodies in search of a normothermic clothed body (see 9A2 above). If death occurs before delousing, delouse the body and clothing by thorough application of insecticides.

4) *Quarantine:* Louse-infested susceptibles exposed to typhus fever should be quarantined for 15 days but may be released directly after application of insecticide with residual effect.

5) *Immunization of contacts:* All immediate contacts.

6) *Investigation of contacts:* Every effort should be made to trace the infection to the immediate source.

7) *Specific treatment:* The tetracyclines or chloramphenicol orally in a loading dose followed by daily doses until the patient becomes afebrile (usually 2 days) and for 1 additional day.

C. Epidemic measures:

1) Delousing: The most important measure for rapid control of typhus, where reporting has been good and cases are

few, is application of insecticides with residual effect to all contacts. Where infection is known to be widespread, systematic application of residual insecticide to all persons in the community is indicated.

2) Immunization: Of persons in contact with cases; vaccination may be offered to entire community.

D. International measures:

1) Telegraphic notification by governments to WHO and to adjacent countries of the occurrence of an outbreak of louse-borne typhus fever in an area previously free of the disease.

2) International travelers: No country currently requires immunization against typhus for entry. Vaccination is recommended for all persons who will work in or visit remote areas where typhus is present.

3) As of January 1, 1971, epidemic louse-borne typhus ceases to be a quarantinable disease under international regulations, but the measures outlined in paragraph (1) above should be continued because it is now a *Disease under Surveillance of WHO,* in accordance with a Resolution of the 22nd World Health Assembly. WHO Reference Centres (see Preface).

TYPHUS, SCRUB

1. Identification—A rickettsial disease frequently characterized by a primary "punched out" skin ulcer (eschar) corresponding to site of attachment of an infected mite. The acute febrile onset follows within several days along with headache, conjunctival injection and lymphadenopathy. Late in the first week of fever a dull red maculopapular eruption appears on the trunk, extends to extremities, and disappears in a few days. Cough and x-ray evidence of pneumonitis are common. Without antibiotic therapy, fever lasts for about 14 days. Fatality in untreated cases varies with locality, from 1 to 40%; consistently higher among older persons. Synonyms: Tsutsugamushi disease, Mite-borne typhus fever. The benign disease seen in some areas of Japan is called Shishito.

Diagnosis is by isolation of the infectious agent by inoculating patient's blood into mice. Fluorescent antibody and complement-fixation tests supplement the Weil-Felix reaction (Proteus OXK) in serologic diagnosis.

2. Occurrence—Eastern and southeastern Asia, northern Australia and adjacent islands, and India; a place disease acquired by man in one of innumerable small, sharply delimited "typhus islands" where rickettsiae, vectors and suitable rodents exist simultaneously. Occupational habits greatly influence sex distribution, but mainly restricted to adult workers who frequent scrub or overgrown terrain. Epidemics occur when susceptibles are brought into endemic areas, especially in military operations, where 20 to 50% of men have been infected within weeks or months.

3. Infectious agent—*Rickettsia tsutsugamushi (Rickettsia orientalis)*.

4. Reservoir—Infected larval stages of *Leptotrombidium akamushi, Leptotrombidium deliensis* and related species (varying with locality). Infection is maintained in mites by transovarian passage and possibly by a mite-wild rodent-mite cycle.

5. Mode of transmission—By the bite of infected larval mites; nymphs and adults do not feed on vertebrate hosts.

6. Incubation period—Usually 10 to 12 days; varies from 6 to 21.

7. Period of communicability—Not directly transmitted from man to man.

8. Susceptibility and resistance—Susceptibility is general. An attack confers prolonged immunity against the homologous strain of *R. tsutsugamushi* but only transient immunity against heterologous strains. Heterologous infection within a few months results in mild disease but such infection after a year produces the typical illness. Second and even third attacks of naturally acquired scrub typhus occur among persons who spend their lives in endemic areas. No currently available vaccine is effective.

9. Methods of control—

A. Preventive measures:

1) Prevent contact with infected mites, and eliminate mites and rodents from particular sites.

2) Personal prophylaxis against the mite vector is by use of clothes and blankets impregnated with miticidal chemicals (benzyl benzoate), and application of mite repellents (N-diethyl-m-toluamide), to exposed skin surfaces.

3) In military practice selected camp sites are cleared of vegetation with a bulldozer, vegetation is burned and the area sprayed with residual miticidal chemicals (dieldrin, lindane or Malathion, effective for weeks or months). Rodent control measures are also instituted.

B. Control of patient, contacts, and the immediate environment:

1) *Report to local health authority:* In selected endemic areas, with clear distinction from endemic and epidemic typhus; in many countries not a reportable disease, Class 3A (see Preface).

2) *Isolation:* None.

3) *Concurrent disinfection:* None.

4) *Quarantine:* None.
5) *Immunization of contacts:* None.
6) *Investigation of contacts:* None.
7) *Specific treatment:* One of the tetracycline antibiotics or chloramphenicol orally in a loading dose followed by divided doses daily until patient is afebrile (average 30 hours). If treatment is instituted within the first 3 days, recrudescence can be prevented by a 2nd course given on the 6th day after termination of the initial course.

C. Epidemic measures:

1) Rigorously employ procedures described in 9A2 and 9A3 in the affected area.
2) Daily observation for fever and appearance of primary lesions of all persons at risk; institute treatment at first indication of illness.

D. International measures: WHO Reference Centres (see Preface).

WHOOPING COUGH (PERTUSSIS)

1. Identification—An acute bacterial disease involving the trachea, bronchi and bronchioles. The initial catarrhal stage has an insidious onset, with an irritating cough which gradually becomes paroxysmal, usually within 1 to 2 weeks, and lasts for 1 to 2 months. Paroxysms are characterized by repeated violent cough; each series of paroxysms has many coughs without intervening inhalation, followed by a characteristic crowing or high-pitched inspiratory whoop and frequently ending with the expulsion of clear, tenacious mucus. Young infants and adults often do not have the typical paroxysm. Fatality in U.S.A. is low, less than 0.5%; approximately 70% of deaths are among children under 1 year of age, with further concentration in those under 6 months. Recent epidemics in less developed countries had a reported fatality of 15%.

The infectious agent is readily recovered, during the catarrhal and early paroxysmal stages, by nasopharyngeal swab and suitable culture; fluorescent antibody technique appears promising as a diagnostic aid.

Parapertussis is an allied disease clinically indistinguishable from pertussis. It is usually milder and occurs relatively infrequently. Identification is by immunologic differences between *Bordetella parapertussis* and *B. pertussis*.

2. Occurrence—A common disease among children everywhere, regardless of race, climate, or geographic location. In large communities, incidence is generally highest in late winter and early spring; in smaller communities, seasonal incidence is variable. There has been a marked decline in incidence and mortality during the past two decades, chiefly in communities fostering active immunization and having good medical care. In many less developed countries, incidence continues high and whooping cough is among the most lethal of the common communicable diseases of childhood.

3. Infectious agent—*Bordetella pertussis,* the pertussis bacillus.

4. Reservoir—Man is the reservoir.

5. Mode of transmission—By direct contact with discharges from laryngeal and bronchial mucous membranes of infected persons by droplet spread; or indirectly, by contact with articles freshly soiled with discharges of infected persons.

6. Incubation period—Commonly 7 days, almost uniformly within 10 days, and not exceeding 21 days.

7. Period of communicability—Highly communicable in the early catarrhal stage, before paroxysmal cough. Thereafter communicability gradually decreases and becomes negligible for ordinary nonfamilial contacts in about 3 weeks despite persisting spasmodic cough with whoop. For control purposes, the communicable stage extends from 7 days after exposure to 3 weeks after onset of typical paroxysms.

8. Susceptibility and resistance—Susceptibility is general; there is no evidence of temporary passive immunity in young infants born of immune mothers. Predominantly a childhood disease, incidence is highest under 7 years of age. Numerous inapparent and missed atypical cases occur. One attack confers definite and prolonged immunity, although exposed adults occasionally have second attacks. Fatality is higher in females than in males, at all ages.

9. Methods of control—

A. *Preventive measures:*

1) Active immunization of all susceptible preschool children is a proven effective procedure for control of pertussis. Plain or alum adjuvant vaccines may be used alone or mixed with diphtheria and tetanus toxoids. In U.S.A., 3 doses of a triple alum adjuvant vaccine (DTP), administered intramuscularly at intervals of 4 to 8 weeks, is commonly used for simultaneous immunization. In general, routine immunization can be started at 2 to 3 months of age. When primary immunization is properly carried out in infancy, a single booster dose of multiple antigen is advised 1 year later and again before entering school. Infants in institutions and in households with other susceptible children, particularly when whooping cough is prevalent in the community, should have active immunization by 2 to 3 months of age.

2) Educational measures to inform the public and particularly parents of infants of the dangers of whooping cough and of the advantage of immunization in infancy.

B. Control of patient, contacts, and the immediate environment:

1) *Report to local health authority:* Case report obligatory in most states and countries, Class 2B (Preface).

2) *Isolation:* Separation of patient from susceptible children and exclusion from school and public places for the recognized period of communicability. Isolation of children over 2 years of age is often impractical; and even for those under 2, should not be practiced at the expense of fresh air in the open when weather permits.

3) *Concurrent disinfection:* Discharges from the nose and throat and articles soiled therewith. Terminal cleaning.

4) *Quarantine:* Exclusion of nonimmune children from school and public gatherings for 14 days after last exposure to a household or similar case; such precaution may be omitted if exposed nonimmune children are observed throughout each school day to detect the first sign of infection. It is especially important that children under 3 years of age be protected from exposure to known or suspected whooping cough contacts.

5) *Protection of contacts:* Passive immunization with immune serum globulin (human) has not proved to be effective. Young unvaccinated children exposed to infection should be carefully observed and given tetracyclines on appearance of the earliest symptoms.

6) *Investigation of contacts:* Carriers in the exact sense of the term are not known; search for missed and atypical cases among contacts is indicated.

7) *Specific treatment:* Tetracycline antibiotics and chloramphenicol given early shorten the period of communicability but, unless given in the earliest stages of the disease, do not modify the clinical manifestations.

C. Epidemic measures: A search for unrecognized and unreported cases to protect preschool children from exposure and to assure adequate medical care for exposed infants.

D. International measures: Active immunization of susceptible infants and young children traveling to other countries, if not already protected; review need of booster dose for those previously inoculated.

WOLHYNIAN FEVER (TRENCH FEVER)

1. Identification—A nonfatal, febrile, self-limited, often relapsing illness of protean manifestations and greatly varying severity. Headache, malaise, and pain and tenderness, especially in the shins, beginning either suddenly or slowly, together with fever, which may be relapsing, typhoid-like, or limited to a single short febrile episode lasting for several days. Splenomegaly is common. Transient macular rash may be present at some time. Subsequent course is extremely variable. Inapparent infection may occur; rickettsemia may last for months with or without repeated recurrence of symptoms. Synonyms: Five-day or Quintana fever.

Laboratory diagnosis is by culture of causative organism from patient's blood on blood agar under 5% CO_2 tension in air. Microcolonies are visible after 2 weeks of incubation at 37 C. Infection results in detectable rise of complement-fixing antibodies to *Rickettsia quintana*.

2. Occurrence—Epidemics occurred in World Wars I and II in Europe among troops living under crowded unhygienic conditions. Sporadic cases in areas of endemic foci probably go unrecognized.

Endemic foci of infection have been detected in Poland, Russia, Mexico, Ethiopia and North Africa. The organism probably can be found wherever man and the human body louse coexist.

3. Infectious agent—*Rickettsia quintana* (probably identical with *R. weiglii, R. pediculi* and *R. wolhynica*).

4. Reservoir—Man is the only known reservoir. Intermediate host is the body louse, *Pediculus humanus humanus*, in which the organism multiplies for the duration of the insect's life, extracellularly, within the gut lumen. No transovarial transmission in the louse.

5. Mode of transmission—Man is infected by inoculation of infected louse's feces through skin damaged by either the bite of the louse or other means. Infected lice excrete infectious feces for duration of life (average life span approximately 5 weeks after hatching from egg), beginning 5–12 days after ingestion of the infecting blood meal. Nymphal stages may become infected. Lice tend to leave abnormally hot (febrile) or cold (dead) bodies in search of a normothermic clothed body.

6. Incubation period—Generally 7–30 days.

7. Period of communicability—Symptomless rickettsemia may last for weeks, months or years. No direct transmission from man to man.

8. Susceptibility and resistance—Susceptibility is general. After infection, the degree of protective immunity to either infection or disease is unknown.

9. Methods of control—

A. *Preventive measures:* Delousing procedures will destroy the vector and block transmission to man. Dusting of clothing and body with an effective lousicide.

B. *Control of patient, contacts, and the immediate environment:*

1) *Report to local health authority:* Cases should be reported so that an evaluation of the lousiness of the population

may be made and appropriate measures taken, since lice also transmit epidemic typhus and relapsing fever. Class 3B (Preface).

2) Isolation: None.

3) Concurrent disinfection: Louse-infested clothing should be treated to kill the lice.

4) Quarantine: None.

5) Immunization of contacts: None.

6) Investigation of contacts and source of infection: Search for the presence of the human body louse in clothing and on the bodies of people at risk.

7) Specific treatment: Tetracycline and chloramphenicol not yet adequately tested in clinical cases; probably effective.

C. Epidemic measures: Systematic application of residual insecticide to all persons in the affected population and their clothing (see 9A above).

D. International measures: WHO Reference Centres (see Preface).

YAWS

1. Identification—A chronic relapsing nonvenereal treponematosis characterized by hypertrophic, granulomatous, or ulcerative destructive lesions of the skin and cartilage (gangosa), and by destructive and hypertrophic changes in bone. Three to 6 weeks after exposure a papule appears at the site of inoculation, eventually developing into a papilloma ("mother yaw"). In several weeks to months, and often before the initial lesion has healed, mild constitutional symptoms appear; also a generalized eruption of papules, some developing into typical frambesial (raspberry) lesions, in successive crops and lasting several months. Papillomata may appear on palms and soles (crab yaws), also hyperkeratoses in both early and late stages. The late stage often develops some years after the last early lesions, with characteristic destructive lesions of skin and bone. Early and late lesions tend to heal spontaneously, but may relapse. Between these active phases infection is latent; thus there is a latent early stage from which early relapses occur, and a latent late stage with late lesions and relapses. Central nervous system, eyes, aorta and viscera are not involved; yaws is never congenitally acquired; rarely, if ever, fatal. Synonyms: Frambesia tropica, Pian, Bouba, Parangi.

Diagnosis is confirmed by dark-field examination of exudates from lesions. Serologic tests for syphilis are reactive with the same frequency in yaws as in syphilis, becoming positive during the initial stage, remaining positive during the early stage and tending to become negative after many years of latency, even without specific therapy.

2. Occurrence—Primarily in rural tropics and subtropics; the lowest social and economic groups have the highest rates. Predominantly a childhood disease; males outnumber females. Particularly common in equatorial Africa, the Philippines, Southeast Asia, Indonesia and throughout the South Pacific Islands; endemic foci in Caribbean area, in parts of Brazil, Colombia, Venezuela, Peru, Ecuador, Panama and British Guiana. Incidence is decreasing in many areas.

3. Infectious agent—*Treponema pertenue,* a spirochete.

4. Reservoir—Man and possibly higher primates.

5. Mode of transmission—Principally by direct contact with exudates of early skin lesions of infected persons. Indirect transmission by contaminated scratching and piercing articles and by flies on open wounds is probable, but of undetermined importance.

6. Incubation period—From 2 weeks to 3 months; generally 3 to 6 weeks.

7. Period of communicability—Variable; may extend intermittently over several years while moist lesions are present; the infectious agent is not usually found in late ulcerative lesions.

8. Susceptibility and resistance—No evidence of natural or racial resistance. Infection results in immunity to homologous and heterologous strains; heterologous immunity develops more slowly and probably not completed until 1 year. The role of superinfection in nature is not well defined, and may be unimportant. Immunity to yaws appears to protect against syphilis.

9. Methods of control—

- A. *Preventive measures:* The following are applicable to yaws and to other nonvenereal treponematoses. By present techniques the infectious agents in all are morphologically identical, but it is unlikely that the differences in clinical syndromes result from epidemiologic factors.

    1) General health promotional measures; health education about treponematosis, better sanitation, and improved social and economic conditions over a period of years will reduce incidence.
    2) Organization of intensive control activities on a community basis, to include analysis of the specific local problem, clinical examination of entire populations, and mass treatment of patients with active lesions, latent cases and contacts, where a high prevalence justifies such measures. Periodic surveys and continuous surveillance are essential to successful results.
    3) Provision of facilities for early diagnosis and treatment on a continuing plan, whereby the mass control campaign (9A2 above) is eventually consolidated into permanent local health services providing early diagnosis and treat-

ment to patients, and contact investigation and health education to the community.

4) Treatment of disfiguring and incapacitating late manifestations, and surveys for latent cases, since many subsequently relapse, with infective lesions, to maintain the
disease in the community.

B. Control of patient, contacts, and the immediate environment:

1) *Report to local health authority:* In selected endemic areas;
in many countries not a reportable disease, Class 3B (see
Preface). Differentiation of venereal and nonvenereal
treponematoses with proper reporting of each has particular importance in evaluation of mass campaigns and in the
consolidation period thereafter.

2) *Isolation:* None; avoid intimate contact, flies and contamination of the environment until lesions are healed.

3) *Concurrent disinfection:* Care in disposal of discharges and
articles contaminated therewith.

4) *Quarantine:* None.

5) *Immunization of contacts:* Not applicable; prompt institution of a course of treatment (see 9B7 below).

6) *Investigation of contacts:* All familial contacts should be
treated; those with no active disease should be regarded
as latent cases and treated. In areas of low prevalence,
treat all active cases, all children, and close contacts of
infectious cases.

7) *Specific treatment:* Penicillin. For patients with active
disease a single intramuscular injection of procaine penicillin G in oil with 2% aluminum monostearate (PAM) or
benzathine penicillin G (Bicillin); half-doses for children
under 15 and for latent cases and contacts.

C. Epidemic measures: Active mass treatment programs in areas
of high prevalence. Essential features are (1) that a high
percentage of the population be examined through field survey; (2) that treatment of active cases be extended to the
segments of the population with demonstrated prevalence of
active yaws; and (3) that periodic surveys be made at yearly
intervals for 1 to 3 years, with surveillance and integration
of activities into the established rural public health activities
of the country.

D. International measures: To protect countries against risk of
reinfection where active mass treatment programs are in
progress, adjacent countries in the endemic area should institute suitable measures against yaws. Movement of infected
persons across frontiers may need supervision. See Syphilis
9D, p. 247. WHO Reference Centres (see Preface).

DEFINITIONS

DEFINITIONS

(Technical meaning of terms used in the text)

1. *Carrier*—A carrier is an infected person (or animal) that harbors a specific infectious agent in the absence of discernible clinical disease and serves as a potential source of infection for man. The carrier state may occur in an individual with an infection inapparent throughout its course (commonly known as *healthy carrier*), or during the incubation period, convalescence, and postconvalescence of an individual with a clinically recognizable disease (commonly known as *incubatory carrier* or *convalescent carrier*). Under either circumstance the carrier state may be of short or long duration (*temporary carrier* or *chronic carrier*).

2. *Chemoprophylaxis*—The administration of a chemical, including antibiotics, to prevent the development of an infection or the progression of an infection to active manifest infectious disease. *Chemotherapy*, on the other hand, refers to use of a chemical to cure a clinically recognizable infectious disease or to limit its further progress.

3. *Cleaning*—The removal by scrubbing and washing, as with hot water, soap or suitable detergent, of infectious agents and of organic matter from surfaces on which and in which infectious agents may find favorable conditions for surviving and multiplying.

4. *Communicable disease*—An illness due to a specific infectious agent or its toxic products which arises through transmission of that agent or its products from a reservoir to a susceptible host—either directly, as from an infected person or animal, or indirectly, through the agency of an intermediate plant or animal host, vector, or the inanimate environment (see 44, Transmission of infectious agents).

5. *Communicable period*—The time or times during which the infectious agent may be transferred directly or indirectly from an infected person to another person, from an infected animal to man, or from an infected man to an animal, including arthropods.

    In diseases such as diphtheria and scarlet fever, in which mucous membranes are involved from the first entry of the pathogen, the period of communicability is from the date of first exposure to a source of infection until the infecting microorganism is no longer disseminated from the involved mucous membranes, i.e., from the period before the prodromata until termination of a carrier state, if this develops. Most diseases are not communicable during the early incubation period or after full recovery.

    In diseases such as tuberculosis, syphilis and gonorrhea, the communicable state may exist at any time over a long and sometimes intermittent period when unhealed lesions permit the discharge of infectious agents from the surface of the skin or through any of the body orifices.

288

In diseases transmitted by arthropods, such as malaria and yellow fever, the periods of communicability are those during which the infectious agent occurs in infective form in the blood or other tissues of the infected person in sufficient numbers to permit vector infection. A period of communicability is also to be distinguished for the arthropod vector—namely, that time during which the agent is present in the tissues of the arthropod in such form and locus (*infective state*) as to be transmissible.

6. **Contact**—A person or animal that has been in such association with an infected person or animal or a contaminated environment as to have had opportunity to acquire the infection.

7. **Contamination**—The presence of an infectious agent on a body surface; also on or in clothes, bedding, toys, surgical instruments or dressings, or other inanimate articles or substances including water, milk and food. Contamination is distinct from *pollution,* which implies the presence of offensive but not necessarily infectious matter in the environment.

8. **Disinfection**—Killing of infectious agents outside the body by chemical or physical means directly applied.
   Concurrent disinfection is the application of disinfective measures as soon as possible after the discharge of infectious material from the body of an infected person, or after the soiling of articles with such infectious discharges, all personal contact with such discharges or articles being prevented prior to such disinfection.
   Terminal disinfection is application of disinfective measures after the patient has been removed by death or to a hospital, or has ceased to be a source of infection, or after isolation practices have been discontinued. Terminal disinfection is rarely practiced; terminal cleaning generally suffices (see 3, Cleaning), along with airing and sunning of rooms, furniture and bedding. It is necessary only for diseases spread by indirect contact; steam sterilization of bedding is desirable after smallpox.

9. **Disinfestation**—Any physical or chemical process serving to destroy undesired small animal forms, particularly arthropods or rodents, present upon the person, the clothing, or in the environment of an individual, or on domestic animals (see 25, Insecticide, and 39, Rodenticide). Disinfestation includes delousing for infestation with *Pediculus humanus humanus,* the body louse. Synonyms include the term *disinsection* when insects only are involved.

10. **Endemic**—The habitual presence of a disease or infectious agent within a given geographic area; may also refer to the usual prevalence of a given disease within such area. *Hyperendemic* expresses a persistent intense transmission, usually applied to malaria.

11. **Epidemic**—The occurrence in a community or region of a group of illnesses (or an outbreak) of similar nature, clearly in excess of normal expectancy and derived from a common or a propagated source. The number of cases indicating presence of an epidemic

will vary according to the infectious agent, size and type of population exposed, previous experience or lack of exposure to the disease, and time and place of occurrence; epidemicity is thus relative to usual frequency of the disease in the same area, among the specified population, at the same season of the year. A single case of a communicable disease long absent from a population (as smallpox, in Boston) or first invasion by a disease not previously recognized in that area (as American trypanosomiasis, in Arizona) is to be considered sufficient evidence of an epidemic to require immediate reporting and full field investigation. (See 36, Report of a disease, par. 3.)

12. *Fatality Rate*—Usually expressed as a percentage of the number of persons diagnosed as having a specified disease who die as a result of that illness. This term is most frequently applied to a specific outbreak of acute disease in which all patients have been followed for an adequate period of time to include all attributable deaths. *Fatality rate* must be clearly differentiated from *mortality rate* (see Definition 28).

13. *Fumigation*—Any process by which the killing of animal forms, especially arthropods and rodents, is accomplished by the use of gaseous agents (see 25, Insecticide, and 39, Rodenticide).

14. *Health Education*—Health education is the process by which individuals and groups of people learn to promote, maintain or restore health. To be effective, the methods and procedures used to achieve this aim must take account of the ways in which people develop various forms of behavior, of the factors that lead them to maintain or to alter their acquired behavior, and of the ways in which people acquire and use knowledge. Therefore, education for health begins with people as they are, with whatever interests they may have in improving their living conditions. It aims at developing in them a sense of responsibility for health conditions, as individuals and as members of families and communities. In communicable disease control, health education commonly includes an appraisal of what is known by a population about a disease; an assessment of habits and attitudes of the people as they relate to spread and frequency of the disease; and the presentation of specific means to remedy observed deficiencies.

15. *Host*—A man or other living animal, including birds and arthropods, affording under natural conditions subsistence or lodgment to an infectious agent. Some protozoa and helminths pass successive stages in alternate hosts of different species. Hosts in which the parasite attains maturity or passes its sexual stage are *primary* or *definitive hosts;* those in which the parasite is in a larval or asexual state are *secondary* or *intermediate hosts.*

16. *Immune person*—A person (or animal) that possesses specific protective antibodies or cellular immunity as a result of previous infection or immunization, or is so conditioned by such previous specific experience as to respond adequately with production of

antibodies sufficient to prevent illness following exposure to the specific infectious agent of the disease. Immunity is relative; an ordinarily effective protection may be overwhelmed by an excessive dose of the infectious agent or an unusual portal of entry (cf. 38, Resistance).

17. *Inapparent infection*—The presence of infection in a host without occurrence of recognizable clinical signs or symptoms. Inapparent infections are only identifiable by laboratory means. Synonym: *subclinical* infection.

18. *Incidence rate*—A quotient, with the number of cases of a specified disease diagnosed or reported during a stated period of time as the numerator, and the number of persons in the population in which they occurred as the denominator. This is usually expressed as cases per 1,000 or 100,000 per annum. This rate may be expressed as age- or sex-specific, or as specific for any other population, characteristic or subdivision (see 27, Morbidity rate).

Attack rate, or *case rate,* is an incidence rate often used for particular populations, observed for limited periods and under special circumstances, as in an epidemic. The *secondary attack rate* in communicable disease practice expresses the number of cases among familial or institutional contacts occurring within the accepted incubation period directly following exposure to a primary case, in relation to the total of such contacts; may be restricted to susceptible contacts when determinable. *Case rate* expresses the incidence of clinically recognized cases; *infection rate* the sum of manifest and inapparent cases.

19. *Incubation period*—The time interval between exposure to an infectious agent and appearance of the first sign or symptom of the disease in question.

20. *Infected person*—A person who harbors an infectious agent and who has either manifest disease (see 31, Patient or sick person) or inapparent infection (see 1, Carrier). An *infectious person* is one from whom the infectious agent can be naturally acquired.

21. *Infection*—The entry and development or multiplication of an infectious agent in the body of man or animals. Infection is not synonymous with infectious disease; the result may be inapparent (see 17, Inapparent infection) or manifest (see 23, Infectious disease). The presence of living infectious agents on exterior surfaces of the body, or upon articles of apparel or soiled articles, is not infection but contamination of such surfaces and articles (see 7, Contamination).

22. *Infectious agent*—An organism, chiefly a microorganism but including helminths, that is capable of producing infection or infectious disease.

23. *Infectious disease*—A disease of man or animals resulting from an infection (see 21).

24. *Infestation*—By infestation of persons or animals is meant the lodgment, development and reproduction of arthropods on the surface of the body or in the clothing. Infested articles or premises are those which harbor or give shelter to animal forms, especially arthropods and rodents.

25. *Insecticide*—Any chemical substance used for the destruction of arthropods, whether applied as powder, liquid, atomized liquid, aerosol, or as a paint spray; residual action is usual. The term *larvicide* is generally used to designate insecticides applied specifically for destruction of immature stages of arthropods; *imago-cide* or *adulticide,* to designate those applied to destroy mature or adult forms.

26. *Isolation*—The separation, for the period of communicability, of infected persons or animals from others, in such places and under such conditions as will prevent the direct or indirect conveyance of the infectious agent from those infected to those who are susceptible or who may spread the agent to others (cf. 34, Quarantine).

27. *Morbidity rate*—An *incidence* rate (see Definition 18) used to include all persons in the population under consideration who become ill during the period of time stated.

28. *Mortality rate*—A rate calculated in the same way as an incidence rate (see Definition 18), using as a numerator the number of deaths occurring in the population during the stated period of time, usually a year. A *total* or *crude* mortality rate utilizes deaths from all causes, usually expressed as deaths per 1,000, while a *disease-specific* mortality rate includes only deaths due to one disease and is usually reported on the basis of 100,000 persons.

29. *Molluscicide*—A chemical substance used for the destruction of snails.

30. *Pathogenicity*—The capacity of an infectious agent to cause disease in a susceptible host.

31. *Patient or sick person*—A person who is ill; here limited to a person suffering from a recognizable attack of a communicable disease.

32. *Personal hygiene*—Those protective measures, primarily within the responsibility of the individual, by which to promote health and to limit the spread of infectious diseases, chiefly those transmitted by direct contact. Such measures encompass (a) keeping the body clean by sufficiently frequent soap and water baths; (b) washing hands in soap and water immediately after voiding bowels or bladder and always before handling food and eating; (c) keeping hands and unclean articles, or articles that have been used for toilet purposes by others, away from the mouth, nose, eyes, ears, genitalia, and wounds; (d) avoiding the use of common or unclean eating, drinking or toilet articles of any kind, such as cutlery and crockery, drinking cups, towels, handkerchiefs, combs, hairbrushes, and pipes; (e) avoiding exposure of other persons to spray from the nose and mouth as in coughing,

sneezing, laughing or talking; (f) washing hands thoroughly after handling a patient or his belongings.

33. *Prevalence rate*—A quotient using as the numerator the number of persons sick or portraying a certain condition, in a stated population, *at a particular time,* regardless of when that illness or condition began, and as the denominator the number of persons in the population in which they occurred. For example, the prevalence rate of ringworm of the foot in a class of boys when examined on a certain day could be 25 per 100. Or, the prevalence rate of a positive serological test in a survey during which blood samples were collected from a population could be 10 per 1,000 positive.

34. *Quarantine*—
   1) **Complete quarantine:** The limitation of freedom of movement of such well persons or domestic animals as have been exposed to a communicable disease, for a period of time not longer than the longest usual incubation period of the disease, in such manner as to prevent effective contact with those not so exposed (cf. 26, Isolation).
   2) **Modified quarantine:** A selective, partial limitation of freedom of movement of persons or domestic animals, commonly on the basis of known or presumed differences in susceptibility, but sometimes because of danger of disease transmission. It may be designed to meet particular situations. Examples are exclusion of children from school; or exemption of immune persons from provisions required of susceptible persons, such as contacts acting as food handlers; or restriction of military populations to the post or to quarters.
   3) **Personal surveillance:** The practice of close medical or other supervision of contacts in order to promote prompt recognition of infection or illness but without restricting their movements.
   4) **Segregation:** The separation for special consideration, control or observation of some part of a group of persons or domestic animals from the others to facilitate control of a communicable disease. Removal of susceptible children to homes of immune persons, or establishment of a sanitary boundary to protect uninfected from infected portions of a population, are examples.

35. *Repellent*—A chemical applied to the skin or clothing or other places to discourage (1) arthropods from alighting on and attacking an individual; and (2) other agents, such as worm larvae, from penetrating the skin.

36. *Report of a disease*—An official report notifying appropriate authority of the occurrence of a specified communicable or other disease in man or in animals. Diseases in man are reported to the local health authority; those in animals to the livestock, sanitary or agriculture authority. Some few diseases in animals also transmissible to man are reportable to both authorities. Each

health jurisdiction declares a list of reportable diseases appropriate to its particular needs (see Preface). Reports also should list suspect cases of diseases of particular public health importance—ordinarily those requiring epidemiologic investigation or initiation of special control measures.

When a person is infected in one health jurisdiction and the case is reported from another, the authority receiving the report should notify the other jurisdiction, especially when the disease requires examination of contacts for infection, or of food and water as possible vehicles.

In addition to routine report of cases of specified diseases, special notification is required of all epidemics or outbreaks of disease, including diseases not on the list declared reportable (see 11, Epidemic).

37. *Reservoir of infectious agents*—Any human beings, animals, arthropods, plants, soil, or inanimate matter in which an infectious agent normally lives and multiplies and on which it depends primarily for survival, reproducing itself in such manner that it can be transmitted to a susceptible host.

38. *Resistance*—The sum total of body mechanisms which interpose barriers to the progress of invasion or multiplication of infectious agents, or to damage by their toxic products.

   a. Immunity—That resistance usually associated with possession of antibodies having a specific action on the microorganism concerned with a particular infectious disease or on its toxin. *Passive immunity* is attained either naturally, by maternal transfer, or artificially, by inoculation of specific protective antibodies [convalescent or immune serum, or immune serum (gamma) globulin (human)] and is of brief duration (days to months). *Active immunity* lasting months to years is attained either naturally, by infection, with or without clinical manifestations, or artificially, by inoculation of fractions or products of the infectious agent or of the agent itself, in killed, modified or variant form.

   b. Inherent resistance—An ability to resist disease independently of antibodies or of specifically developed tissue response; it commonly rests in anatomic or physiologic characteristics of the host; it may be genetic or acquired, permanent or temporary.

39. *Rodenticide*—A chemical substance used for the destruction of rodents, generally through ingestion (cf. 13, Fumigation).

40. *Source of infection*—The person, animal, object or substance from which an infectious agent passes immediately to a host. Source of infection should be clearly distinguished from source of contamination, such as overflow of a septic tank contaminating a water supply, or an infected cook contaminating a salad. (Cf. 37, Reservoir.)

41. *Surveillance of disease*—As distinct from surveillance of persons

(see 34, par. 3), surveillance of disease is the continuing scrutiny of all aspects of occurrence and spread of a disease that are pertinent to effective control. Included are the systematic collection and evaluation of (a) morbidity and mortality reports; (b) special reports of field investigations, of epidemics and of individual cases; (c) isolation and identification of infectious agents by laboratories; (d) data concerning the availability and use of vaccines and toxoids, immune globulin, insecticides, and other substances used in control; (e) information regarding immunity levels in segments of the population, and (f) other relevant epidemiologic data. The procedure applies to all jurisdictional levels of public health, from local to international.

42. *Susceptible*—A person or animal presumably not possessing sufficient resistance against a particular pathogenic agent and for that reason liable to contract a disease if or when exposed to the disease agent.

43. *Suspect*—A person whose medical history and symptoms suggest that he may have or be developing some communicable disease.

44. **Transmission of infectious agents**—Any mechanism by which a susceptible human host is exposed to an infectious agent. These mechanisms are

   a. Direct transmission: Direct and essentially immediate transfer of infectious agents (other than from an arthropod in which the organism has undergone essential multiplication or development) to a receptive portal of entry by which infection of man may take place. This may be by touching, as in kissing or sexual intercourse (direct contact); or by the direct projection of droplet spray onto the conjunctivae, or onto the mucous membranes of the nose or mouth during sneezing, coughing, spitting, singing or talking (usually not possible over a distance greater than 3 feet) (droplet spread); or, as in the systemic mycoses, by direct exposure of susceptible tissue to soil, compost or decaying vegetable matter that contains the agent and where it normally leads a saprophytic existence.

   b. Indirect transmission:
   1) VEHICLE-BORNE—Contaminated materials or objects such as toys, handkerchiefs, soiled clothes, bedding, surgical instruments or dressings (indirect contact); water, food, milk, biological products including serum and plasma, or any substance serving as an intermediate means by which an infectious agent is transported and introduced into a susceptible host through a suitable portal of entry. The agent may or may not have multiplied or developed in or on the vehicle before being introduced into man.
   2) VECTOR-BORNE—*(a) Mechanical:* Includes simple mechanical carriage by a crawling or flying insect through soiling of its feet or proboscis, or by passage of organisms through its gastrointestinal tract. This does not require multi-

plication or development of the organism. *(b) Biological:* Propagation (multiplication), cyclic development, or a combination of these (cyclopropagation) is required before the arthropod can transmit the infective form of the agent to man. An incubation period (extrinsic) is required following infection before the arthropod becomes *infective*. Transmission may be by saliva during biting, or by regurgitation or deposition on the skin of agents capable of penetrating subsequently through the bite wound or through an area of trauma following scratching or rubbing. This is transmission by an infected nonvertebrate host and must be differentiated for epidemiological purposes from simple mechanical carriage by a vector in the role of a vehicle. An arthropod in either role is termed a *vector*.

3) AIRBORNE—The dissemination of microbial aerosols with carriage to a suitable portal of entry, usually the respiratory tract. Microbial aerosols are suspensions in air of particles consisting partially or wholly of microorganisms. Particles in the 1 to 5 micron range are quite easily drawn into the lungs and retained there. They may remain suspended in the air for long periods of time, some retaining and others losing infectivity or virulence. Not considered as airborne are droplets and other large particles, which promptly settle out (see a. Direct transmission, above); the following are airborne, their mode of transmission indirect:

  (a) Droplet nuclei: Usually the small residues which result from evaporation of droplets emitted by an infected host (see above). Droplet nuclei also may be created purposely by a variety of atomizing devices, or accidentally, in microbiology laboratories or in abattoirs, rendering plants, autopsy rooms, etc. They usually remain suspended in the air for long periods of time.

  (b) Dust: The small particles of widely varying size which may arise from contaminated floors, clothes, bedding, other articles; or from soil (usually fungus spores separated from dry soil by wind or mechanical stirring).

45. Zoonosis—An infection or an infectious disease transmissible under natural conditions between vertebrate animals and man.

INDEX